*Perioperative and* 

**University of Trieste**
**School of Anaesthesia and Intensive Care**
**APICE School of Critical Care Medicine, Trieste, Italy**

*Editors:* A. GULLO, G. BERLOT

*Associate Editors:* U. LUCANGELO, T. PELLIS

A. Gullo • G. Berlot (Eds)

# Perioperative and Critical Care Medicine

## Educational Issues 2004

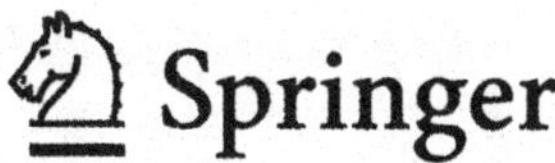 Springer

Antonino Gullo
Giorgio Berlot
Department of Perioperative Medicine
Intensive Care and Emergency
Trieste University School of Medicine
Trieste, Italy

springeronline.com

© Springer-Verlag Italia 2004
Originally published by Springer-Verlag Italia, Milano in 2004

ISBN 978-88-470-0278-4     ISBN 978-88-470-2135-8 (eBook)
DOI 10.1007/978-88-470-2135-8

Library of Congress Cataloging-in-Publication Data: applied for



Typesetting: gramma multimedia, Milan, Italy

Cover design: Simona Colombo, Milan, Italy

# Foreword

by S. Guaschino
*Dean, Trieste University School of Medicine*

The society we live in is in continual development and has a number of priorities for improving the standards of communication. The scientific sector in particular thrives on the exchange of information, which is the foundation of progress itself. The channels through which this interaction takes place are many and are aimed at optimising teaching methodology. Researchers and scholars, research centres and the places of higher learning themselves are increasingly aware of the growing importance of universities, which, thanks to their intrinsic ability to renew themselves, have taken on a vital central and propulsive role. Communication develops as a result of free exchange, debate and analysis of the materials available and the study of the various references sources. With the advent of information systems, the teaching methodology has assumed a decisive role, both in terms of the quantity of data available and the quality of the information. Distance learning is a new and important opportunity for the immediate future.

The Anaesthesia and Critical Care School of Trieste has promoted this interesting and highly relevant initiative by drawing together teaching material from the academic year 2003/2004. Numerous international lecturers have contributed to this valuable achievement. In addition, a large part of the material is the fruit of a real consortium between the various Italian Schools of Anaesthesia. The College of Professors of Anaesthesia and Critical Care, the Directors of the Schools and an international board of lecturers have made possible this project, which was proposed by Antonino Gullo, Giorgio Berlot, Umberto Lucangelo and Thomas Pellis. The new school in Trieste, the recently established joint Cattinara University Hospital, is another favourable undertaking. The aim is to "export" the Trieste model, one that is rich in traditions and modern objectives, both of which play a vital part in training.

On behalf of the Faculty of Medicine I would like to express my deep appreciation for this important initiative.

# Foreword

by R. Proietti
*President, Italian College of Anaesthesiologists*

This "Educational Year Book 2004" is proof of the validity and modernity of a training project that the Trieste school has supported for years with commendable determination and outstanding results. Given the plan of the Year Book and the qualifications of its authors, the aims of its editor are clear: to gather together experience of the highest quality and of undisputed relevance.

These aims have been thoroughly achieved. Now it is the task of the Directors of the School of Specialisation in Anaesthesia and Intensive Care, under the guidance of Dr. Antonino Gullo, to nurture the seed which has been sown and to help it thrive and bear fruit. Because this volume is not an endpoint but rather a beginning, it is also an invitation to experts in the field to solidly cooperate in order to improve the quality of training and offer our students sound study materials.

# Foreword

by F. Zɪɢʀɪɴᴏ
*General Director, Trieste University Hospital*

My sincere congratulations to Professor A. Gullo and his colleagues for having provided the Anaesthesia and Critical Care School with such a fine publication. The book offers a broad panorama of recent progress in the fields of perioperative medicine, critical care and end-of-life care. The chapter focussing on quality and standards of care is particularly noteworthy.

I trust that the medical staff of the Cattinara Hospital pay particular attention to the standards of health-care quality and that the quality of health care they provide is always of the highest level.

In March 2004, the Hospital and the University of Trieste reached a high level of agreement and cooperation with the creation of the new joint University Hospital of Trieste. The mission of the University Hospital is patient satisfaction, which is to be achieved through the provision of high-quality medical care and the training of graduates and postgraduates with the highest level of proficiency, integrity and skill.

I am certain that the Educational Year Book 2004 will contribute to achieving these aims in the fields of anaesthesia and critical care.

I wish Professor Gullo continued success in the study of anaesthesia and critical care, in the training of highly skilled professionals in the field, and in his devotion to science.

# Aims of the Volume and Acknowledgements

This editorial project has been undertaken for trainees and teachers, with the aim of offering them an additional instrument and a source of reference for the teaching and training performed during the year.

The volume is a selection of lessons, seminars, courses and up-dates carried out throughout the previous year by a number of teachers. The teaching staff of the Trieste School, together with colleagues from other institutions, has put together the contents, which are focused on the current issues in the field of Perioperative and Critical Care Medicine in order to develop methodology in teaching and research.

*The publication is acknowledged by:*

**The University of Trieste and the University Hospital of Trieste**

**The National Board of Directors of the Schools of Anaesthesia and Intensive Care:**
Felice Agrò, Raffaele Alvisi, Bruno Amantea, Sergio Boncinelli, Antonio Braschi, Francesco Bruno, Andrea Candiani, Maurizio Chiaranda, Maria Chiefari, Francesco Della Corte, Giorgio Della Rocca, Gianfranco Di Nino, Guido Fanelli, Francesco Foti, Luciano Gattinoni, Gian Piero Giron, Francesco Giunta, Stefano Ischia, Salvatore Mangione, Alberto Pasetto, Vito Aldo Peduto, Antonio Pesenti, Rodolfo Proietti, Marco Ranieri, Letterio Santamaria, Clelia Siani, Giuseppe Susini, Giorgio Torri, Rosalba Tufano, Michele Tupputi, Giustino Varrassi

**The International Board of University Teachers which cooperates with The Trieste School:**
José Otavio Costa Auler (Brazil), Lluis Blanch (Spain), Julian Bion (UK), Geoffrey J. Dobb (Australia), Misa Dzoljic (The Netherlands), Raúl J. Gazmuri (USA), Burkhard Lachmann (The Netherlands), Philip D. Lumb (USA), Michael Parr (Australia), Joseph Rupreht (The Netherlands), Wanchun Tang (USA), Jean-Louis Vincent (Belgium), Max Harry Weil (USA), Michael Zimpfer (Austria), Walter Zin (Brazil)

# Table of Contents


*EDUCATION*

**Chapter 1 – Educational Challenges: Past, Present and Future**
P. LUMB . . . . . . . . . . . . . . . . . . . . . . . . . . . . . . . . . . . . . . . . . . . . . . . . . . . . . . . 3

*QUALITY AND STANDARDS OF CARE*

**Chapter 2 – Quality Has its Price – Costs of Anaesthesiological Care**
M. KLIMEK . . . . . . . . . . . . . . . . . . . . . . . . . . . . . . . . . . . . . . . . . . . . . . . . . . . 11

**Chapter 3 – The Best Weaning after Cardiac Transplantation**
J.O. COSTA AULER J. . . . . . . . . . . . . . . . . . . . . . . . . . . . . . . . . . . . . . . . . . . . . . 17

*BASICS*

**Chapter 4 – Basic Physics for Anaesthesia and Intensive Care**
U. LUCANGELO, S. PASCOTTO, P. ACCARDO . . . . . . . . . . . . . . . . . . . . . . . . . . 29

*FOCUS*

**Chapter 5 – To Tube or Not To Tube? A Critical Point in Emergency and Trauma**
G. BERLOT . . . . . . . . . . . . . . . . . . . . . . . . . . . . . . . . . . . . . . . . . . . . . . . . . . . . . 49

*ADVANCES*

**Chapter 6 – Recent Observations on Pharmacological. Interventions During CPR**
G. CAMMARATA, M.H. WEIL . . . . . . . . . . . . . . . . . . . . . . . . . . . . . . . . . . . . . . 55

*PERIOPERATIVE MEDICINE*

**Chapter 7 – Respiratory Mechanics and Lung Parenchyma Remodelling in Acute Respiratory Distress Syndrome**
W.A. ZIN, P.R.M. ROCCO . . . . . . . . . . . . . . . . . . . . . . . . . . . . . . . . . . . . . . . . . 61

**Chapter 8 – Pulmonary Diseases of Interest for Anaesthesiologists**
F. Ciani . . . . . . . . . . . . . . . . . . . . . . . . . . . . . . . . . . . . . . . . . . . . 73

**Chapter 9 – Paediatric Respiratory Diseases**
A. Sarti, C. Dell'Oste . . . . . . . . . . . . . . . . . . . . . . . . . . . . . . . . . 83

**Chapter 10 – Informed Consent: Origin, Controversies, Contradictions and Sociological Aspects**
A. De Monte . . . . . . . . . . . . . . . . . . . . . . . . . . . . . . . . . . . . . . . . 99

**Chapter 11 – Total Intravenous Anesthesia and Respiratory System**
A. Pasetto, L. Rinaldi . . . . . . . . . . . . . . . . . . . . . . . . . . . . . . . . 113

**Chapter 12 – Determining a Rationale for the Choice of Neuromuscular Blocking Agents in Anaesthesia Practice**
T. Pellis . . . . . . . . . . . . . . . . . . . . . . . . . . . . . . . . . . . . . . . . . . 123

**Chapter 13 – Recovery Room**
Y. Leykin . . . . . . . . . . . . . . . . . . . . . . . . . . . . . . . . . . . . . . . . . 133

**Chapter 14 – Post-operative Respiratory Complications**
Y. Leykin, S. Milesi . . . . . . . . . . . . . . . . . . . . . . . . . . . . . . . . . . 145

## INTENSIVE CARE

**Chapter 15 – Debate on Cardiac Resynchronisation Therapy**
M. Zecchin, G. Sinagra . . . . . . . . . . . . . . . . . . . . . . . . . . . . . . . . 159

**Chapter 16 – Acute Pulmonary Embolism: Hemodynamic Aspects and Treatment**
G. Della Rocca, C. Coccia, I. Reffo . . . . . . . . . . . . . . . . . . . . . . . 167

**Chapter 17 – Pulmonary Infections in the Intensive Care Unit**
A. Luzzani, E. Polati, S. Bassanini . . . . . . . . . . . . . . . . . . . . . . . 183

**Chapter 18 – Intravascular Catheter- Related Infections: An Update on Epidemiology and Prevention**
M. Viviani, R. Dezzoni, L. Silvestri, H.K.F. van Saene . . . . . . . . . . . . . . . . . . 205

## PALLIATIVE CARE

**Chapter 19 – Challenges in End-of-Life Care**
F.M. Rubulotta, L. Serra, A. Gullo . . . . . . . . . . . . . . . . . . . . . . . . 221

**Subject Index** . . . . . . . . . . . . . . . . . . . . . . . . . . . . . . . . . . . . . 233

# List of Contributors

*Accardo P.*
Department of Physics, Trieste
University, Trieste, Italy

*Auler J.O.C.*
Anesthesia and Critical Medicine,
Director of Anesthesia and Surgical ICU,
Heart Institute, Incor, Hospital das
Clínicas, School of Medicine, São Paulo
University, Brazil

*Bassanini S.*
Department of Anesthesia and Intensive
Care, Verona University, Ospedale Civile
Maggiore, Verona, Italy

*Berlot G.*
Department of Perioperative Medicine,
Intensive Care and Emergency, School of
Anaesthesia and Intensive Care,
Cattinara University Hospital, Trieste,
Italy

*Cammarata G.L.*
Institute of Critical Care Medicine, Palm
Springs, USA *and* Department of
Perioperative Medicine, Intensive Care
and Emergency, Cattinara University
Hospital, Trieste, Italy

*Ciani F.*
Pneumology Unit, Cattinara University
Hospital, Trieste, Italy

*Coccia C.*
Department of Anaesthesia and Intensive
Care, Udine University Hospital, Udine,
Italy

*De Monte A.*
Department of Anaesthesia and
Emergency Department, Ospedale Civile,
Tolmezzo, Italy

*Della Rocca G.*
Department of Anaesthesia and Intensive
Care, Udine University, Udine, Italy

*Dell'Oste C.*
Department of Anaesthesia and Intensive
Care, Scientific Research Institute,
Children Hospital "Burlo Garofolo",
Trieste, Italy

*Dezzoni R.*
Department of Perioperative Medicine,
Intensive Care and Emergency, Trieste,
School of Anaesthesia and Intensive
Care, Cattinara University Hospital,
Trieste, Italy

*Guaschino S.*
Dean, Trieste University School of
Medicine, University of Trieste, Italy

*Gullo A.*
Department of Perioperative Medicine,
Intensive Care and Emergency, School of
Anaesthesia and Intensive Care,
Cattinara University Hospital, Trieste,
Italy

*Klimek M.*
Department of Anaesthesia and Intensive
Care, Erasmus University Medical
Centre, Rotterdam, The Netherlands

*Leykin Y.*
Department of Anaesthesia and Intensive Care, S. Maria degli Angeli Hospital, Pordenone, Italy

*Lucangelo U.*
Department of Perioperative Medicine, Intensive Care and Emergency, School of Anaesthesia and Intensive Care, Cattinara University Hospital, Trieste, Italy

*Lumb P.*
Department of Anaesthesiology, Keck School of Medicine, USC, Los Angeles, United States

*Luzzani A.*
Department of Anesthesia and Intensive Care, Verona University, Ospedale Civile Maggiore, Verona, Italy

*Milesi S.*
Department of Anaesthesia and Intensive Care, S. Maria degli Angeli Hospital, Pordenone, Italy

*Pascotto S.*
Department of Perioperative Medicine, Intensive Care and Emergency, School of Anaesthesia and Intensive Care, Cattinara University Hospital, Trieste, Italy

*Pasetto A.*
Emergency and Surgical Department, Modena and Reggio Emilia University. Modena, Italy

*Pellis T.*
Department of Anaesthesia and Intensive Care, S. Maria degli Angeli Hospital, Pordenone, Italy

*Polati E.*
Department of Anesthesia and Intensive Care, Verona University, Ospedale Civile Maggiore, Verona, Italy

*Proietti R.*
Insituite of Anaesthesiology and Intensive Care, Università Cattolica del Sacro Cuore, University School of Medicine, Rome, Italy

*Reffo I.*
Department of Anaesthesia and Intensive Care, Udine University Hospital, Udine, Italy

*Rocco P.M.*
Laboratory of Pulmonary Investigation, Carlos Chagas Filho Biophysics Institute, Federal University of Rio de Janeiro, Centro de Ciências da Saúde, Ilha do Fundão, Rio de Janeiro, Brazil

*Rubulotta F.*
Department of Perioperative Medicine, Intensive Care and Emergency, School of Anaesthesia and Intensive Care, Cattinara University Hospital, Trieste, Italy *and* Medical Intensive Care Unit (MICU) Brown University, Rhode Island Hospital, Providence, USA

*Sarti S.*
Department of Anaesthesia and Intensive Care, Scientific Research Institute, Children Hospital "Burlo Garofolo", Trieste, Italy

*Serra L.*
Department of Perioperative Medicine, Intensive Care and Emergency, School of Anaesthesia and Intensive Care, Cattinara University Hospital, Trieste, Italy

*Silvestri L.*
Department of of Anaesthesia and Intensive Care, Gorizia Hospital, Italy

*Sinagra G.*
Cardiology Centre, Cattinara University Hospital, Trieste, Italy

*van Saene H.K.F.*
Department of Microbiology,
Department of Clinical Microbiology,
Alder Hey Children's Hospital, NHS
Trust, Liverpool, UK

*Viviani M.*
Department of Perioperative Medicine,
Intensive Care and Emergency, School of
Anaesthesia and Intensive Care,
Cattinara University Hospital, Trieste,
Italy

*Weil M.H.*
Institute of Critical Care Medicine, Palm
Springs, CA  The Keck School of
Medicine of the University of Southern
California, Los Angeles, USA

*Zecchin M.*
Cardiology Centre, Cattinara University
Hospital, Trieste, Italy

*Zigrino F.*
General Director, University Hospital of
Trieste, Trieste, Italy

*Zin W.A.*
Laboratory of Respiration Physiology
Carlos Chagas Filho Biophysics Institute,
Federal University of Rio de Janeiro,
Centro de Ciências da Saúde, Ilha do
Fundão, Rio de Janeiro, Brazil

# Abbreviations

| | |
|---|---|
| A-aDO$_2$ | Oxygen Alveolo-Arterial Difference |
| ABA | American Board of Anesthesiology |
| ACAD | Allograft Coronary Artery Disease |
| ACC/AHA | American College of Cardiology/American Heart Association |
| ACPE | Acute Cardiogenic Pulmonary Edema |
| AF | Atrial Fibrillation |
| ALI | Acute Lung Injury |
| ANS | Autonomic Nervous System |
| APACHE | Acute Physiology and Chronic Health Evaluation |
| ARDS | Acute Respiratory Distress Syndrome |
| ATS | American Thoracic Society |
| BAL | Broncho-Alveolar Lavage |
| BIS | Biospectral Index System |
| BSI | Bloodstream Infection |
| BTS | British Thoracic Society |
| BVM | Bag-Valve mask |
| CABG | Coronary Artery Bypass Graft |
| CAD | Coronary Artery Disease |
| CAP | Community Acquired Pneumonia |
| CARE-HF | Cardiac Resynchronization in Heart Failure |
| CC | Closing Capacity |
| CHF | Congestive Heart Failure |
| CMV | Citomegalovirus |
| CNS | Coagulase Negative Staphylococcus |
| CO | Cardiac Output |
| COMPANION | Comparison of Medical Therapy, Pacing and Defibrillation in Chronic Heart |
| COPD | Chronic Obstructive Pulmonary Disease |
| CPAP | Continuous Positive Airway Pressure |
| CPB | Cardiopulmonary Bypass |
| CPIS | Clinical Pulmonary Infection Score |
| CR-BSI | Catheter-Related Bloodstream Infection |
| CRP | C-Reactive Protein |
| CRT | Cardiac Reysnchronization Therapy |
| CVC | Central Venous Catheters |
| DCA | Dichloroacetate |
| DLCO | Diffusing Capacity Lung Carbon Monoxide |
| DNR | Do Not Resuscitate |

| | |
|---|---|
| DRSP | Drug Resistant Streptococcus Pneumoniae |
| DVT | Deep Vein Thrombosis |
| E | Tissue Elastance |
| EAST | Eastern Association for the Surgery of Trauma |
| ECM | Extracellular Matrix |
| ECMO | Extracorporeal Membrane Oxygenation |
| ED | Emergency Department |
| EDV | End Diastolic Volume |
| EF | Ejection Phase |
| EF=SV/EDV | Ejection Phase Index of Contractility |
| EMT | Emergency Medicine Technicians |
| ERS | European Respiratory Society |
| ESPVR | End Systolic Pressure Volume Relation |
| $\eta$ | Viscosity coefficient |
| FEV | Forced Expiratory Volume |
| FEV1 | Forced Expiratory Volume 0.1 |
| Fi | Force of Inertia |
| FiO2 | Inspired Fraction of Oxygen |
| FRC | Functional Residual Capacity |
| Fv | Force of Viscosity |
| GCS | Glasgow Coma Scale |
| HAP | Hospital Acquired Pneumonia |
| HEMS | Helicopter Emergency Medical System |
| HETA | Hydroxyeicosatetraenoic Acid |
| HFOV | High Frequency Oscillatory Ventilation |
| HICPAC | Hospital Infection Control Practices Advisory Committee |
| HLA | Human Leukocyte Antigen |
| HPV | Hypoxic Pulmonary Vasoconstriction |
| ICU | Intensive Care Unit |
| IFN | Interferon |
| IGF-I | Insulin-like Growth Factor-I |
| IL 13 | Interleukin 13 |
| IL-1 beta | Interleukin 1- 1 beta |
| IL-4 | Interleukin - 4 |
| IVD | Intra-Vascular Device |
| LAP | Let Atrial Pressure |
| LBBB | Left Bundle Branch Block |
| LMA | Laryngeal Mask Airways |
| LMWH | Low Molecular Weight Heparins |
| LV | Left Ventricle |
| LVAD | LV Assist Device |
| LVEDV | Left Ventricle End Diastolic Volume |
| MI | Myocardial Infarction |
| MICU | Medical Intensive Care Unit |
| MIRACLE | Multicenter Insync Randomised Clinical Evaluation |
| MLC | Myosin Light Chain |
| MMPs | Matrix Metalloproteinases |
| MODS | Multi-Organ Dysfunction Syndrome |

| | |
|---|---|
| MRSA | Methicillin Resistant Staphylococcus Aureus |
| MSSA | Methicillin-Sensitive Staphylococcus Aureus |
| MUSTIC | Multisite Stimulation in the Cardiomyopathy |
| NMBA's | Neuromuscular Blocking Agents |
| NO | Nitric Oxide |
| NYHA | New York Heart Association |
| OSA | Obstructive Sleep Apnoea |
| P | Pressure |
| PA | Pulmonary Artery |
| PaCO2 | Carbon Dioxide Tension |
| PADSS | Post-Anaesthesia Discharge Scoring System |
| PAO2 | Alveolar Oxygen Partial Pressure |
| PaO2 | Arterial Oxygen Tension |
| PaO2/FiO2 | Arterial Oxygen Pressure/Fraction of Inspired Oxygen |
| PAOP | Pulmonary Artery Occlusion Pressure |
| PAP | Pulmonary Artery Pressures |
| PCT | Procalcitonin |
| PDGF | Platelet-Derived Growth Factor |
| PE | Pulmonary Embolism |
| PEEP | Positive End Expiratory Pressure |
| $PGE_2$ | Prostaglandin $E_2$ |
| PNX | Pnewmothorax |
| PONV | Post-Operative Nausea and Vomiting |
| PPH | Primary Pulmonary Hypertension |
| PSB | Protective Specimen Brushing |
| PTCA | Percutaneous Transluminal Coronary Angioplasty |
| PVR | Pulmonary Vascular Resistance |
| R | Tissue Resistance |
| RBBB | Right Bundle Branch Block |
| RR | Recovery Room |
| RV | Right Ventricle |
| RVAD | RV Assist Device |
| $\varrho$ | Density of the fluid |
| SAPS | Simplified Acute Physiology Score |
| SARS | Severe Acute Respiratory Syndrome |
| SDD | Selective Digestive Decontamination |
| SIRS | Systemic Inflammatory Response Syndrome |
| SR | Sarcoplasmic Reticulum |
| SUPPORT | Study to Understand Prognoses and Preferences for Outcome and Risk of Treatment |
| SVC | Superior Vena Cava |
| T | Temperature |
| TDI | Tissue Doppler Imaging |
| TGF | Transforming Growth Factor |
| TI | Tracheal Intubation |
| TIMPs | Tissue Inhibitors of Metalloproteinases |
| TIVA | Total Intravenous Anesthesia Techniques |
| TNF | Transforming Nuclear Factor |

| | |
|---|---|
| UFH | Unfractioned Heparin |
| V | Volume |
| V/Q | Ventilation/Perfusion |
| VAD | Ventricular Assist Devices |
| VAP | Ventilator Associated Pneumonia |
| VC | Vital Capacity |
| Vc | Critical Velocity |
| VDCC | Voltage-Dependant Calcium Channels |
| VF | Ventricular Fibrillation |
| VT | Tidal Volume |
| VTE | Venous Thromboembolism |

# EDUCATION

# Educational Challenges: Past, Present and Future

P. Lumb

The challenge for teachers has always been not only to maintain scientific accuracy and intellectual honesty regarding subject matter but also to codify and disseminate it in a manner that can be reproduced and assimilated over distance and time. Inherent in the process is the requisite updating of information thereby avoiding stagnation and retaining an immediacy of purpose, irrespective of societal or political constraints. New techniques and curricula are often regarded with suspicion, and the task for any new educational institution is to develop scientific, intellectual and professionally enduring credibility. The current undertaking embodied in this textbook represents a bold initiative to establish an educational and scientific forum composed of multinational, multidisciplinary and multicultural experts who share a commitment to the care of the critically ill and injured patients admitted to hospitals and clinics worldwide.

In a recent discussion of the issues facing research universities in the 21st century, University of Southern California scholars identified three major trends that will determine the strategic initiatives necessary to ensure a viable and aggressive future academic presence. First, it is apparent that society will look to research universities for solutions to its most intractable and pressing problems; this will demand innovation as well as the exploration and exploitation of new scientific horizons. Second, global competition will be the forge in which academic mettle will be tempered, and only a few institutions will be capable of defining international academic excellence. Third, the global marketplace with instant access to information services and increased consumer sophistication and education will lead to a learner-oriented educational paradigm rather than today's environment in which the institution demands and expects the student's presence on a unique and identifiable campus. Distance learning and the opportunity to reach across national, political and cultural barriers will define the future learning paradigm, and institutions and organizations that do not compete successfully in this environment are unlikely to survive.

With specific attention to the challenges facing medical educators in the decades ahead, it is important to recognize and understand the significant changes already taking place in "traditional" programs. No longer are unique courses in anatomy, physiology and pharmacology deemed appropriate. Dependence on computer facilitated dissections and "case-based learning" scenarios, in which the educational focus is based on patient data rather than on amassing specific discipline-based knowledge from which a cohesive plan is formulated, has become the norm rather than the exception. Curricular changes have swept across most American medical schools, and the concept of "life-long" learning has been inculcated into the educational paradigm. The impact of such changes is patently obvious to anyone who has been actively engaged in medical practice during the time in which new technologic, therapeutic and diagnostic initiatives have been introduced. Nonetheless, recertification and credentialing programs have not been adopted warmly by the medical profession; rather they have become the mandated plea from an educated public to ensure the most appropriate and timely care from a profession that is perceived as being largely unregulated. This is a far cry from the reputation enjoyed by our predecessors.

In order to match these initiatives, credentialing and certifying organizations are incorporating traditional outcome assessment into a new and creative graduate medical education curriculum. In the United States, the residency training program requires its graduates to obtain competency to the level expected of a new practitioner in the following six areas (ACGME guidelines):
- Patient care that is compassionate, appropriate and effective for the treatment of the health problems and the promotion of health.
- Medical knowledge about established and evolving biomedical, clinical and cognate (e.g. epidemiological and social-behavioral) sciences, and the application of this knowledge to patient care.
- Practice-based learning that includes investigation and evaluation of the physician's own approach to patient care, as well as appraisal and assimilation of scientific evidence and improvements in patient care.
- Interpersonal and communication skills that result in effective information exchange and teaming with patients, their families, and other health professionals.
- Professionalism, as manifested through a commitment to carrying out professional responsabilities, adherence to ethical principles, and sensitivity to a diverse patient population.
- Systems-based practice, as manifested by actions that demonstrate an awareness of and responsiveness to the larger context and system of health care, and the ability to effectively call on system resources to provide care that is of optimal value.

It is important for the individual training program to define the experiences necessary to demonstrate proficiency in each of those areas.

Not only is the curriculum in such an endeavor important; the training program must demonstrate that it can effectively assess learner performance throughout the educational continuum and utilize results of such assessments to modify teaching/learning techniques thereby improving clinical and intellectual skills. Assessment and remediation plans should include:

- Use of dependable measures to assess trainees' competence in patient care, practice-based learning and improvement, interpersonal and communication skills, as well as professionalism and systems-based practice.
- Mechanisms for providing regular and timely performance feedback to trainees.
- A process involving use of assessment results to achieve progressive improvements in trainees' competence and performance.

Consistent with current attempts to ensure self-assessment and improvement, the training program must also demonstrate an internal evaluation process through which the following issues are addressed:

- How to use trainee performance and outcome assessment results in evaluating the training program's own effectiveness.
- How to improve the training program  based on resident and performance assessment results together with other program evaluation results.

The onus is not only on the primary educational environment or specialty training program, but also on licensing authorities, who are increasingly accountable and who are required to set continuing performance standards for certified practitioners.  The American Board of Anesthesiology employs successful completion of both written and oral examinations to determine appropriate credentials and knowledge base for specialty certification. The written test is objective and evaluates standard clinical skills. The oral examination has evolved into an assessment of certain professional qualities and attributes that the Board feels are essential components and requisite skills that must be present prior to specialty certification. The Board evaluates candidates in the following four areas for consistency in demonstrating the attributes of a certified practitioner (ABA guidelines for examiners):

- Mature medical judgment applicable to the solution of medical problems in the practice of anesthesiology, in making decisions and in the application of said decisions.
- Adaptability, as evidenced by the ability to recognize complications and respond appropriately to changing medical and clinical situations.
- Application of knowledge, as demonstrated by the ability to assimilate and analyze relevant data in order to achieve a rational and timely treatment plan, even when faced with rapidly changing conditions.
- Competence in logically organizing and effectively communicating targeted information about specific issues that, although vested in general medicine, are relevant to anesthetic practice and of paramount importance to ensuring safe and effective patient care.

Setting standards is a difficult task; there is a high degree of variability in the application of evidence-based regimens to patient care, and medicine remains a bastion of individual clinician prerogatives despite indications that more algorithmic therapeutic approaches would deliver an improved, cost-effective patient outcome. Unfortunately, despite numerous advances in educational theory, resistance to behavioral change remains a key impediment to translating therapeutic efficiencies into clinical realities. It is in this area that the professional organization can and should play a major role by providing an accountable forum in which therapeutic innovation and change can be discussed, evaluated and implemented. Peer-reviewed publications as well as published expert opinion and practice standards provide some of the most forceful arguments for therapeutic change and practice modification. International conferences that stimulate recognized specialty leaders to discuss openly and completely contentious therapeutic challenges offer a readily accessible forum through which medical progress can be accomplished and made accessible.

The Mediterranean School promoted by the Department of Anesthesiology in Trieste, provides such a forum and its goal is to become a well-respected international leader in distance learning of anesthesia and intensive-care medicine. Drawing from traditional paradigms, the school balances its mission in the cradle of intellectual civilization with the reality that currently existing international organizations ignore much of the developing world and the specific problems associated with under-funded and over-committed intellectual, technologic and therapeutic resources. The educational motives for medical schools, specialty programs and professional societies are different and the target audiences equally diverse and poorly defined. Government agencies are poorly equipped to understand specialty prerogatives, and new therapeutic options have made previous licensing laws obsolete. Furthermore, technologic advances have raised ethical questions unthinkable only a few years ago, and globalization has made it important that culturally responsive therapeutic initiatives are understood and practiced internationally. Physicians must be culturally aware, intellectually honest, scientifically sound and technically capable of meeting the increasingly international challenges facing our institutions daily. The recent SARS outbreak demonstrated that medicine can be practiced without the constraints of national prerogatives and borders hampering the flow of necessary therapeutic information between colleagues in order to effect rapid improvements in quarantine, therapy, early diagnosis and ultimate cure. The learning paradigm is fast evolving, and academic institutions must keep pace in order to make the changes necessary to remain relevant in the future.

What is the future of the medical conference with its lecture, panel and scientific presentation format? Despite concern that these modes of education are doomed, the venue remains popular. Increasingly, the challenge is to provide stimulating and demonstrably effective learning experiences for the participants. Course evaluations and demonstration of both competence and knowledge gained provided by more than a certificate of attendance will be the standard. In this competitive arena, the Mediterranean School strives to develop the curriculum, presence and effective outcomes that are necessary to succeed. Its international focus and heritage will prevent complacency, ensure credibility and scientific integrity, stimulate far-reaching discussion and controversy, enjoin collaboration and create a forum in which future best practices can be elucidated.

The past is prologue. In the field of medical education, scientific integrity has ultimately persevered despite occasionally slavish devotion to outmoded methodologies and "core knowledge" bases. Each of us is indebted to the work of former mentors, none perhaps better known than Sir William Osler. Although expressed within a context of arrogance that, despite the source is unwarranted and unfounded, this debt is made clear in the following statement:

I am sorry for you, young men (and women) of this generation. You will do great things. You will have great victories, and standing on our shoulders, you will see far, but you can never have our sensations. To have lived through  revolution, to have seen a new birth of science, a new dispensation of health, reorganized medical schools, remodeled hospitals; a new outlook for humanity, is not given to every generation.

[from W. Osler, *Essays*]

Rather, it is important to understand, as did Machiavelli, the importance of understanding the difficulty in changing perceptions, behaviors and practices.

There is nothing more difficult to plan, more doubtful of success, not more dangerous to manage than the creation of a new order of things... Whenever his enemies have the ability to attack the innovator they do so with the passion of partisans, while the others defend him sluggishly, so that the innovator and his party alike are vulnerable.

[from N. Machiavelli, *The Prince*]

It took over 250 years for citrus to be used in the treatment of scurvy; it took less than 2 months for the medical community to be sensitized to the importance of SARS. Future medical education will embrace the technologies of communication and information dissemination as well as more traditional activities. The medical meeting place will continue in the form of a Socratic environment in which medical opinion can be tempered, questioned, developed and enacted.

# QUALITY AND STANDARDS OF CARE

# Quality Has its Price – Costs of Anaesthesiological Care

M. KLIMEK

## Introduction

The daily life of the anaesthesiologist is marked by budget deficits on the one hand and costly opportunities for better patient care on the other. Many of the new methods, drugs and devices offer a secondary profit or cost reductions if one considers the whole hospital or even the whole health system. Of course, it is still possible to perform anaesthesia with ether alone, but the price of treating vomiting patients with delayed recovery and severe wound pain might be much higher than the expenses for e.g. propofol, fentanyl and/or an epidural catheter together.

Reducing costs, improving quality of care and increasing clinical production – these are the challenges most anaesthesiological departments are confronted with. This survey will make an attempt at focusing on some of the aspects concerning these challenges.

## Who Pays for What?

Before thinking about costs of anaesthesiological care, one should define the tasks of the Department of Anaesthesiology: providing perioperative care for patients undergoing any procedure. Teaching hospitals have the additional task of teaching and training students, nurses and/or residents, and – in the case of an academic hospital – performing research and publishing the results.

These tasks can only be fulfilled with a certain budget, which might be provided by the hospital administration as a fixed amount of money. In some countries, the Department of Anaesthesiology has the possibility to create (additional) income of its own by billing for (parts of) the clinical service provided by the department. In this case, production and income are closely related and production might even be stimulated if the generated income is higher than the costs.

However, in most systems anaesthesiological care is an essential *secondary* cost factor for all surgical disciplines. Secondary cost factor means that there is no direct external reimbursement for anaesthesiological care, but – as for radiological or laboratory examinations – an internal reimbursement.

How can the productivity (and much more difficult, but not less important: quality) of anaesthesiological care be estimated? How can it be made transparent and how can it be communicated – with the surgeons and the board of directors – so that adequate reimbursement for the anaesthesiological performance, not only in the OR, but, e.g. also for reanimations or placing i.v. lines in difficult patients, is provided?

Apart from pain therapy, no patient comes to a hospital in need of the anaesthesiologist alone. We are not "first-line specialists", but instead have a facilitating role for other disciplines. This is an important issue when considering the opportunities to generate income for an anaesthesiology department: Who pays for what? The surgeon, for a certain number of procedures? The surgeon, for a certain number of hours of anaesthesiological care? The hospital administration, which decides how many hours may be used by which surgical discipline? What about the costs for preoperative visits? Is there a standard price or will it depend on, e.g. age and ASA-classification of the patient? What about the monitoring needed for a special procedure? It makes a great difference whether the surgeon performs 150 inguinal hernia repairs or 150 Whipple procedures if the anaesthesia department is paid simply by the number of procedures! What about the costs of postoperative pain treatment? Is the PCA-pump billed by the anaesthesiologists or by the surgeons? Who pays for the drugs needed to refill it? Who cares for the acute-pain service? What about packed red blood cells? Blood loss is caused by the surgeon, the packed cells are ordered and transfused by the anaesthesiologist. These are just a few questions showing the basic problems with distributing the money within a hospital to reimburse for anaesthesia care.

However, the anaesthesiology department also produces costs of its own: What about the costs for a chest-X-ray that is requested by the anaesthesiologist for a patient undergoing knee surgery? Especially in those cases where extra costs in anaesthesiological care produce a cost reduction in other parts of the hospital, the means of internal reimbursement should be evident: e.g. the intraoperative use of warming devices increases the speed of recovery and lowers the risk of bleeding problems and wound infections; however, they are expensive. Who should pay for them? The surgeon, who needs less blood transfusions and antibiotics to treat his patients on the ward?

Another example: disposable infusion pumps are a useful device for postoperative pain therapy in patients undergoing day-care surgery with peripheral neural blockade by a small catheter. However, they are very expensive. Who should pay for them? The surgeon, who needs to prescribe fewer analgesics? The patient, who is extraordinarily happy with this trendy and useful but not mandatory technique? The hospital administration, because providing such an effective type of postoperative pain treatment promotes the image of the hospital?

Watcha *et al.* [1] pointed out another problem: using preoperative 50 mg rofecoxib means about $5 more direct costs per patient than 2 g acetaminophen. However, the total costs to reach full perioperative patient satisfaction are more than twice as high after acetaminophen as after rofecoxib (209 vs. 92 $). How can an anaesthesia department get at least partially reimbursed for the money we save on the general wards by using more expensive drugs in the OR?

## Training, Learning and Teaching

And what about the costs for non-patient-related activities of an anaesthesia department? Is it economically reasonable, to close ORs to perform simulator training with some staff members in order to improve their skills in difficult airway management? Facing the need of continuous medical education, the need of teaching the teachers and the need of faculty development, it is mandatory to create budgets for participating in courses in all fields of interest. This might also be done by organising a course within the department! Investing in simulation techniques and training will reduce the number of complications and claims; however, it is hard to find, e.g. an insurance company to pay for it.

Depending on the health system, anaesthesia departments receive extra money for the training and teaching of residents. Residents are something between cheap workers and an expensive burden, depending on the energy a department puts into training and teaching them. If the residents' lessons are scheduled during OR working hours, there is a serious impact on OR productivity; if they are scheduled in the evening, the knowledge transfer might be minimal.

Finding the right amount of supervision and bedside-teaching for the residents is another problem: if the residents are directed too much, a residency program becomes unattractive, if the residents experience too much independence, they become dangerous. Posner and Freund [2] recently published that second years residents have a higher relative risk for critical incidents, escalation of care, and operational inefficiencies. This can be translated easily into higher costs for the hospital.

The experienced anaesthesiologist is more cost-effective in the provision of anaesthesia care than a non medically directed nurse-based service [3]. Cost-effectiveness estimates between 4,410-38,778 dollars per year of life saved are very strong arguments to keep the level of training high and to limit nurse-based services to the absolute minimum needed for providing care even in rural areas with no better alternatives.

One aspect should also be considered: in the competition between the hospitals to get the best personnel, next to salary all kinds of facilities for personal development will become more important. Departments with modern IT-equipment and simulation facilities, offering courses, performing top research and participating in international scientific exchange will be able to attract the talented. Investing in these fields means investing in the future.

## Quality Has its Price – The Patient's View

A recently published study asked patients by a computer-generated questionnaire about their willingness to pay for the avoidance of anaesthesia-related adverse events during the perioperative period [4]. Patients seemed quite motivated to pay for "high quality-anaesthesia": $ 34 for the avoidance of intraoperative awareness, $ 50 for the avoidance of postoperative pain, $ 33 for the avoidance of nausea and vomiting and $ 20 for the avoidance of postoperative grogginess (all data: median). This raises some ethical dilemmas: what may be expected as a basic standard of perioperative care? Will there be a future with a kind of "business- or economy-class" anaesthesia, in which the patient can order some levels of perioperative care quality? Should we ask patients to pay for being BIS-monitored, even if we see no real indication to do so?

The Australian Society of Anaesthetists offers a position statement, in which, next to the informed consent for the anaesthesiological procedure, an informed "financial consent" is required [5]. This consent includes an estimate of the total costs of anaesthesia care and, where possible, some indication of the likely out-of-pocket-costs, i.e. those not paid by a third party.

## Simple Measures to Take

Cost reduction can easily be achieved in many areas of anaesthesiology. The following measures have turned out to be effective:

- *Avoid drug wastage* [6]: drawing up drugs in several syringes (split doses) if the contents of the vial are likely to be used on more than one patient. The cost-effectiveness of routine prophylactic preparation of cardiac resuscitation drugs must be called into question. Depending on the actual hospital drug-acquisition costs, savings up to $ 10 per case is possible. Another method of avoiding drug wastage is the use of monitors, like BIS or Narcotrend, to hasten recovery and minimise drug usage [7].

- *Create transparency* [8]: creating cost-consciousness by the distribution of price-lists for certain drugs, tubes and catheters and their therapeutic alternatives will make cost-efficiency a part of daily clinical decision-making. Is the use of Woodbridge tubes justified for every patient operated on in the prone position? Can we create an escalation protocol for the treatment of nausea, or must every patient get his serotoninantagonist immediately? Which hypnotic, opioid or muscle-relaxant are we to choose? Who does not know the price, will not take efforts to save the money.

- *Price dealing*: it is useful to deal with representatives of different medical companies and to be open about concurrent offers. I am repeatedly surprised by the creativity of some representatives in finding a way of being able to make their product cheaper.

- *Create "economical awareness"*: in our department, we informed the medical staff and the nurses with one short notice about the fact that 500 ml saline solution is about 50% cheaper than 500 ml Ringer's solution. Without any further measures, this information led to a still persisting reduction of costs for infusion fluids of about 1000 € month! However, it has also been reported that "price tags" have no effect on drug usage [9].

- *Increase in productivity*: a higher patient-turnover on the OR by better planning [10], choosing those drugs with faster pharmacokinetics [11] and avoiding unnecessary "experimental" procedures by unsupervised surgical residents [12] have turned out to be cost-saving. As soon as productivity in the OR is directly coupled with the income of an anaesthesia department, responsible planning should be taken over by the anaesthesia department, too.

In conclusion, it should be the aim of each anaesthesia department to be able to create an income of its own by clinical and scientific activities. Next to this, an intra-hospital reimbursement strategy must be developed. A re-distribution of the budgets has to take place, since (expensive) modern anaesthesia leads to more effective (cheaper) patient care on the general wards. This demands a pro-active attitude, careful documentation of all activities, cost-awareness and ongoing investment in the clinical (and academic) development of the staff. Quality has its price, but quality is also sparing costs by avoiding complications – this must be communicated to surgeons, the hospital administration, health insurance providers, the government and, of course, the patients.

# References


1. Watcha MF, Issioui T, Klein KW, White PF (2003) Costs and effectiveness of Rofecoxib, Celecoxib, and Acetaminophen for preventing pain after ambulatory otolaryngologic surgery. Anesth Analg 96:987-994
2. Posner KL, Freund PR (2004) Resident training level and quality of anesthesia care in a university hospital. Anesth Analg 98:437-442
3. Abenstein JP, Hall Long K, McGlinch BP, Dietz NM (2004) Is physician anesthesia cost-effective? Anesth Analg 98:750-757
4. Gan TJ, Ing RJ, de L Dear G, Wright D, El-Moalem HE, Lubarsky DA (2003) How much are patients willing to pay to avoid intraoperative awareness? J Clin Anesth 15:108-112
5. http://www.asa.org.au/ArticleDetails.asp?A=1708
6. Weinberg MB (2001) Drug wastage contributes significantly to the cost of routine anesthesia care. J Clin Anesth 13:491-497
7. Kreuer S, Biedler A, Larsen R, Altmann S, Wilhelm W (2003) Narcotrend monitoring allows faster emergence and a reduction of drug consumption in propofol-remifentanil anesthesia. Anesthesiology 99:34-41
8. Snyder-Ramos SA, Bauer M, Martin E, Motsch J, Böttiger BW (2003) Accessible price lists at the anaesthesiologist's working place enhance cost consciousness as a part of process and cost optimization. Anaesthesist 52:154-161
9. Horrow JC, Rosenberg H (1994) Price stickers do not alter drug usage. Can J Anaesth 41:1047-1052
10. Strum DP, Vargas LG, May JH, Basheim G (1997) Surgical suite utilization and capacity planning: a minimal cost analysis model. J Med Syst 21:309-322
11. Puura AI, Rorarius MC, Manninen P, Hopput S, Baer GA (1999) The costs of intense neuromuscular block for anesthesia during endolaryngeal procedures due to waiting time. Anesth Analg 88:1335-1339
12. Koperna T (2003) How long do we need teaching in the operating room? The true costs of achieving surgical routine. Langenbecks Arch Surg (Epub ahead of print)

# Chapter 3

# The Best Weaning after Cardiac Transplantation

J.O. COSTA AULER J.

## Introduction

Since the first human-to-human *heart transplant* was performed, in 1967, by Christiaan Barnard [1], remarkable progress in this field has been achieved. Heart transplantation nowadays is efficiently performed worldwide with high rates of success: 3175 cases in the year 2000, reported by 321 centers according to reports of International Society for Heart and Lung Transplantation Registry [2]. Improvement of surgical and anesthetic techniques, as well as *perioperative care*, associated with new immunosuppressive strategies, newer antibiotics planning, improved donor and recipient selection, and graft preservation, have improved results considerably. After transplantation, the average 1-year survival rate is 79.96% and the average 5-year survival rate is about 66%, considering that these survival rates continue to improve. Pre-transplant risk factors are related to the degree of hemodynamic instability of the *donor*, as well as to the poor general-health conditions of the recipient. An added factor affecting survival is the level of human leukocyte antigen (*HLA*)-matching between donor and recipient. The literature reports a progressive reduction in the risk of failure after heart transplantation with better HLA matching. Graft dysfunction prevails as a cause of death during the first month after cardiac transplantation. This is because the patient requires more intensive and invasive care with a subsequently higher risk of infection and rejection; an otherwise inefficiently functioning heart compromises others organs, mainly renal and liver function, which limits the doses of *immunosuppressive drugs*. According to the literature, acute rejection and infection are the predominant causes of death from the first month to one year after heart transplantation (42.21 and 14.30%, respectively) [2]. The most significant problem limiting survival after one year is still chronic rejection (20.46% from 3 to 5 years), which appears as a progressive allograft coronary artery disease (*ACAD*). This is followed by graft failure (18.56% from 3 to 5 years) and malignancy (15.87% from 3 to 5 years post-transplant) [2]. The immediate management of cardiac transplant recipients is challenging and warrants, beside the basic intensive-care, the administration of immunosuppressive therapies, knowledge of the physiology of the transplanted heart and acute rejection management. Most postoperative management success may be attributed to careful selection of recipient and donor, as well as to protection of the graft against prolonged ischemia. This article aims, based on our institutional experience of 258 cases of adult heart transplant in the last 15 years, to discuss the general aspects of heart transplantation as well as pharmacological and ventilatory support following heart transplantation.


## General Considerations

### Indications for Cardiac Transplantation

Cardiac transplantation is reserved for a selected group of patients with end-stage heart disease and a poor response to medical therapy or other surgical alternatives. The prognosis for 1-year survival of patients considered for a heart transplant, without transplantation, should be less than 75%. Over 90% of adult patients presented for heart transplantation have ischemic dilated heart or *cardiomyopathy* (46.07 *vs* 45.10%), and typically have symptoms at rest *NYHA* (New York Heart Association) class IV. A subgroup of patients with NYHA class III (symptoms with limited exercise) presenting with maximal oxygen consumption values equal or less than 14 ml/kg per minute, may also be considered as potential candidates, due to the elevated 1-year mortality [2]. In our patients there is also a subgroup with terminal heart failure due to chronic *Chagas disease* (48 patients, 18.60%). There are several contraindications for cardiac transplantation: *age* seems to be the most controversial. Although the upper age limit for recipients is between 55 and 65 years, survival expectancy and quality of life in selected older patients is equivalent to that of younger recipients [3]. This was confirmed when we analyzed the age of recipients in the year 2000: 50.20% were 50-64 years of age followed by 27.15% of recipients with ages ranging from 35 to 49 years in the same period [2].

Another point of paramount importance is related to the recipients' previous "cutoff" values of pulmonary vascular resistance *(PVR)*. A fixed PVR greater than 6 Wood units or a transpulmonary gradient higher than 15 mmHg, which does not respond to vasodilators such as *oxygen, sodium nitroprusside, milrinone* or *prostaglandin*, was formerly considered a contraindication for orthotopic cardiac transplantation in most centers around the world [4, 5]. Fundamentally, high PVR values in patients with *heart failure* have been considered as a passive consequence of high pressure back from the left atrium toward the pulmonary circulation as a result of mitral insufficiency in cases of ventricular and annulus dilation. Nevertheless, PVR commonly remains elevated after transplantation with a tendency to decrease gradually, although the moment of its resolution is still unclear. Delgado *et al.* [6] showed that the PVR index is the hemodynamic parameter most related to early mortality after heart transplantation. According to these Authors, the hemodynamic profile of the pulmonary system after transplantation is partially dependent on the level of pulmonary pressure before surgery, at least during the first year after the procedure. Non-*insulin* dependent *diabetes mellitus* may be considered a relative contraindication, depending on the presence of significant end-organ damage, such as *nephropathy, retinopathy* or *neuropathy*. On the other hand, insulin-dependent patients usually are considered as risk recipients because of their severe organ injury. In conclusion, ambulatory patients who have NYHA class III to IV and who are refractory to optimized medical treatment seem the most likely to benefit from cardiac transplant. However, hospital-admitted patients with severe heart failure and supported with inotropic drugs or even mechanical or ventricular assist devices (*VAD*), are likely to benefit from transplant if their organs are relatively healthy and if they are free from sepsis or any sort of infection [7, 8].

## Donor Selection

The availability of donor organs remains the main restrictive factor to *heart transplantation*. In the year 2002, 22,733 transplants of different organs were performed from 11,633 donors, but there is still a waiting list of 80,675 recipients [9]. Once a potential cardiac donor has been identified and all legal processes related to organ donation have been considered, a meticulous protocol of exams must be done. First of all, a record of the previous condition of health and the life-habits of the donor should be obtained. As the majority of potential organ-donors are victims of trauma and have been subjected to critical conditions, a general record of these conditions, principally, the degree of hemodynamic stability and the amount of circulatory supportive therapeutics, should be obtained. Also, laboratory data, including viral serologies, should be requested. Specific exams, such as EKG, thoracic X-ray and especially echocardiography, are of fundamental importance. *Coronary angiography* should be considered when the donors age is > 50 years or in the presence of history of tobacco use, diabetes, or another risk factor for coronary obstruction. Donor and recipient ABO compatibility is essential, and histocompatibility-antigen matching should be taken into account. A random panel of pooled lymphocytes representing the histocompatibility antigens in the community is used to test the recipient for anti-human-lymphocyte antigen antibodies that may ignite hyperacute rejection soon after the graft has been implanted. Recipient cellular toxicity in response to several lymphocytes is indicated by a reactive antibody titer higher than 10-15%. In this case, a prospective negative T-cell crossmatch between the recipient and donor sera is obligatory before transplantation [10, 11]. A positive crossmatch, even if performed retrospectively, is an absolute contraindication to transplantation. Prospective HLA matching, although ideal, is not routinely performed due to current allocation criteria and restrictions on ischemic time of the allograft. Cytomegalovirus (*CMV*)-negative donors for CMV-negative recipients should be used whenever possible. A significant consideration is size matching between donor and recipient. Acceptable size-matching is guided by similar weight between both, but the presence of higher PVRS in recipients requires hearts grafts with more preload recruitment capacity. In this particular condition it is preferable that donors are larger than recipients. Central *diabetes insipidus,* which develops in more than 50% of donors because of *pituitary dys-*

*function* and which causes massive diuresis that may lead to hypovolemia and electrolyte disturbances, may be controlled with low doses of *vasopressin* [12, 13]. It is important to consider evidence of *myocardial dysfunction* after *brain death*, severe enough to preclude the heart for transplantation in a significant number of cases. Birks *et al.* [14] investigated *caspases,* involved in the terminal part of the apoptotic pathway, in dysfunctional non-available donor hearts and their relation to inflammatory markers compared to well-functioning hearts used in recipients. These Authors concluded that caspases were elevated in dysfunctional donor hearts compared to hearts with preserved ventricular function. This fact may establish a possible link to inflammatory activation, endorsing the concept that brain death ignites inflammatory activation which can lead to apoptosis with an important effect on heart function. Finally, once considered as potential donors, due to the loss of central regulatory mechanisms, these patients are subjected to hypothermia, hypotension and several electrolyte disturbances that require intensive-care treatment until the moment of the donation.

## Recipient Anesthesia

A successful heart-transplant program requires the active participation of expert anesthesiologists who are familiar with complex *cardiothoracic anesthesia* techniques and *cardiopulmonary bypass*. The standard protocol for cardiac anesthesia is used for *heart transplantation*. Usually, heart transplantation is an emergency and "full-stomach" precautions should be taken into account. Long-term congestive heart failure promotes down-regulation of cardiac beta-1 receptors and there is a partial uncoupling of these receptors from adenylate cyclase. At the same time, altered ratios of inhibitory stimulatory signal-transduction proteins decrease receptor sensitivity to beta agonists. These factors, associated with a high circulatory dependency of increased *preload* and *afterload,* may lead the recipient heart to a poor tolerance of potent inhaled anesthetics and a sudden decrease in systemic resistance [15]. Anesthesia induction and maintenance should be carefully tailored, preferably by utilizing a *BIS* (biospectral index system) to guide the dose. Our practice is based on *hypnomidate* and small doses of *fentanyl* or *sufentanil* as induction agents, in association with *isofluorane* or *sevofluorane* as well as muscle-relaxation agents with fast elimination for maintenance. All patients are monitored with central venous lines, Foley catheters, radial artery catheters, central temperature probes, pulmonary artery catheters and transesophageal echocardiography. The *pulmonary artery catheter* is retracted during heart removal and graft anastomosis and then advanced again into the pulmonary artery at the end of the surgical procedure. Long-term anticoagulation of the recipient, such as during thromboembolic prophylaxis, or a deficiency in the coagulation system due to generalized hypoperfusion, consequent to congestive heart failure, may cause a significant disturbance in coagulation after cardiopulmonary bypass (*CPB*). Anti-fibrinolytics, such as *aprotinin* or *aminocaproic acid,* have been routinely used to reduce the risk of hemorrhage after CPB. In conclusion, due to impairment of systolic and diastolic function and consequent lower ejection fraction, the recipient should be carefully managed before CPB. Complete hemodynamic monitoring and judicious use of inotropic and vasodilators agents are indicated to obtain a cardiac output necessary to maintain organ perfusion from the initiation of anesthesia until CPB. Hemodynamic support is continued after CPB, when the transplanted heart is allowed to beat. However, the transplanted heart presents physiologic characteristics that require special attention, discussed below.

## Physiology of the Denervated Heart

At the time of cardiac transplant surgery, the donor's heart is completely denervated. Orthotopic implantation of the donor's heart is currently performed using the bicaval anastomotic technique, using the following anastomoses: *left atrium, inferior vena cava, pulmonary artery, aorta*, and *superior vena cava*. Due to this technique, the autonomic nerve connection is totally disrupted. The function of the recently transplanted heart is strongly influenced by the previous PVR of the recipient and the presence of total denervation. Performance may be also aggravated by ischemic/reperfusion injury caused by the foregoing graft ischemia. Ischemia induces diastolic dysfunction, which requires higher atrial filling pressures than normal. Characteristically, the cardiac allograft may present several degrees of impaired contractility and systolic dysfunction [16]. As a consequence of the lack of direct innervation, the transplanted heart may show an exacerbated chronotropic and inotropic response to the systemic infusion of adrenergic agents. This fact, often referred to as an exaggerated sensitivity to catecholamines, seems to result from the associated loss of sympathetic and parasympathetic innervation [17]. The inotropic supersensitivity seems to be a consequence of loss of pre-synaptic re-uptake and the depletion of endogenous pre-synaptic catecholamine stores [18]. Gerber *et al.* [19] showed that chronotropic supersensitivity, in turn, appears to result from the loss of the afferent vagal nerve tone that mediates baroreflex activity, responsible for slowing the heart rate when arterial pressure increases. The practical consequence of denervation is the necessity of catecholamine infusion after transplantation. Due to the exaggerated chronotropic and energetic response mainly to beta-agonists, the doses of exogenous catecholamine should be carefully adjusted to avoid these side effects, described in the literature. The same Authors evidenced that transplanted recipients exhibit a larger fall in contractile effectiveness and significant oxygen wasting during *dobutamine* infusion, when compared to normal volunteers. The fall in myocardial efficiency, as induced by dobutamine, correlated with increased heart rate and presented as the same effect, i.e., chronotropic supersensitivity observed in volunteers under *atropine* effect. This result may be caused by the loss of inhibitory parasympathetic innervation [19]. Stark and colleagues *et al.* [20], in tyramine response studies, demonstrated that reinnervation in transplanted hearts may occur 1 year after transplantation, but the maximum responses to catecholamines remain depressed.

## Immediate Postoperative Management

The standard care for cardiac-transplanted patients in the immediate postoperative period obeys the same pattern employed for patients who have undergone cardiac surgery. Additional protection against infection is added to the general care, and patients may be admitted to a special ICU area. Early complications after *cardiac transplantation* include acute and hyperacute rejection; low cardiac output, more commonly due to right ventricle failure; arrhythmias; pulmonary and systemic hypertension and renal failure. Early infection may occur, mainly pulmonary infection due to common bacteria, while opportunistic, viral and fungal infections become more frequent after a couple of weeks. Although rare, hyperacute rejection caused by preformed recipient cytotoxic antibodies against donor heart antigens, is a cause of global graft failure. Most of the time this is life-threatening, requiring urgent *plasmapheresis* and, in critical situations, a re-transplant [8].

In our protocol, as soon as the anastomosis is completed and the heart starts to beat, a complete hemodynamic profile and an echocardiographic evaluation of cardiac function is obtained. Depending on the heart function, specifically, the right ventricle performance, as well as the PVR and pulmonary artery values, a direct beta-adrenergic agonist is started. Routinely, a drip of dobutamine (5.0-20 µg/kg per minute) or *epinephrine* (1.0-5.0 µg per minute) is the first option. In the presence of evident right-ventricle dysfunction, *milrinone* can be included (0.3-0.75 µg/kg per minute). *Sodium nitroprusside* often is required additionally in order to offset peripheral and pulmonary vasoconstriction. Right ventricle dysfunction associated with elevated pulmonary vascular resistance is a significant problem immediately after CPB. Inflammatory mediators released during CPB may aggravate previous pulmonary hypertension of the recipient. There is no specific treatment of severe pulmonary hypertension due to the lack of a selective pulmonary vasodilator. Inhaled *nitric oxide*, phosphodiesterase inhibitors, intravenous *prostaglandin E1*, *nitroglycerin*, *isoproterenol*, high levels of inspired oxygen, mechanical ventilation with adequate alveolar recruitment to minimize ventilatory/perfusion mismatching all may contribute to controlling pulmonary hypertension crisis and consequently right ventricle failure. An  increase in pulmonary artery pressure in the first hours after transplantation may reflect low capacity of vasoreactivity in the pulmonary system, which means that pressure becomes flow dependent. Elevated right atrial pressure, above 15 mmHg, may be evidence of right ventricle dysfunction; if confirmed by echocardiography, this may require more aggressive drug therapy, including vasodilator agents. Right atrial pressures above 20 mmHg are associated with a rapid decline in renal function due to low cardiac output [21]. Due to the lack of a selective pulmonary vasodilator, nitric oxide, an endothelium-derived factor that produces relaxation of the vascular smooth muscle, has been used. In 10 patients after heart transplantation we observed a beneficial effect of inhaled nitric oxide, by decreasing PVR, transpulmonary gradient and increasing cardiac index, demonstrating that nitric oxide acts mainly on the pulmonary system [22]. The immunosuppressive regimen, typically consisting of *cyclosporine, azathioprine* and *methylprednisolone,* is adjusted according to biochemical exams and/or serum values. Tacrolimus is a macrolide antibiotic that shares many pharmacological properties with cyclosporine. Several studies have compared the immunosuppressive results of tacrolimus and cyclosporine, related to survival and rejection, but the results of clinical trials are inconclusive [23]. Acute *rejection* can be manifested with signals of low cardiac output, arrhythmias, and fever. Most of the episodes are insidious, and right ventricular endomyocardial biopsy remains the gold standard for the diagnosis of acute rejection. This is done by means of a percutaneous approach through the right internal jugular vein.

The weaning of vasoactive drugs is performed according to hemodynamic and echocardiographic data. In general, after 2-4 days only a small dosage of *dobutamine* or *epinephrine* is maintained, and then a few days later the vasoactive drugs are completely withdrawn guided by echocardiography and clinical signals. Invasive monitoring is removed as soon as stable hemodynamic condition is reached, on average 48-72 after transplantation. In our practice, we subsequently maintain only a central venous line during the first week after transplantation. If the patient is then free from major complications, he or she is discharged from the ICU.

## Respiratory Management

Patients submitted to *heart transplantation* are treated with the same protocol used in patients undergoing major cardiothoracic surgery. Routinely, they are maintained in volume-controlled ventilation (6–8 ml/Kg, with low PEEP, around 5 cm of water and an inspired oxygen fraction of 60%). Upon admission, a chest roentgenogram is obtained to place an *endotracheal tube* and to check mediastinal and/or pleural drains position as well as to verify lung expansion. Depending on the $PaO_2/FiO_2$ ratio, if lower than 150 mmHg, a pressure-controlled modality is started to maintain an expired tidal volume of 6-8 ml/kg. At the same time, alveolar recruitment maneuvers, comprising CPAP 20 to 30 cm $H_2O$, 20 s, repeated every two or three hours, are employed until the $PaO_2/FiO_2$ ratio is restored to adequate. Ideal PEEP is calculated utilizing the best compliance, set at 2 cm up to the best point. Due to the delicate balance between right ventricle ejection fraction and the pulmonary system, all these maneuvers should be carefully performed. The incidence of pulmonary complications in heart transplant recipients has not been completely studied. Lenner *et al.* [24] reported pulmonary complications in 159 consecutive adult *orthotopic heart transplantations* performed in 157 patients. In their retrospective review, 47 of 157 recipients (29.9%) had 81 types of pulmonary complications, *pneumonia* being the most common. They concluded that patients who have pulmonary complications after transplantation have a higher mortality than patients without pulmonary complications. The influence of cardiac allograft vasculopathy has also been investigated. Schwaiblmair *et al.* [25] , following 120 patients 2-137 months after orthotopic transplantation, showed that, in patients with significant cardiac allograft vasculopathy, there is a decrease in exercise capacity, reduced oxygen uptake and ventilation-perfusion mismatch.

In conclusion, heart transplantation has evolved from an experimental procedure to a well accepted therapy for selected patients with heart failure refractory to medical treatment. The success of the procedure depends on several factors: one of them is well-structured support in the immediate post-operative period.

# References


1. Barnard CN (1967) The operation. A human cardiac transplant: an interim report of a successful operation performed at Groote Schuur Hospital, Cape Town. S Afr Med J 41:1271-1274
2. Hosenpud JD, Bennett LE, Keck BM et al (2000) The Registry of the International Society of Heart and Lung Transplantation: seventeenth official report – 2000. J Heart Lung Transplant 19:909-931
3. Olivari MT, Antolick A, Kaye MP et al (1988) Heart transplantation in elderly patients. J Heart Transplant 7:258-264
4. Stinson EB, Griepp RB, Schroeder JS et al (1972) Hemodynamic observations one and two years after cardiac transplantation in man. Circulation 45:1183-1194
5. Griepp RB, Stinson EB, Dong E Jr et al (1971) Determinants of operative risk in human heart transplantation. Am J Surg 122:192-197
6. Delgado JF, Gomez-Sanchez MA, Saenz de la Calzada C et al (2001) Impact of mild pulmonary hypertension on mortality and pulmonary artery pressure profile after heart transplantation. J Heart Lung Transplant 20:942-948
7. Marks JD, Karwande SV, Richenbacher WE et al (1992) Perioperative mechanical circulatory support for transplantation. J Heart Lung Transplant 11:117-128
8. Edmunds HL Jr (1997) Heart transplant. In: Cardiac surgery in the adult. New York: McGraw-Hill chapter 49
9. (2003) The International Society for Heart and Lung Transplantation. ISHLT Registries. Overall heart and adult heart transplantation statistics. Available at: http://www.ishlt.org/regist_slides_2002/slides_web_heart_adult.ppt.   Accessed February 14
10. Loh E, Bergin JD, Couper GS, Mudge GH Jr (1994) Role of panel-reactive antibody cross-reactivity in predicting survival after orthotopic heart transplantation. J Heart Lung Transplant 13:194-128
11. Jarcho J, Naftel DC, Shroyer JK et al (1994) Influence of HLA mismatch on rejection after heart transplantation: a multiinstitutional study. The Cardiac Transplant Research Database Group. J Heart Lung Transplant 13:583-595
12. Frist WH, Fanning WJ (1990) Donor management and matching. Cardiol Clin 8:55-71
13. Davis FD (1987) Coordination of cardiac transplantation: patient processing and donor organ procurement. Circulation 75:29-39
14. Birks EJ , Yacoub MH, Burton PS et al (2000) Activation of apoptotic and inflammatory pathways in dysfunctional donor hearts. Transplantation 70:1498-1506
15. Chetham PM (2000) Anesthesia for heart or single or double lung transplantation in the adult patient. J Card Surg 15:167-174
16. Renlund GD (1998) Cardiac transplantation. In: Topol EJ (ed) Comprehensive cardiovascular medicine. Philadelphia: Lippincott-Raven Publishers 2701-2723

17.  von Scheidt W, Böhm M, Schneider B et al (1992) Isolated presynaptic inotropic b-adrenergic supersensitivity of the transplanted denervated human heart in vivo. Circulation 85:1056-1063

18.  Schwaiger M, Hutchins GD, Kalff V et al (1991) Evidence for regional catecholamine uptake and storage sites in the transplanted human heart by positron emission tomography. J Clin Invest 87:1681-1690

19.  Gerber BL, Bernard X, Melin JA et al (2001) Exaggerated chronotropic and energetic response to dobutamine after orthotopic cardiac transplantation. J Heart Lung Transplant 20:824-832

20.  Stark RP, McGinn AL, Wilson RF (1991) Chest pain in cardiac-transplant recipients. Evidence of sensory reinnervation after cardiac transplantation. N Engl J Med 324:1791-1799

21.  Miller WL (1997) Heart transplantation in critical care. In: Civetta J, Taylor RW, Kirby R (eds) Critical Care. 3ª ed. Philadelphia: Lippincott Williams & Wilkins Publishers 1333-1340

22.  Auler Jr JOC, Carmona MJC, Bocchi AE et al (1996) Low doses of inhaled nitric oxide in heart transplant recipients. J Heart Lung Transplant 15:443-450

23.  Kobashigawa JA (1999) Postoperative management following heart transplantation. Transplant Proc 31:2038-2046

24.  Lenner R, Padilla ML, Teirstein AS et al (2001) Pulmonary complications in cardiac transplant recipients. Chest 120:508-513

25.  Schwaiblmair M, von Scheidt W, Uberfuhr P et al (1999) Lung function and cardiopulmonary exercise performance after heart transplantation: influence of cardiac allograft vasculopathy. Chest 116:332-339

# BASICS

# Basic Physics for Anaesthesia and Intensive Care

U. Lucangelo, S. Pascotto, P. Accardo

The correct use of sophisticated devices by the anaesthetist for life support and the monitoring of vital functions require the understanding of several basic laws of physics. By way of example, we examine two extremely important topics: the gas laws, which are fundamental for understanding the physiology of respiratory exchange and inhalation anaesthesia, and fluid dynamics, which is a principle common to cardiovascular and respiratory function. For a more specific analysis of the physical applications, the reader is invited to refer to specialist articles (echocardiography, aortic and thoracic acoustic imaging, neuromuscular monitoring, infrared spectroscopy, etc.).

## The Gas Laws

The ideal gas laws [1] show the interrelations between volume ($V$), pressure ($P$), temperature ($T$) and quantities of gas, and they are applied to diluted gases at temperatures above boiling point. The *boiling point* of a gas is the temperature at which, at a standard pressure, the gas condenses to the liquid state. The boiling point can be increased by increasing the pressure, up to a critical temperature above which the gas cannot change to the liquid state regardless of the amount of pressure applied. The closer the temperature is to the boiling point, the greater the error will be in using the gas laws.

## Boyle's Law

If the temperature and the quantity of gas are constant, the volume ($V$) of a gas is inversely proportional to the pressure ($P$):

$$V = \frac{1}{P} \ \text{ or } \ PV = \text{constant}$$

Therefore, doubling $V$ halves $P$ and vice versa.

## Charles's Law

If the pressure and quantity of gas are constant, the volume is proportional to the temperature:

$$\frac{V}{T} = \text{constant}$$

## Gay-Lussac's Law

If the volume and quantity of gas are constant, the pressure is proportional to the temperature:

$$\frac{P}{T} = \text{constant}$$

With an increase in temperature, gases expand and the volume increases, according to the following relationship:

$$Vt = V_0(1+at)$$

where   $Vt$ = the volume of the gas at a certain temperature (in °C)
        $V_0$ = the volume of the gas at 0 °C
        $a$  = gas expansion coefficient at constant pressure (1/273)

The quantity of gas is measured in moles. A *mole* is one gram multiplied by the molecular weight of a substance (therefore, its molecular weight expressed in grams). According to Avogadro's law, 1 mole of any (ideal) gas always occupies 22.4 l ($22.4 \times 10^3$ cm³) under conditions of constant pressure and temperature. For example, the molecular weight of oxygen is 32, therefore 1 mole of oxygen equals 32 grams of oxygen and occupies 22.4 l.

The concepts outlined so far are combined in the *ideal gas law* (or *ideal gas equation of state*), which states that the pressure of a gas is directly proportional to the temperature and number of molecules constituting it, and inversely proportional to the volume in which it is contained:

$$PV = nRT$$

where   $n$ = the quantity of gas expressed in moles
        $R$ = the Boltzmann constant (or universal gas constant, identical for all
            ideal gases)
        $T$ = the absolute temperature of the gas in degrees Kelvin ($T = t + 273$)

The important message contained in this formula is that the pressure is directly proportional to the number of moles, which is equivalent to the number of molecules present. If a gas, such as oxygen, is in a cylinder, the pressure gauge gives an accurate estimate of the quantity of gas contained within it.

According to convention, the volumes of blood gas are measure in STPD, or standard temperature (0 °C or 273 K) and pressure (760 mmHg or 1 atm) dry.

Gas volumes in respiration, by contrast, are measured in BTPS, or body temperature (37 °C), ambient pressure and saturated with water vapour (47 mmHg).

## Dalton's Law of Partial Pressure

The pressure of a gas mixture is the sum of the partial pressures of the individual components of the mixture. In other words, the pressure exerted by each gas is the same as that which it would exert if it occupied the container alone:

$$P = P_1 + P_2 + P_x$$

The ideal gas law can be similarly reformulated:

$$P = \frac{n_1 RT}{V} + \frac{n_2 RT}{V} + \frac{n_x RT}{V}$$

The pressure of water vapour does not follow Dalton's law because under normal atmospheric conditions it is mainly dependent on temperature. Therefore, when calculating the partial pressure of a gas where water vapour is present, the total barometric pressure needs to be corrected before calculating the partial pressure of each gas.

## Graham's Law

The diffusion velocity ($v$) of a gas is inversely proportional to the square root of its molecular mass:

$$v = \sqrt{\frac{1}{PM}}$$

## Henry's Law (Gas Diffusion Law)

The concentration ($C$) of a gas dissolved in a solution is directly proportional to its external partial pressure ($P$) and inversely proportional to the absolute temperature ($T$) of the gas-liquid system:

$$C = \frac{\alpha P}{T}$$

where $\alpha$ = the Ostwald solubility coefficient.

For the diffusion of a gas through a tissue, such as the alveolar membrane, Fick's law is used, which reformulates some of the concepts considered in the previous two laws. The velocity of transfer of a gas through a layer of tissue is directly proportional to the area of tissue ($A$), the difference in partial pressure of the gases on either side ($P_1 - P_2$) and the gas diffusion constant, and inversely proportional to the thickness of the tissue (5):

$$V = \frac{A\delta\left(P_1 - P_2\right)}{s}$$

where $\alpha$ = the diffusion constant = $\dfrac{\alpha}{\sqrt{PM}}$

This is why $CO_2$ diffuses across the alveolar-capillary barrier much more rapidly than $O_2$, because its solubility is 22 times greater, whereas its molecular weight is only slightly greater (44 vs. 32).

The concepts outlined so far are also important for understanding the action of volatile anaesthetics. The solubility of a volatile anaesthetic is described by the blood-gas partition coefficient, which describes the relationship between the concentration of the anaesthetic in the blood and the concentration in the alveolar air, under conditions of equilibrium between the two phases, and constant temperature and pressure.

The greater the solubility of an inhalation anaesthetic, the less is its speed of action, given that it dissolves rapidly in the blood. This creates a low alveolus/blood gradient and therefore a low blood/brain gradient, with consequent reduced action. For this reason, an inhalation anaesthetic is more powerful the less soluble it is.

Despite being highly insoluble in blood, nitrogen monoxide is twenty times more soluble than nitrogen, the main gas present in air (79%). During induction with nitrogen monoxide, upon reaching the alveoli the gas diffuses according to the concentration gradient more rapidly than nitrogen, and the other gases present become concentrated in a reduced space (concentration effect). Furthermore, if another anaesthetic agent is present, its effective concentration increases (second gas effect). During the anaesthesia recovery period, however, the opposite effect occurs: the nitrogen monoxide is quickly eliminated, leaving greater space for the other gases, among which is $O_2$, causing dilution hypoxia.

Volatile halogenated anaesthetics are vapours (and not gases) in that they are present in liquid form at ambient temperature. For anaesthetic purposes, a vaporiser – a device which transforms the anaesthetic from the liquid to the vapour state – is used. Passing through the vaporiser is a mixture of carrier gases in which a controllable quantity of the anaesthetic is released.

The change from a liquid to a gaseous phase requires work, and therefore a consumption of energy. If the energy required is not supplied externally through the administration of heat, the work is performed at the expense of the kinetic energy of the molecules of the liquid, which undergoes gradual cooling.

The *evaporation heat* is the quantity of heat to be administered per unit mass of a liquid, at a certain temperature, in order to transform the liquid into saturated vapour at the same temperature. This problem is avoided by modern precision vaporisers, which are equipped with metal blades that vary the resistance at the entrance of the vaporisation chamber with respect to its internal temperature. The reduction of resistance under conditions of reduced temperature enables an increase in flow.

## Fluid dynamics

Fluids include gases and liquids and have two important properties: density and pressure. The density ($\varrho$) is the mass ($m$) per unit volume ($V$):

$$\varrho = \frac{m}{V}$$

and in the international system of units of measurement (SI) it is measured in kg/m³.

The pressure ($p$) is the force ($F$) which a fluid exerts on a surface ($A$):

$$p = \frac{F}{A}$$

Fluids take the shape of the container they are held in, because they cannot support a shear force, that is, a force tangential to their surface. They can, however, support a normal (perpendicular) force to their surface; that force per surface unit is, of course, pressure.

The SI unit of measurement of pressure is the Newton (N) per square metre, known as the Pascal (Pa). Because the Pascal is a very small unit, the commonly used measurement is the kilopascal (kPa). Another unit of measurement is the bar, which is a multiple of the Pascal:

$$1 \text{ bar} = 10^5 \text{ Pa}$$

The atmosphere (atm) is the average pressure of the atmosphere at sea level, and it is almost equal to the bar:

$$1 \text{ atm} = 1.013 * 10^5 \text{ Pa} = 760 \text{ torr}$$

The torr (named after Evangelista Torricelli, who invented the mercury barometer in 1674) is the pressure of a column of mercury of 1 mm (mmHg):

$$1 \text{ torr} = 133.3 \text{ Pa} = 1.36 \text{ cmH}_2\text{O}$$

The centimetre of water ($\text{cmH}_2\text{O}$) is a unit of measurement which has a better definition than mmHg:

$$1 \text{ cmH}_2\text{O} = 98 \text{ Pa}$$

It is used solely for the measurement of the pressure in the airways, because the viscosity of air is low and the pressure gradient required to overcome the resistance within the conducting airways is in the order of the mmHg.

The manometer is an instrument used for measuring the pressure of fluids, such as arterial blood, and it consists of a tube containing mercury (or water). The weight of the column of liquid is used to equilibrate the pressure exerted against it, and the height reached by the column indicates the pressure to be measured. If a column of liquid with a transverse section $A$ and a height $h$ has a volume $V=Ah$ and a weight $mg= \varrho Ahg$, then it exerts a force at its base equal to its weight and a pressure $p = \varrho hg$. The pressure of the manometer, therefore, only depends on the density of the fluid used and the vertical height of the column.

A fundamental characteristic of fluids is described in *Pascal's law of fluid pressures* (Blaise Pascal 1623-1662) [2]: pressure applied anywhere to a body of fluid causes a force to be transmitted equally in all directions; the force acts at right angles to any surface in contact with the fluid. This principle lies at the basis of the Heimlich manoeuvre, by which a sharp increase in pressure applied to the abdomen is transferred to the throat, causing the expulsion of food particles from the trachea. Another example in which this principle is applied is a water bed, which uniformly distributes the body's weight thus reducing decubitus pain.

The easiest fluids to study are ideal fluids, which have a number of characteristics in contrast with real fluids. An ideal or perfect fluid is one which is:
- *Incompressible*: its density is constant regardless of changes in pressure. In reality, gases are easily compressed, whereas liquids are not.
- *Inviscid*: the viscosity of a fluid is the measurement of its resistance to flow, which is similar to the friction that occurs due to the contact of two solid bodies. Viscosity is responsible for shear forces between one layer and another of the fluid in motion. When these forces can be assumed to be zero, the fluid is said to be inviscid.
- *Irrotational*: each element of the fluid moves without undergoing rotation.
- *Laminar*: a moving fluid has laminar motion when the velocity in a point of the fluid is dependent only on its position and does not change neither in time, direction nor intensity. A fluid will have, by contrast, turbulent motion when the velocity changes in time and vortices are formed [3].

Under conditions of laminar flow, the elements of a fluid move following non-intersecting *streamlines.* The velocity in each point is the tangent to the streamline at that point. The fluid moves staying within a flow tube, which is determined by the sum of all of the streamlines passing through the points of a closed curve.

## Equation of Continuity [2]

In a fluid undergoing laminar flow, the flow rate remains constant; that is, the product of the area of the section through which the flow passes multiplied by the velocity is constant:

(1) $$A_1 v_1 = A_2 v_2$$

To demonstrate this equation, consider a tube with abrupt variations in the area of the section in which a perfect fluid is moving. $A_1$ and $A_2$ are two areas of normal sections of the tube and $v_1$ and $v_2$ are the velocities of the fluid passing through those sections. If in a certain time interval $\Delta t$ the fluid in $A_1$ travels a distance $x_1$, in the same time interval the fluid in $A_2$ will travel a distance $x_2$. Once the velocity of a fluid is given by the distance travelled in a time interval:

$$v_1 = \frac{x_1}{\Delta t} \quad \text{and} \quad v_2 = \frac{x_2}{\Delta t}$$

the shift will be:

$$x_1 = v_1 \Delta t \quad \text{and} \quad x_2 = v_2 \Delta t$$

In addition, the volumes of fluid in the two tracts are given by the relationship between the area of the section through which the fluid passes and the distance travelled:

$$V_1 = A_1 x_1 \quad \text{and} \quad V_2 = A_2 x_2$$

and therefore:

$$V_1 = A_1 v_1 \Delta t \quad \text{and} \quad V_2 = A_2 v_2 \Delta t$$

Under conditions of laminar flow, the quantities of fluid which pass through sections $A_1$ and $A_2$ in $\Delta t$ have equal volumes because, by definition, no fluid can leave or enter through the walls. The flow rate ($Q$) will also be constant:

$$Q_1 = Q_2 = \quad \text{constant}$$

The flow rate of a tube is the volume of fluid which passes through a normal section of the tube in a unit of time:

$$Q_1 = \frac{V_1}{\Delta t} \quad \text{and} \quad Q_2 = \frac{V_2}{\Delta t}$$

and the relationship between section area and velocity is constant:

$$A_1 v_1 = A_2 v_2$$

This is the basis of *Leonardo's law* [2]: the mean velocity of a fluid through a normal tube section is inversely proportional to the area of the section. If the tube narrows, the streamlines draw closer together and the velocity of the fluid increases.

In physiology, the equation of continuity can be applied in an approximate manner to the movement of air through the bronchial tree. The bronchial tree is characterised by an irregular dichotomous ramification, through which the section area increases at each generation of airways, despite the formation of branches continually smaller in diameter and shorter in length.

Another application of the law is in pulmonary vascularisation. Pulmonary blood-flow can be considered constant in time. Therefore, its velocity is greater in the arteries and the arterioles, where the section area is greater, than it is in the pulmonary capillary network. This reduction in velocity has the physiological advantage of lengthening the time for gas exchange through the alveolar-capillary membrane.

## Bernoulli's Theorem [2, 3, 4]

This theorem takes its name from the mathematician and physicist Daniel Bernoulli (1700-1782) and it is the principle of conservation of mechanical energy applied to a fluid in motion. It states that, for each element of a perfect fluid in movement in a gravitational force field, the sum of the pressure energy, the kinetic energy (due to movement) and the potential energy (due to the force of gravity) times a unit of volume is constant:

(2)
$$\varrho + \frac{1}{2}\varrho v^2 + \varrho g h = E \quad \text{(constant)}$$

That sum corresponds to the mechanical energy which is conserved in laminar movement, given that there are no viscous forces.

Let us return now to the perfect fluid flowing in a tube under stationary conditions. A certain quantity of fluid $m$ ($= \varrho/V$) enters one end ($A_1$) of the tube and the same quantity exits the other end ($A_2$) after having travelled a distance $\Delta x$ in a time interval $\Delta t$. The height, velocity and pressure of the fluid at the entrance are $h_1$, $v_1$ and $p_1$, whereas at the exit they are $h_2$, $v_2$ and $p_2$.

The pressure difference at the two ends of the tube determines a force which, according to Newton's second law ($F = ma$), causes an acceleration ($a$) of the fluid. In other words, the force required to increase the velocity is guaranteed by the reduction in pressure. Therefore, if the potential energy is considered constant, an increase in velocity is accompanied by a reduction in pressure, and viceversa.

The pressure force $F_1$ exerted on $A_1$ promotes the movement of the fluid, whereas the force $F_2$ exerted on $A_2$ opposes movement. If $L_1$ and $L_2$ are, correspondingly, the work performed:

$$L_1 = F_1 \Delta x = p_1 S_1 \Delta x = p_1 V$$

$$L_2 = - F_2 \Delta x = - p_2 S_2 \Delta x = - p_2 V$$

then the overall work ($L$) will be:

$$L = L_1 + L_2 = p_1 V - p_2 V$$

The change in the velocity at the ends of the tube correspond to the change in kinetic energy ($\Delta K$):

$$\Delta K = \frac{1}{2} m \left( v_2^{\,2} - v_1^{\,2} \right) = \frac{1}{2} \varrho V \left( v_2^{\,2} - v_1^{\,2} \right)$$

whereas the change in potential energy ($\Delta U$) is equal to:

$$\Delta U = mg \left( h_2 - h_1 \right) = \varrho g V \left( h_2 - h_1 \right)$$

The overall change in kinetic energy ($\Delta K$) and potential energy ($\Delta U$) corresponds to the work ($L$) performed by the external forces on the volume of fluid considered:

$$L = \Delta K + \Delta U$$

It can be stated that:

(3)
$$p_1 V - p_2 V = \frac{1}{2}\varrho V \left(v_2^{\,2} - v_1^{\,2}\right) + \varrho g V \left(h_2 - h_1\right)$$

or:

$$p_1 + \frac{1}{2}\varrho v_1^{\,2} + \varrho g h_1 = p_2 + \frac{1}{2}\varrho v_2^{\,2} + \varrho g h_2$$

Given that the reference is to any two sections of fluid, this relationship can also be written as Eq. (2):

$$p + \frac{1}{2}\varrho v^2 + \varrho g h = E \qquad \text{(constant)}$$

With slight approximation, Bernoulli's theorem is also valid for marginally viscous real fluids that flow in tubes with reasonably large sections. In the case of a viscous fluid, a part of the work performed by the forces in action does not contribute to increasing the kinetic energy, in that it is dissipated as heat due to friction.

The theorem can explain the situation in which for some reason an airway narrows: the pressure of the flow within the airway decreases and this contributes to a further narrowing of the pathological airway, as in the case of sleep apnoea syndrome.

There are numerous applications for Bernoulli's theorem, such as the lift an aeroplane wing receives. The lower surface of the wing is flat, whereas the upper surface is convex. This divides the air into two currents which pass one above the wing and one below and then meet up again. The current passing above the wing travels a greater distance, and will therefore be faster. As a consequence the pressure exerted above the wing will be less than the pressure exerted below. This imbalance in pressure creates the lift the plane receives (Fig. 1).

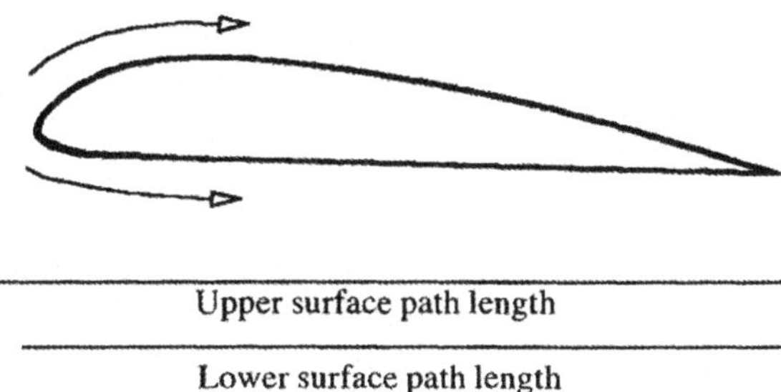


**Fig. 1.** Representation of the wing of an aeroplane

Another important application of this theorem is the *Venturi tube* (Giovanni Venturi, 1767), which is a tube in which a section is narrowed. Its purpose is to measure the flow rate in a tube and it is therefore inserted horizontally into a section of the tube itself. The velocity of the fluid flowing inside is approximately constant in all the points of a normal section of the axis of the tube, so the equation of continuity ($p_1v_1 = p_2v_2$) is valid. As can be seen in Fig. 2, the flow passing through section $A_1$ has a lesser velocity $v_1$ than the velocity $v_2$ of the flow passing through section $A_2$ in correspondence to the narrowing.

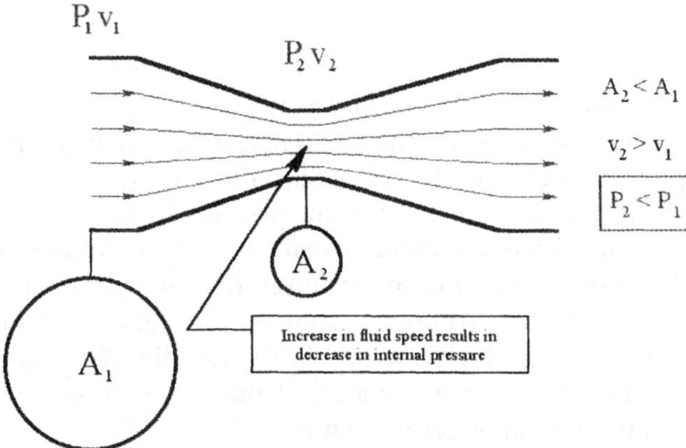


**Fig. 2.** Venturi tube (from http://hyperphysics.phy-astr.gsu.edu/hbase/hframe.htm). P, Pressure; v, velocity; A, area

According to Bernoulli's theorem, the pressure in $A_1$ is greater than the pressure in $A_2$, and this can be measured by inserting a manometer in correspondence with the two sections. Given that the two sections are at the same height ($h_1 = h_2$), Eq. (3) becomes:

$$p_1 - p_2 = \frac{1}{2}\varrho\left(v_2^{\,2} - v_1^{\,2}\right)$$

and inserting Eq. (1):

$$v_1 = \frac{v_2 A_2}{A_1}$$

we arrive at:

$$p_1 - p_2 = \frac{1}{2}\varrho v_2^{\,2}\left(1 - \frac{A_2^{\,2}}{A_1^{\,2}}\right)$$

From here the velocity of the flow at the level of the narrowing can be calculated:

$$v_2 = \sqrt{\frac{2\left(p_1 - p_2\right)}{\varrho\left(1 - \frac{A_2^{\,2}}{A_1^{\,2}}\right)}}$$

and therefore the flow rate of the tube ($Q = Av$).

The Venturi tube operates on the general principle that the pressure in a narrowed region is lower than the pressure in the main tube. If the velocity of flow in the tube is sufficiently high, then the pressure in the narrow region may be lower than atmospheric pressure; this fact is exploited in the carburetor of an automobile. In the chamber of the carburetor, the fuel is under the effects of atmospheric pressure. The carburetor vaporises the liquid fuel and forces it up a tube, where air passes, which narrows in the middle. This narrow section accelerates the mixture of air and fuel, and the acceleration causes a fall in pressure, which in turn vaporises more fuel [5].

The Venturi principle is also the basis for the functioning of the mask for the administration of high-flow oxygen, known as the Venturi mask or ventimask. The oxygen is supplied to the mask at a low-flow velocity; at the entrance to the mask, however, it is drawn into a narrow hole, and this passage generates high-velocity flow. The flow of gas produced in its turn draws ambient air into the mask. By adjusting the diameter of the hole, the $O_2$ can be appropriately diluted with ambient air, obtaining $FiO_2$ [6] (Fig. 3).

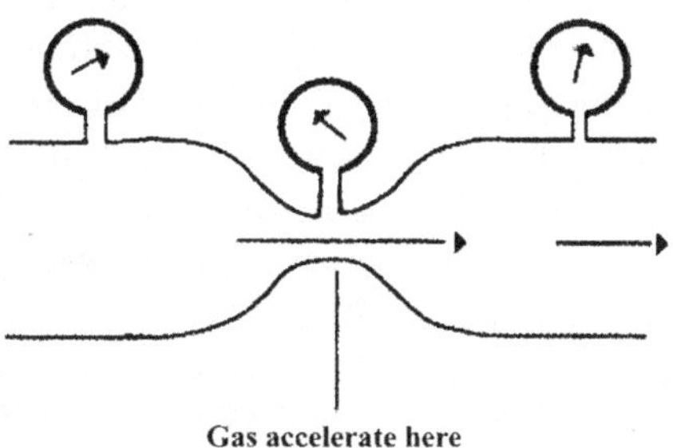



*a) The Bernoulli effect, with a flow of gas passing through a narrow tube. Note how the pressure falls at the narrow point.*

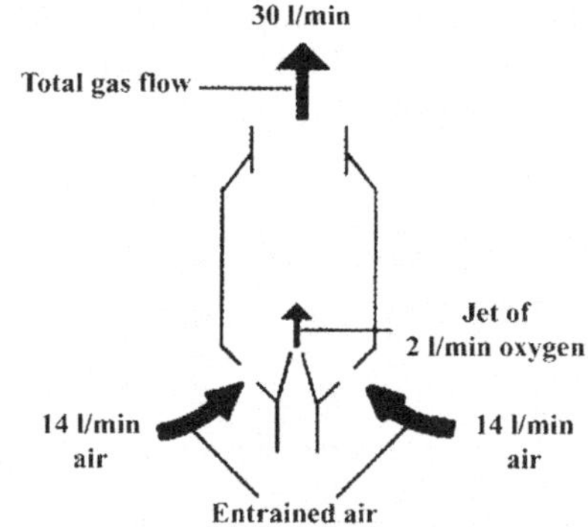



*b) Venturi valve - a low flow of oxygen, 2l/min passing through a narrow tube draws in 28l/min air, the hole size ensures the correct mixture of oxygen and air.*

**Fig. 3a.** The Bernoulli effect, **b** representation of the Venturi mask

It has been demonstrated, however, that the ventimask, rather than functioning according to the Venturi principle, functions according to the principle of jet mixing. The variation of the flow of oxygen through the hole modifies the pressure only at the level of the narrowing, and this slight pressure gradient is insignificant for the air inlet. The flow of oxygen in movement, upon meeting still ambient air, generates a viscous force which transports with it the nearby laminar flows of air to a degree proportional to the flow velocity. The entrance of air, therefore, practically takes place at constant pressure, as a result of the viscosity of the fluid, and each pressure variation is a consequence of the mixing process [5, 7].

## Viscosity

A real liquid can be considered incompressible to a fair degree of approximation, but it always presents a certain viscosity, a certain force of internal friction. Consider a fluid in movement under conditions of laminar flow along a horizontal cylindrical tube. If the liquid were perfect, the pressure would be the same in all of the sections, whereas in the case of a real liquid the pressure decreases in the direction of movement, and between two sections of liquid there is always a pressure difference, known as pressure (or head) loss. This loss is typical of frictional or dissipative forces, the intensity of which is determined by a property known as viscosity. The viscosity of liquids is influenced by the van der Walls cohesive forces between the molecules and is reduced with heat, whereas the viscosity of gases derives from the collision between particles of gas which move rapidly and increase their velocity with heat.

One of the effects of viscosity is that the velocity of each particle of fluid depends on the distance from the axis of the tube. Laminar flow is characteristically made up of a series of concentric layers whose velocity ($V_m$) increases from the layer nearest the edge towards the centre of the tube (Fig. 4).

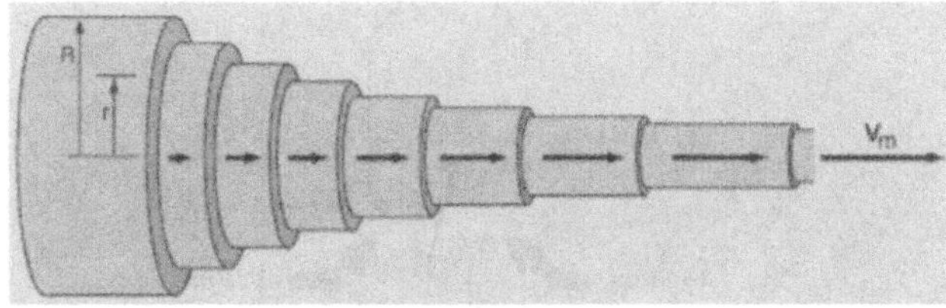

**Fig. 4.** Laminar flow (from http://hyperphysics.phy-astr.gsu.edu/hbase/hframe.htm). *R*, Radius of the layer nearest the edge; *r*, radius of a layer nearer the centre. *Arrows* indicate the vector of the flow velocity along the axis of the tube

All laminar movement is regulated by Poiseuille's law: under conditions of laminar movement the flow rate ($Q$) of a tube is directly proportional to the radius ($r$) raised to the fourth power and the pressure difference between the two ends of the tube ($\Delta p$), and inversely proportional to the viscosity coefficient ($\eta$) and the length of the tube ($l$):

$$(4) \qquad\qquad Q = \frac{\pi r^4 \Delta p}{8 \eta l}$$

The fact that the radius of the tube appears raised to the fourth power in this formula is important when a quantity of liquid needs to be transferred rapidly through a large tube. With blood transfusions, for example, increasing the diameter of the needle is preferable to increasing the height of the bag with respect to the needle. Doubling the diameter of the needle increases the flow rate sixteen times. In contrast, halving the diameter increases the resistance sixteen times [7].

This fact also explains how arterial stenosis of 20% can reduce blood flow by as much as 60%, and how vasodilatation is much more effective in increasing arterial pressure as a compensation mechanism for peripheral hypoperfusion.

If the fluid velocity is increased, the laminar motion becomes turbulent, with the direction of the velocity at one point changing from instant to instant. This leads to the creation of vortices, or small areas of flow which close in on themselves and maintain their own individual motion within the tube. Initially, significant kinetic energy is associated with the vortices which then due to internal friction is dissipated in heat and the vortices dissolve. With the same pressure difference between the two ends of the tube, therefore, the flow rate is less than it would be under conditions of laminar motion, and Poiseuille's law is no longer applicable.

The critical velocity $(v_c)$ above which the motion becomes turbulent depends on the viscosity coefficient, the density of the fluid and the radius of the tube:

$$v_c = \frac{\text{Re}\,\eta}{\varrho r}$$

Re is Reynold's number, an absolute number derived from the relationship between the force of inertia $(F_i)$, dependent on the absolute density of the fluid $(\varrho)$, and the force of viscosity $(F_v)$, dependent on the viscosity coefficient $(\eta)$:

$$F_i \simeq \frac{\varrho v^2}{2r}$$

$$F_v \simeq \frac{\eta v}{4r^2}$$

$$\text{Re} = \frac{F_i}{F_v} = \frac{\varrho r v}{\eta}$$

Therefore, the transition to turbulent motion takes place when there is a considerable increase in the forces of inertia with respect to the viscous forces.

Real liquids can be divided into Newtonian and non-Newtonian liquids according to whether their viscosity remains constant or not [8]. A Newtonian liquid has a Reynold's number around 2,000: the motion will be laminar if Re < 2,000, turbulent if Re > 3,000 and instable for Re values between 2,000 and 3,000.

Those values can also be considered valid for blood under normal conditions, even though it is a non-Newtonian liquid. The blood viscosity coefficient increases with haematocrit, whereas it decreases in capillaries with a diameter less than a millimetre (Fahraeus-Lidqvist effect). An explanation for this feature is that in the capillaries blood has bubble motion, in which almost all of the plasma is found between one erythrocyte and another, therefore the apparent viscosity tends towards zero. Furthermore, in small vessels the erythrocytes, being large cells, tend to accumulate in the faster central part of the flow, such that there are few cells near the vessel walls that contribute to wall friction.

In many vessels with normal levels of arterial pressure, turbulence is practically absent, and the blood flow can be well described with Poiseuille's law. Only in the central part of the aorta does the blood flow reaches critical velocity and becomes turbulent.

Poiseuille's law can also be applied to gas flow in the airways. In this case $\Delta p$ indicates the pressure difference between the intrathoracic pressure and the pressure of the external environment. During free breathing, with the exception of the superior extra-pulmonary airways, the motion can be considered laminar in all regions. With an increase in ventilation, motion becomes turbulent in the trachea and the main bronchi, where the velocity is highest, whereas in the distal ramifications, due to the increase in the total section, the velocity decrease and the motion returns to being laminar. In the regions around the bifurcations there are transition areas, characterised by tracts of laminar motion and tracts of turbulent motion [8].

Fluids apply resistance to the motion of a body immersed in them. The layer of fluid around the surface of the body in movement is the boundary layer, whose motion is given by the Reynold's number. At low Re values, viscous forces prevail and the motion in the boundary layer is laminar. At high Re values, the forces of inertia prevail (with consequent pressure variations) and the entire boundary layer is turbulent. For intermediate Re values, the motion is laminar in the near-surface layer and turbulent immediately thereafter.

## Stokes's Law

The resistance encountered by a body immersed in a fluid in laminar motion is due to a force ($F$) proportional to the velocity ($v$) and the radius ($r$) of the body:

$$F = 6\pi\eta v r$$

In the case of turbulent motion, the formula is:

$$F = \frac{1}{2} c S \varrho v^2$$

where there is a coefficient dependent on the shape of the body and where $S$ is the maximum section of the body.

The flowmeter in anaesthetic devices utilises several of the principles described above. It consists of a vertical tube, whose section increases from bottom to top, and a coil or rotameter on its inside. The space between the rotameter and the wall of the tube is known as the annular space and is considered equivalent to a circular canal having the same transverse area. With an increase in the flow supplied, the rotameter rises and the annular space increases owing to the widening of the tube. The rotameter reaches a point of equilibrium for a given flow volume when the pressure raising it equals its weight. The reduction in pressure which is created via the annular space is maintained constant for any position of the rotameter (such devices are therefore called constant-pressure flowmeters). What does change is the type of dependence of the flow on that pressure difference.

At low flows the annular space is long and narrow, and therefore the flow is laminar, dependent on the viscosity of the gas and regulated by Poiseuille's law. At high flows, however, the annular space is wide and short, and the flow is turbulent, dependent on the density of the gas and regulated by Graham's law (the velocity of a gas is inversely proportional to the square root of its density).

Given that the changes of the area of the transverse section of flow are abrupt and not gradual, Bernoulli's theorem does not accurately describe this type of flow. The flow above the rotameter is very turbulent, and the turbulence dissipates the kinetic energy in heat. However, the introduction of an empirical constant (discharge coefficient), which varies with the shape of the hole and the Reynold's number, makes the application of the law possible [9, 10].

# References


1.  Giannazzo E (1998) Lezioni di biofisica e tecnologie biomediche, Piccin. Padua
2.  Holliday D, Resnick R, Walker J (1998) Fondamenti di fisica. Ambrosiana, Milan, ch 16
3.  Panitteri M, Barcio S, Corsello A (1972) Fisica per licei scientifici. Paravia, Turin, ch 13
4.  Rosati S (1978) Fisica generale. Ambrosiana, Milan, ch 17
5.  Scacci R (1979) Air entrainment mask: jet mixing is how they work; the Bernoulli and Venturi principles are how they don't. Resp Care 24:928-931
6.  Marino PL (1999) Terapia intensiva. Masson, Milan, pp 390-391
7.  Miller RD (1993) Trattato di anestesia. Delfino, Rome, p 2399
8.  Burns DM, MacDonald SGG (1998) Fisica per studenti di biologia e medicina. Zanichelli, Bologna, ch 9
9.  Miller RD (1993) Trattato di anestesia. Delfino, Rome, ch 9 e 32
10. Romano E (1997) Anestesia generale e speciale, UTET, Turin, p 193

# FOCUS

# Chapter 5

# To Tube or Not To Tube?
# A Critical Point in Emergency and Trauma

G. BERLOT

The brief history of *critical care medicine* has been marked by some hotly debated issues, including the "crystalloid-colloid controversy", the "stay and play vs. scoop and run" approach to severely injured patients, and the utility of obtaining above normal levels of cardiovascular and oxygenation variables. Basically, despite the relevance of the debated points and the high scientific ranks of the advocates of the different approaches, no study has been able to demonstrate conclusively that one given therapeutic behaviour is always the best option for all patients. In other words, an up-to-date reader of the scientific journals dealing with these issues can hardly draw a firm conclusion on the strategy to adopt in his daily clinical work. The very same considerations apply to the on-the-scene tracheal intubation (*TI*) of trauma patients, the role of which has been recently questioned by a number of studies mainly from the USA and Canada, in which a worse outcome was demonstrated in patients treated with on-the-scene TI. I find this particularly disturbing, because when I was young trainee I was taught (and I presently teach to my younger colleagues) that early TI can make the difference between life and death in trauma patients. On the side of life, needless to say.

It is worthwhile to recall that immediate TI of trauma patients has two main goals, namely (a) the prevention and/or the treatment of *hypoxaemia,* which is rather common in the immediate posttraumatic phase [1] and which is considered, along with arterial hypotension, the main cause of secondary brain injury [2]; and (b) the prevention of *aspiration* in patients unable to protect their airways [3]. Despite these advantages, different Authors have demonstrated that patients intubated at the scene of the accident had a worse prognosis than patients who received TI up on their arrival at the Emergency Department (*ED*). In a poorly randomized study performed on a paediatric population, Gausche *et al.* [4] demonstrated that both survival and neurological outcome were similar in patients who were treated with bag-valve mask (*BVM*) and those who underwent tracheal intubation on the scene; interestingly, TI was successful in only 57% of children in whom it was attempted and several misplacements or dislodgements of the tube occurred in this group. In other terms, in this patient population TI apparently proved more harmful than good. In another study [5] comparing major trauma patients treated with BVM or TI performed by emergency medicine technicians (*EMT*) without the assistance of sedatives and muscle relaxants a remarkably better outcome was demonstrated in the BVM group. In the TI group, the mortality exceeded 90%. However, it must be remarked that the feasibility of TI without drugs is a strong indicator of a grim prognosis [6], thus making it difficult to conclude positively that TI is harmful in itself. Recently, Di Bartolomeo *et al.* [7] demonstrated that the outcome of severely head-injured patients was not affected by either the levels of intervention (advanced trauma care performed by experienced anaesthetists involved in the Helicopter Emergency Medical System (*HEMS*) vs. expanded basic life support performed by registered nurses) or the type of transportation to the ED (helicopter vs. ground ambulance); the Authors attributed this result to the high level of training of the ground ambulance teams, who were specifically trained in trauma care. Regardless of the relevant role played by highly trained personnel working in the ground ambulances, these results are in sharp contrast with those of a previous study from the same group in which a remarkably better outcome was demonstrated in patients treated by the HEMS [8]. If these studies clearly indicate that on-the-scene TI may be harmful or ineffective in term of outcome improvement, other investigators have demonstrated the exact opposite: Winchell *et al.* [9] reported a better outcome in tracheally intubated patients with impending or established apnoea associated with a depressed level of consciousness compared with patients treated with BVM only (the mortality rate was 26.0% and 36.0%, respectively). Interestingly again, the rate of successful TI was only slightly higher than 50%, and this could have contributed to the higher mortality in patients in which TI could not be performed who were treated with the BVM. Another study demonstrated that the introduction of physicians specifically trained in critical care medicine in a helicopter transport team previously manned by paramedics was associated with both an increased rate of on-the-scene TI (51% vs. 10%) and with an overall improvement of the outcomes [10]. As stated above, it is difficult to draw definite conclusions from these conflicting studies, yet some considerations can be made.

Firstly, as underlined by a recent statement of the Eastern Association for the Surgery of Trauma (*EAST*) [11], the maintenance of *oxygenation* and the prevention of *asphyxia* are the cornerstones of the treatment of trauma victims unable to breath spontaneously and/or at risk of aspiration. Although different devices have been developed and used to this end, including laryngeal mask airways (*LMA*) and combitubes, TI remains the gold standard against which all these approaches must be challenged. However, its use is not risk-free and requires an appropriate level of manual skill and the safe use of drugs whose actions and side effects must be known and recognized. According to the aforementioned studies, in trauma patients TI appears safe and cost-effective in terms of outcomes, provided that (a) it is performed by highly trained professionals, able either to secure the airways in a short time in the vast majority if not all patients; and (b) the same individuals must be able to adopt alternative measures, i.e. LMA, *crycothiroctomy, (cricothyrotomy? cricothoracotomy? cricothyroidotomy?)* etc., when TI proves unfeasible. These operative capabilities apply to physicians specially trained in the management of the airways. In this setting, anaesthetists appears to be the best candidates for this role, as their syllabus includes from the very early days of training a full knowledge of the drugs and the techniques to keep the airways open and clear from secretions.

Secondly, a safe and rapid TI might not be sufficient for preventing death or disabling neurological consequences: in trauma patients, other conditions exist which may contribute to these poor outcomes. Indeed, in an earlier study, Stocchetti *et al.* [12] demonstrated that roughly 10% of in-hospital early post-traumatic deaths were clearly preventable and that the underlying causes were hypoxaemia or hypotension occurring alone or in association. It should be borne in mind that both conditions may be caused by a *pneumothorax (PNX)*, whose deleterious effects can be precipitated by the mechanical ventilation used after TI. It follows then that, although appropriate management of the airway remains an absolute priority, this is only the beginning, and the on-the-scene subsequent care of trauma patients must be performed by professionals specifically trained in the recognition and treatment of these harmful conditions. In settings where emergency care is provided by professionals with heterogeneous training and background (trained police officers and fire fighters, volunteers, etc.), these goals are hardly accomplished. Conversely, when skilled physicians are involved, these complications are fully diagnosed and treated. In a recent study comparing the effect of different approaches on the outcome of trauma patients [13], TI and PNX drainage were performed in 91% and 25% of patients treated by HEMS-operating *anaesthetists* as compared with much lower rates of these procedures performed by ground ambulance teams which, in the vast majority of cases, did not include such professionals. In our region, similar rates of TI and PNX drainage by means of a small-sized *thoracotomy* performed in the pre-flight phase have been accomplished by anaesthetists operating in the regional HEMS.

Finally, the TI-BVM controversy should not be considered a component of the wider "scoop and run" vs. "stay and play" debate. Although there is no doubt that in the presence of active bleeding the definitive care must be supplied in the surgical theatre, it is not conceivable, even in the most extreme conditions, that an asphyxiating patient could be rushed to the hospital without securing the airways and looking for other immediate life-threatening injuries. This also applies to situations in which multiple patients must be triaged and cared for simultaneously. In a recent paper dealing with the treatment of the victims of a terrorist attack in Israel, the only immediate procedures were the TI and the needle decompression of PNX, which were performed either on-the-scene or en route to the ED [14]. Again, these manoeuvers require specific training which cannot be acquired only theoretically or with minimal practice. Actually, a suboptimal level of both basic and advanced training could account for the negative results present in some studies dealing with the high rate of complications of TI performed by medics [15] and the worse outcome of patients in whom a considerable pre-ED time was spent in attempting to establish an intravenous line [16].

In conclusion, there is no firm evidence that TI is associated with detrimental effects, provided it is performed by trained physicians with a full knowledge of the TI-related drugs, the related complications and the available alternatives. In other terms, the TI vs. BVM controversy appears more a philosophical discussion than a real scientific debate.

# References


1. Stocchetti N, Furlan A, Volta F (1996) Hypoxaemia and arterial hypotension at the accident scene. J Trauma 40:764-767
2. Ravussin P, Bracco D, Moeschler O (1999) Prevention and treatment of secondary brain injury. Curr Opin Crit Care 5:511-516
3. Gillahm M, Parr JA (2002) Resuscitation for major trauma. Curr Opin Crit Care 15:167-172
4. Gausce M, Lewis RJ, Stratton SJ et al (2000) Effect of out-of-hospital pediatric endotracheal intubation on survival and neurologic outcome. JAMA 283:783-790
5. Eckstein M, Chan L, Schneir A et al (2000) Effect of prehospital advanced life support on outcomes of major trauma patients. J Trauma 48:643-648
6. Lockey D, Davies G, Coats T (2001) An observational study of the survival of trauma patients who have pre-hospital tracheal intubation without anesthesia or muscle relaxants. Br Med J 323:1410
7. Di Bartolomeo S, Sanson G, Nardi G et al (2001) Effects of 2 patterns of prehopsital care on the outcome of patients with severe head injury. Ann Surg 136: 1293-1300
8. Nardi G, Massarutti D, Muzzi R et al (1994) Impact of emergency medical helicopter service on mortality for trauma in north east Italy: a regional prospective audit. Eur J Emerg Med 1:69-77
9. Winchell RJ, Hoyt DB (1997) Endoctracheal intubation on the scene improves survival in patients with severe head injury. Arch Surg 132:592-597
10. Garner A, Rashford S, Lee A, Bartolacci R (1999) Addition of physicians to paramedics helicopter services decreases blunt trauma mortality. Aust N Z J Surg 69:697-701
11. Dunham CM, Barraco RD, Clark DE et al (2003) Guidelines for emergency tracheal intubation immediately after traumatic injury. J Trauma Inj Infect and Crit Care 55:162-179
12. Stocchetti N, Pagliarini G, Gennari M et al (1994) Trauma care in Italy: evidence of in-hospital preventable deaths. J Trauma 36:401-405
13. Biewener A, Aschenbrenner U, Rammelt S, Grass R, Zwipp H (2004) Impact of helicopter transport and hospital level on mortality of polytrauma patients. J Trauma Inj Infect and Crit Care 56:94-98
14. Peleg K, Ahronson-Daniel L, Stein M et al (2004) Gunshot and explosion injuries – characteristics, outcomes and implications for care of terror-related injuries in Israel. Ann Surg 239:311-318
15. Karch SB, Lewis T, Young S et al (1996) Field intubation of trauma patients: complications, indications and outcomes. Am J Emerg Med 14:617-619
16. Sampalis JS, Tamin H, Denis R et al (1997) Ineffectiveness of on-site intravenous line: is prehopsital time the culprit? J Trauma Inj Infect and Crit Care 43:608-617

# ADVANCES

# Recent Observations on Pharmacological Interventions During CPR

G. CAMMARATA, M.H. WEIL

Myocardial dysfunction, accounts for death during the first 72 h after resuscitation from cardiac arrest. When the heart stops beating, ischemic injury of myocytes follows cessation of coronary blood flow. The severity of injury is contingent on the duration of the "no-flow" interval. When ventricular fibrillation (VF) was electrically induced in 20 male pigs and animals were randomized to 4 or 7 min of untreated cardiac arrest, the severity of post-resuscitation myocardial dysfunction was proportional to the duration of untreated VF [1]. This conclusion is also supported by human data reported by Schultz et al. [2]. Even precordial compression fails to fully supply coronary blood flow in amounts that fulfill myocardial oxygen needs during VF [3]. With the aid of esophageal echocardiographic measurements, our research team has demonstrated ischemic contracture of the heart with increased thickness of the interventricular septum and the left ventricular free wall during prolonged CPR. This accounts for the "stony heart" [4]. Compliance of the left ventricle is greatly reduced with progressive reductions in stroke volumes. On a cellular level, the stone heart is best explained by intracellular calcium overload during ischemic injury and probably due to reperfusion.

## The Role of Vasoactive Drugs When Administered During CPR

Endogenous release of adrenergic receptor agonist is a physiologic response to low-flow states including cardiac arrest in both experimental animal models and in human patients [5, 6, 7]. The resulting vasopressor effect may be helpful for initial successful resuscitation, but it adversely affects the balance between oxygen supply and demand, especially when coronary blood flow is critically reduced.

In 1995, we reported that administration of exogenous epinephrine during cardiac arrest, in fact, increases the severity of post-resuscitation myocardial dysfunction and decreases the duration of post-resuscitation survival, when compared with an $\alpha$-agonist such as phenylephrine. When the $\beta$-adrenergic effects of epinephrine were blocked by prior administration of a $\beta_1$-selective blocker in rats, the effects of epinephrine and phenylephrine on outcomes of CPR were comparable [8]. Ditchey and Lindenfeld [9] had previously identified increased myocardial oxygen consumption, due to $\beta$-stimulation, to explain the adverse effects of epinephrine. In a dog model of cardiac arrest and resuscitation, epinephrine significantly increased myocardial lactate production together with decreased myocardial ATP. With critical decreases in myocyte ATP, there is greater severity of ischemic injury and lesser myocyte survival after initial resuscitation with return of spontaneous circulation [10].

Additional effort to define a more optimal adrenergic vasopressor agonist prompted use of a selective $\alpha_1$-agonist, methoxamine. Liversay et al. [11] obtained an effect comparable to epinephrine with methoxamine on myocardial perfusion but without the corresponding increases in myocardial oxygen consumption. More recently, Roberts et al. [12] confirmed that methoxamine produced significantly greater myocardial blood flow during precordial compression, when compared with epinephrine. Additional evidence favoring an alternative to epinephrine was reported by Berg et al. [13], who found an increase in early post-resuscitation death after high doses of epinephrine in a porcine model of cardiac arrest.

The issue is especially important because during the chaotic and disorganized contraction of the heart during VF there are dramatic increases in the myocardial demand for oxygen. Human data reported in a paper by Holmberg et al. [14] was based on the administration of epinephrine in 14,065 patients during cardiac arrest. Among 10,966 resuscitated patients, epinephrine had been administered to 4,566 or 42.4% of cases, but only 156 (3.4%) patients survived one month. This contrasted with 388 (6.3%) survivors of the 6,207 patients who received no epinephrine. Treatment with epinephrine was an independent predictor of lower likelihood of survival (p< 0.0001), independently of gender, incidence of arrhythmias, witnessed or unwitnessed arrest and bystander-CPR. These data are supported by Laurent et al. [15], who repeated that administration of epinephrine was associated with a lower post-resuscitation cardial output in survivors of out-of-hospital cardiac arrest. Gonzales et al. [16] found a decrease in end-tidal carbon dioxide with increased doses of epinephrine, a finding indicative of pulmonary A-V shunting produced by epinephrine subsequently cont by our own group [17].

Because the concentration of endogenous vasopressin was much higher in patients who were successfully resuscitated, Lindner were attracted to vasopressin as a resuscitation drug [18]. Wenzel et al. [19] observed in pigs that vasopressin improved return of spontaneous circulation in comparison with epinephrine and placebo-treated animals. Neurologic deficits in resuscitated animals were minimized and magnetic resonance imaging provided evidence of less cerebral ischemia injury. Prengel et al. [20, 21] observed, also in pigs, that vasopressin significantly improved cerebral oxygen delivery during CPR in association with improved post-resuscitation myocardial function, when compared with epinephrine.

However, we have no objective confirmation on human patients of benefit of vasopressin for CPR excepting a small, single-center study on 40 patients or less. In this study, Lindner [22] found that a significantly larger proportion of patients treated with arginine vasopressin were successfully resuscitated and survived for more than 24 h when compared to patients treated with epinephrine. In a case series of eight patients who had in-hospital cardiac arrest, the Lindner research team used 40 U of vasopressin after standard ACLS after at least one dose of epinephrine, had proven unsuccessful. All patients regained spontaneous circulation, and three were discharged from the hospital neurologically intact [23]. Unfortunately, in a large multicenter study which enrolled 200 patients with ventricular tachycardia or VF, Stiell et al. [24] failed to confirm even a modest trend favoring vasopressin over epinephrine.

As of this writing, neither epinephrine nor vasopressin can be recommended as optimal drugs for CPR.

## β-Adrenergic Blocking Agents

Propranolol, a non-selective β-adrenergic blocking agent, has also been shown, by Maroko et al. [25, 26], to decrease electrocardiographic evidence of ischemic myocardial cell damage in both experimental and clinical settings. Ischemic cells had less mitochondrial swelling in propranolol-pretreated animals. Obeid et al. [27] confirmed that propranolol, preserved ATP stores in ischemic myocardium. In brief, we are now on secure ground that β-adrenergic stimulation is adverse to the ischemic heart and this concept has now been extended to the global ischemic injury of cardiac arrest and resuscitation.

In an isolated heart model, Midei et al. [28] found that β-adrenergic agonists lowered coronary perfusion pressure and decreased myocardial performance after reversal of VF. Ditchey et al. [29] presented experimental evidence in dogs that both resuscitability and post-resuscitation myocardial function were improved after nonspecific β-adrenergic blockade with propranolol. In their model of cardiac arrest, two groups of 11 dogs each received 15 μg/kg of epinephrine after onset of untreated VF. The dose repeated at 4 min after starting CPR. One of the two groups was pretreated with 2 mg/kg propranolol. Coronary perfusion pressure was significantly higher when animals were pretreated with propranolol. In this group, 9 out of 11 dogs were successfully defibrillated but only 6 of 11 in the absence of propranolol pretreatment. The severity of post-resuscitation myocardial dysfunction was minimized when the animals were pretreated with the β-blocking agent. Accordingly, a non-selective β-adrenergic blocking agent reduced the severity of myocardial ischemic injury during CPR without compromising the success of defibrillation attempts. Our own research team confirmed these results in as yet unpublished studies. The administration of propranolol in doses of 1 mg/kg at 15 min prior to inducing VF in rats yielded a significantly better post-resuscitation myocardial function and survival.

The benefits of β-adrenergic blockade for minimizing myocardial ischemic injury in experimental model are now firmly established. Alternatively, the present evidence favors the use of a selective peripherally acting $\alpha_2$ agonist whish does not increase the severity of myocardial ischemic injury during the low flow state of CPR [30, 31].

## References


1. Tang W, Weil MH, Sun S et al (1999) The effect of biphasic and conventional monophasic defibrillation on post-resuscitation myocardial dysfunction. J Am Coll Cardiol 34:815-822
2. Schultz CH, Rivers EP, Feldkamp CS et al (1993) A characterization of hypothalamic-pituitary-adrenal axis function during and after human cardiac arrest. Crit Care Med 21:1339-1347
3. Tang W, Weil MH, Schock RB et al (1997) Phased chest and abdominal compression-decompression: a new option for cardiopulmonary resuscitation. Circulation 95:1335-1340
4. Klouche K, Weil MH, Sun S et al (2002) Evolution of the stone heart after prolonged cardiac arrest. Chest 122:1006-1011
5. Wortsman J, Frank S, Cryer PE (1984) Adrenomedullary response to maximal stress in humans. Am J Med 77:779-784
6. Little RA, Frayn KN, Randall PE et al (1985) Plasma catecholamines in patients with acute myocardial infarction and in cardiac arrest. Q J Med 54:133-140
7. Kern K, Elchisak MA, Sanders AB et al (1989) Plasma catecholamine and resuscitation from prolonged cardiac arrest. Crit Care Med 17:786-791
8. Tang W, Weil MH, Sun S et al (1995) Epinephrine increases the severity of post-resuscitation myocardial dysfunction. Circ 92:3089-3093
9. Ditchey RV, Lindenfeld J (1988) Failure of epinephrine to improve the balance between myocardial oxygen supply and demand during closed-chest resuscitation in dogs. Circulation 78:382-389
10. Jennings RB, Reimer KA, Steenbergen C (1986) Myocardial ischemia revisited: the osmolar load, membrane damage and perfusion. J Mol Cell Cardiol 18:769-780
11. Liversay JJ, Follette D, Fey KH et al (1978) Optimizing myocardial supply/demand balance with alpha-adrenergic drugs during cardiopulmonary resuscitation. J Thorac Cardiovasc Surg 76:244-251
12. Roberts D, Landolfo K, Dobson K, Light RB (1990) The effects of methoxamine on survival and regional distribution of cardiac output in dogs with prolonged ventricular fibrillation. Chest 98:999-1005
13. Berg RA, Otto CW, Kern K et al (1994) High dose of epinephrine results in greater early mortality after resuscitation from prolonged cardiac arrest in pigs: a prospective randomized study. Crit Care Med 22:282-290
14. Holmberg M, Holmberg S, Herlitz J (2002) Low chance of survival among patients requiring adrenaline (epinephrine) or intubation after out-of-hospital cardiac arrest in Sweden. Resuscitation 54:37-45
15. Laurent I, Monchi M, Chiche J et al (2002) Reversible myocardial dysfunction in survivors of out-of-hospital cardiac arrest. J Am Coll Cardiol 40:2110-2116
16. Gonzales ER, Ornato JP, Garnet AR et al (1989) Dose-dependent vasopressor response to phenylephrine during CPR in human beings. Ann Emerg Med 18:920-926
17. Tang W, Weil MH, Gazmuri RJ et al (1991) Pulmonary ventilation/perfusion defects induced by epinephrine during cardiopulmonary resuscitation. Circ 84:2101-2107
18. Lindner KH, Strohmenger HU, Ensinger H et al (1992) Stress hormone response during and after cardiopulmonary resuscitation. Anesthesiology 77:662-668
19. Wenzel V, Lindner KH, Krismer AC et al (2000) Improved survival and neurological outcome with vasopressin after prolonged resuscitation in pigs. J Am Coll Cardiol 35:527-533
20. Prengel AW, Lindner KH, Keller A (1996) Cerebral oxygenation during cardiopulmonary resuscitation with epinephrine and vasopressin in pigs. Stroke 27:1241-1248
21. Prengel AW, Lindner KH, Keller A, Lurie K (1996) Cardiovascular function during the postresuscitation phase after cardiac arrest in pigs: a comparison of epineph-

rine versus vasopressin. Crit Care Med 24:2014-2019
22. Lindner KH, Dirks B, Strohmenger HU et al (1997) Randomized comparison of epinephrine and vasopressin in patients with out-of-hospital cardiac arrest. Lancet 349:535
23. Lindner KH, Prengel AW, Brinkmann A et al (1996) Vasopressin administration in refractory cardiac arrest. Ann Intern Med 124:1061-1064
24. Stiell JG, Hebert P, Wells G et al (2001) Vasopressin versus epinephrine for in-hospital cardiac arrest: a randomized controlled trial. Lancet 358:105-109
25. Gold HK, Leinbach RC, Maroko PR (1976) Propranolol-induced reduction of sing of ischemic injury during acute myocardial infarction. Am J Cardiol 38:689-695
26. Maroko PR, Libby P, Covell JW et al (1972) Precordial S-T elevation mapping: an atraumatic method for assessing alteration in the extent of myocardial ischemic injury. Am J Cardiol 29:223-230
27. Obeid A, Spear R, Mookherjee S et al (1976) The effect of propranolol on myocardial energy stores during myocardial ischemia in dogs. Circ (Suppl)II:II-159
28. Midei MG, Sugiura S, Maughan WL et al (1990) Preservation of ventricular function by treatment of ventricular fibrillation with phenylephrine. J Am Coll Cardiol 16:489-494
29. Ditchey RV, Rubio-Perez A, Slinker BK (1994) Beta-adrenergic blockade reduces myocardial injury during experimental cardiopulmonary resuscitation. J Am Coll Cardiol 24:804-812
30. Klouche K, Weil MH, Sun S et al (2003) A comparison of alpha-methylnorepinephrine, vasopressin and epinephrine for cardiac resuscitation. Resuscitation 57:93-100
31. Sun S, Weil MH, Tang W et al (2001) Alpha-Methylnorepinephrine, a selective alpha2-adrenergic agonist for cardiac resuscitation. J Am Coll Cardiol 37:951-956

# Respiratory Mechanics and Lung Parenchyma Remodelling in Acute Respiratory Distress Syndrome

W.A. ZIN, P.R.M. ROCCO

The first descriptions of acute respiratory distress syndrome appeared in 1967, when Ashbaugh *et al.* [1] described 12 patients with acute respiratory distress, cyanosis refractory to oxygen therapy, decreased lung compliance, and diffuse infiltrates evident on the chest radiograph. It is not defined by a specific pathogenesis, but reflects the lung's non-selective response to numerous insults and precipitating factors. Based on these observations, the term "syndrome", defined as "group of symptoms and signs of disordered function related to one another by means of some anatomic, physiologic, or biochemical peculiarity", was used. Although the term acute respiratory distress syndrome (ARDS) is often used interchangeably with acute lung injury (ALI), by strict criteria ARDS should be reserved for the most severe end of the spectrum [2].

Acute respiratory distress syndrome is a heterogeneous process that results in diffuse alveolar damage. It is associated with a variety of causative factors that can be grouped into two general categories, those associated with direct lung injury through the airways and those associated with indirect lung injury through the blood stream (Table 1) [3, 4]. Direct injury is associated with pneumonia, lung trauma, smoke inhalation, near drowning, and aspiration. Indirect injury is associated with sepsis, blood transfusion, nonthoracic trauma, hypovolemic shock, reperfusion injury, acute pancreatitis, and overdose. More recently, investigators have focused on an extension of the direct factors associated with iatrogenic lung injury induced by mechanical ventilation [5-9]. This new mechanism of injury is referred to as ventilator-associated lung injury. Regardless of whether injury originates within or outside the lung, a systemic inflammatory response is triggered.

Traditionally, ARDS has been divided into three stages: an initial inflammatory phase (exudative) is followed by fibroproliferation, which can lead to established interstitial and intra-alveolar fibrosis, the final phase. The histological features of exudative phase are: (a) hyaline membranes, (b) alveolar collapse, and (c) swollen type I pneumocytes with cytoplasmic vacuoles. The endothelial cells swell, the intercellular junctions widen, and pinocytic vesicles increase, causing disruption in the capillary membrane and resulting in a capillary leak and oedema formation [10, 11]. The proliferative phase was described to begin as early as the third day and was most prominent in the second and third weeks after symptom onset. However, recently, some Authors described increased numbers of myofibroblasts and procollagen-type-I- and III-producing cells ear-

**Table 1.** Recommended criteria for acute lung injury (ALI) and acute respiratory distress syndrome (ARDS) [2]

| | Timing | Oxygenation | Chest radiograph | Pulmonary artery wedge pressure |
|---|---|---|---|---|
| ALI criteria | Acute onset | $PaO_2/FIO_2 \leq 300$ (regardless of PEEP level) | Bilateral infiltrates seen on frontal chest radiograph | $\leq 18$ mmHg when measured or no clinical evidence of left atrial hypertension |
| ARDS criteria | Acute onset | $PaO_2/FIO_2 \leq 200$ (regardless of PEEP level) | Bilateral infiltrates seen on frontal chest radiograph | $\leq 18$ mmHg when measured or no clinical evidence of left atrial hypertension |

ly in the course of ALI, suggesting that the proliferative phase begins much sooner than had been previously appreciated [12-16]. Thus, inflammatory and repair mechanisms occur in parallel rather than in series. Fibroproliferation is a stereotypical reparative reaction to tissue injury, and is characterized by the replacement of damaged epithelial cell by accumulation of mesenchymal cells, in particular interstitial fibroblasts, which migrate, replicate, and secrete extracellular matrix proteins such as collagen; type II cells begin to proliferate and reline the denuded basement membrane; epithelial cells migrate over the surface of the organising granulation tissue and transform the intra-alveolar exudate into interstitial tissue. In the fibrotic phase, extensive remodelling of the lung by sparsely cellular collagenous tissue occurs, air spaces are irregularly enlarged and there is alveolar duct fibrosis. Type III collagen is replaced by type I collagen, leading to a stiff lung over time [17, 18].

Despite recent advances in intensive care, mortality rates persist at 40-60%. In those who survive the initiating insult, the most common causes of death are multi-organ dysfunction syndrome (MODS), sepsis and then respiratory failure [19]. Persistent inflammation is a characteristic feature of sepsis and MODS, while both inflammation and pulmonary fibrosis underlie the respiratory failure in the later phases of ARDS [20]. Thus, fibrosis exerts a significant impact on many patients with ARDS because the decrement in lung compliance and hypoxia leads to ventilator dependence, contributing to a high incidence of sepsis and MODS. Hence, pulmonary fibrosis correlates with outcome in ARDS [21]. Thus, resolution of both inflammation and fibrosis is essential to survival and a full recovery from ARDS.

This article will focus on the alterations in respiratory mechanics because of ARDS remodelling.

Lung static elastance, airway resistance, and viscoelastic/inhomogeneous pressure increase significantly in acute respiratory distress syndrome because of surfactant dysfunction and/or loss of functional capacity due to alveolar flooding [16, 22, 23]. Actually, mechanical dysfunction can result from air-liquid interface and/or tissue changes [24]. The increase in lung resistive pressure can be attributed to a reduction in bronchial calibre caused by fluid in the airways, reflex bronchoconstriction, and/or reduced lung volume. The augment in lung viscoelastic and/or inhomogeneous pressure suggests the presence of heterogeneities that can be due to many different factors, for example, alveoli collapse and overdistension, distortion of patent alveoli, oedema, inflammation with neutrophil and mononuclear cell infiltration, and changes in collagen and elastic fibre contents.

The mechanical properties of pulmonary parenchyma are major determinants of lung physiological function [25-28]. In the lung, these properties are derived from the stress-strain relationship of the pulmonary parenchyma, which depends in turn on the extracellular matrix integrity [29]. Connective tissue cells produce and secrete an array of macromolecules, forming a complex network filling the extracellular space of the submucosa, called the extracellular matrix (ECM) [30]. The ECM not only has a mechanical role in supporting and maintaining tissue structure, but it is also a complex and dynamic meshwork influencing many biologic cell functions such as development, migration, and proliferation. The macromolecules that constitute the ECM are secreted locally, and its composition depends on the cell types, their state of differentiation, and their metabolic status. Molecules comprising ECM consist of fibrous proteins (collagen, elastin) and structural or adhesive proteins (fibronectin and laminin) embedded in a hydrated polysaccharide gel containing several glycosaminoglycans, including hyaluronic acid. When the fibres are deformed, they carry stress and store energy that depends on their size, quantity, and organisation. In all vertebrates, collagen acts as a source of tensile strength to the tissue, whilst elastin and proteoglycans are essential to matrix resiliency.

Tissue mechanical properties can be analysed in oscillating lung parenchymal strips. The advantage of making *in vitro* measurements is that contributions to the mechanical behaviour related to surface film, alveolar flooding, or heterogeneity effects can be excluded. As a result, a direct analysis of the role of fibre-fibre networking within the connective tissue matrix on tissue mechanical properties is ensured [16, 18, 31-33].

Remodelling is defined in the Concise Oxford Dictionary (10th edn, 1999) as model again or differently reconstruct. This is a critical aspect of wound repair in all organs, representing a dynamic process that associates matrix production and degradation in reaction to an inflammatory insult that leads to a normal reconstruction process (model again) or a pathologic one (model differently).

The process of fibrosing alveolitis begins early in the course of ARDS [12-16, 18] and results from a complex interaction between fibroblasts, other lung parenchymal cells, and macrophages. Fibroblasts migrate into areas of acute lung injury and are stimulated to secrete collagen and other matrix proteins.

These cells also release various proteases that have the capacity to degrade and remodel these matrix proteins. Macrophages have been thought to be important in the progression of acute lung injury to fibroproliferative ARDS, as they are present in high numbers and secrete numerous proinflammatory mediators (IL-1 beta, IL-4, and IL-13) and growth factors [transforming growth factor (TGF)-beta, TGF-alpha, tumor necrosis factor (TNF)-alpha, platelet-derived growth factor (PDGF)-like factor, fibroblast growth factor 2 (basic fibroblast growth factor), and insulin-like growth factor-I (IGF-I)] [34-36]. These peptide growth factors influence mesenchymal cell migration, proliferation, and extracellular matrix deposition, thus implicating them in the progression of fibroproliferative lung disorders. The stimuli that activate fibroblasts to remodel the lung are not well defined but likely include components of blood (fibrin), matrix degradation products, and mediators (transforming growth factor beta) that are released from macrophages and lung parenchymal cells. Fibrin provides a provisional matrix for both inflammatory cells and fibroblasts to migrate into the inflamed site, and by binding mediators it acts as a reservoir of fibroproliferative growth factors. Factors and circumstances that determine whether areas of the lung heal with minimal injury or progress to irreversible injury need to be defined [37].

Lung collagen content increases significantly in ARDS. Initially, this consists of type III collagen, which is more flexible and susceptible to breakdown. Later, remodelling leads to the thicker and more resistant type I collagen [17, 18].

In normal alveolar septa, a subepithelial layer of elastic system fibres composed mainly of fully mature elastic fibres confers a great elasticity to the alveolar tissue in normal situations [38]. The amount of elastic fibres increases in line with lung growth [39], and elastin is in fact responsible for alveolar formation [40]. Early in development, the elastic fibre consists of microfibrils that define fibre location and morphology [41, 42]. Over time, tropoelastin accumulates within the bed of microfibrils to form the functional, polymeric protein known as elastin. The elastic system has three components, defined according to crescent amounts of elastin and fibril orientation: (1) oxytalan fibre, composed of a bundle of microfibrils; (2) elaunin fibre, made of microfibrils and a small amount of elastin; and (3) fully developed elastic fibres, consisting of microfibrils and abundant elastin [43].

The occurrence of elastosis has been well studied and demonstrated in animal models of pulmonary fibrosis, and recent studies suggest that elastin gene expression is increased following injury in certain animal models [44, 45]. Despite advances in the understanding of the structural complexity of the elastic system, the interaction between the elastin and microfibril components of the elastin fibre system remains a matter of speculation, mainly in the face of lung remodelling and repair after ARDS.

Rocco *et al.* [16, 18], in a model of acute lung injury induced by paraquat, observed that mild ALI was followed by a late increase in elastic fibre content, whereas the severe lesion presented early elastogenesis. They also analysed the kind of fibre responsible for the elevation of elastin content: the total amount of elaunin and fully developed elastic fibres was not modified by ALI, whereas oxytalan microfibrils content was higher in a severe lesion. They suggested the possibility that the destruction of fully developed fibres by paraquat-induced ALI leads to an increase in the microfibrillar component, because the amount of fully developed fibres was not modified [16, 18].

Previous studies on lung tissue strips challenged with elastase and collagenase showed mechanical changes that agree with the classical model of elastin-dependent elastance and collagen-dependent maximal distension. Elastase decreased both tissue elastance (E) and resistance (R) in a coupled fashion, so the ratio E/R, hysteresivity, was not modified [46]. However, Yuan *et al.* [33] reported in normal animals that both collagen and elastic fibres contribute to tissue elasticity during normal breathing, which contradicts the notion of independent functionality of elastin and collagen fibres. In this line, Rocco *et al.* [16] observed that dynamic elastance increased sigmoidally with the increment in the amount of collagen until a plateau was reached. Tissue resistance augmented with the increment in oxytalan fibre content only in a severe lesion. Thus, they concluded that 24 h after the induction of ALI with paraquat, collagen and oxytalan fibres were important in determining parenchymal mechanics [16].

In a murine model of pulmonary and extrapulmonary ARDS, oscillatory tissue mechanical parameters [resistance, elastance, and hysteresivity ($\eta$)] were also correlated with the content of fibres of the collagenous and elastic system (oxytalan + elaunin + fully developed elastic fibre) of the alveolar septum. R, E, $\eta$ increased similarly in pulmonary and extrapulmonary ARDS, which are accompanied by collagen fibre content augment [47]. Thus, collagen fibre content was already elevated 24 h after tissue damage independent of the aetiology of lung injury, indicating that the biochemical processes implicated in collagen synthesis are indeed able to react very quickly to the aggression (Fig. 1). Collagen types were identified by electron microscopy. Type III collagen appeared early in the course of pulmonary and extrapulmonary ARDS while type I collagen appeared late in pulmonary ARDS [48]. Armstrong *et al.* [49] hypothesized that an imbalance between synthesis and degradation may contribute to the net accumulation of type I collagen in ARDS. They demonstrated that the synthesis of type I procollagen was elevated in subjects with ARDS or ALI, and that the increased synthesis was associated with decreased collagen degradation by collagenase. The profibrotic response occurred early in the course of disease and was associated with the severity of the lung injury and mortality. Elastic system fibres content was also analysed in the murine model of pulmonary and extrapulmonary ARDS. Interestingly, there is a late increase in the amount of elastic fibre [48].

The ECM is a dynamic structure, and equilibrium between synthesis and degradation of ECM components is required for the maintenance of its homeostasis [50].

Although many proteases can cleave ECM molecules, the family of $Zn^{2+}$ matrix metalloproteinases (MMPs) and their inhibitors are likely to be the normal physiologically relevant mediators of ECM degradation [51]. Several sub-

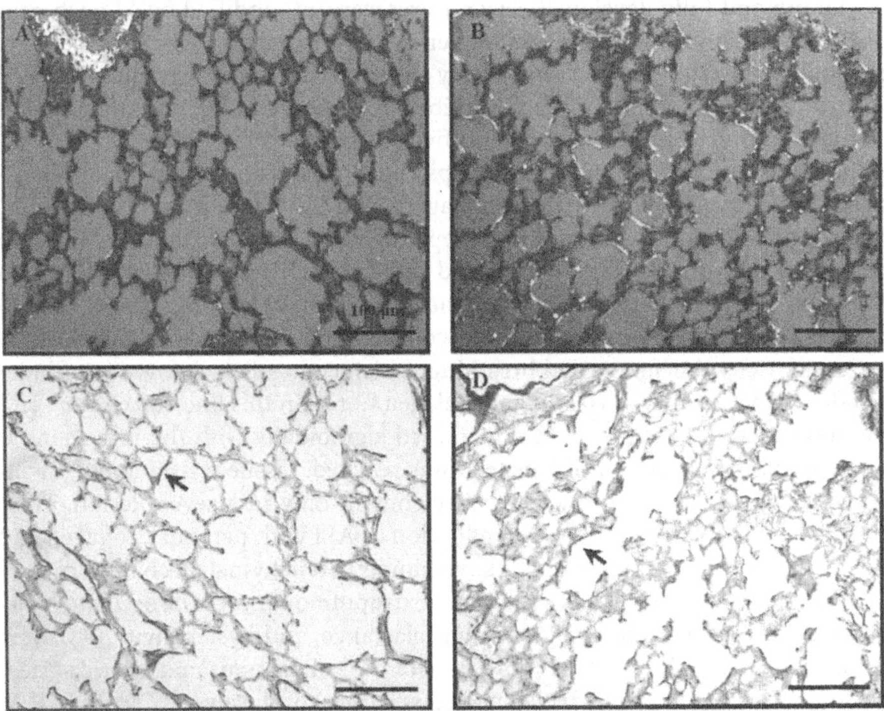

**Fig. 1.** Photomicrographs of parenchymal strips stained with Sirius Red with polarization for collagen in control (**A**) and *E. coli* LPS-treated lung (10 µg, intratracheally, **B**). All brightly birefringent structures, which shine against a dark background, contain collagen molecules (**A, B**). **C, D** representative fields illustrating elastic fiber system distribution in control (**C**) and acute lung injury induced by *E. coli* LPS (10 µg, intratracheally, **D**). Elastic fibres are stained in black within alveolar walls (*arrows*). Photographs were taken at an original magnification of x200 from slides stained by Weigert's resorcin-fuchsin with oxidation

classes of MMPs have been identified, including interstitial collagenases, gelatinases, stromelysins, and membrane-type MMPs. These can degrade many proteins, including collagens, fibronectin, laminin, proteoglycans, entactins, and elastin. MMPs are secreted in a latent form, as inactive proenzymes, and are activated by the loss of the propeptide under physiologic conditions. At least two matrix metalloproteinases (MMP-2 and MMP-9) are elevated in the lungs of patients with ARDS. The proteolytic activity of MMPs is precisely controlled by endogenous physiologic inhibitors, which include the broad-spectrum serum inhibitor alpha$_2$-macroglobulin and a special class of tissue inhibitors of metalloproteinases (TIMPs). Four members of the TIMP family have been characterized and designated as TIMP-1, TIMP-2, TIMP-3, and TIMP-4. The major role of MMPs is the breakdown of basement membrane and ECM in tissue remodelling and angiogenesis. TIMP-1 and TIMP-2 are capable of inhibiting the activities of all known MMPs and, as such, play a key role in maintaining the balance between ECM deposition and degradation in different physiologic processes. Loss of coordination in the expression of proteinases and inhibitors is believed to generate tissue degradation in inflammatory diseases. The restoration of functional connective tissue is a major goal in the wound-healing process. This regenerative event requires the deposition and accumulation of collagenous and noncollagenous ECM molecules as well as the remodelling of ECM by MMPs. Lanchou *et al.* [52] studied the role of MMPs and their natural inhibitors (TIMPs) in the genesis and the evolution of ARDS. They suggested that MMP-9 has an antifibroproliferative role, preventing patients from developing fibrosis by degrading the ECM components that are synthesized by fibroblasts.

Many other potential candidates exist that could attenuate pulmonary fibrosis. Interferon (IFN)-γ inhibits fibroblast collagen synthesis in a murine model of pulmonary fibrosis [53]. Prostaglandin E2 (PGE2) inhibits the response of mesenchymal cells to profibrotic cytokines, and is diminished in the lungs of patients with pulmonary fibrosis [54].

## Conclusions

The mechanical properties of pulmonary parenchyma are major determinants of lung physiological function. Elastic and collagen fibres are the main structural components of pulmonary connective tissue matrix, but their elastic properties are essentially different. They form a continuous network throughout the lung that provides the forces necessary for passive expiration. Because the ECM is considerably altered in ARDS, knowledge of the composition and distribution of the ECM at different stages of the disease may offer further understanding of the pathogenesis of ARDS. An overall increase of collagen expression in ARDS has been well documented. However, the functional significance of increased elastin production in this disorder is not yet known. Additionally, there are only few reports describing the mechanical interactions between ECM elements and how they influence pulmonary mechanics, especially tissue hysteretic properties.

## References

1. Ashbaugh DG, Bigelow DB, Petty TL et al (1967) Acute respiratory distress syndrome. Lancet 2:319-323
2. Bernard GR, Artigas A, Bringham KL et al (1994) The American-European consensus conference on ARDS: definitions, mechanisms, relevant outcomes, and clinical trial coordination. Am J Respir Crit Care Med 149:818-824
3. Matthay MA (1999) Conference summary: acute lung injury. Chest 116:119-126
4. Ware LB, Matthay MA (2000) The acute respiratory distress syndrome. N Engl J Med 342:1334-1339
5. Webb HH, Tierney DF (1974) Experimental pulmonary edema due to intermittent positive pressure ventilation with high inflation pressures: protection by positive end-expiratory pressure. Am Rev Respir Dis 110:556-565
6. Parker JC, Townsley MI, Rippe B et al (1984) Increased microvascular permeability

in dog lungs due to high peak airway pressure. J Appl Physiol 57:1809-1816

7.  Dreyfuss D, Soler P, Basset G et al (1988) High inflation pressure pulmonary edema: respective effects of high airway pressure, high tidal volume, and positive end-expiratory pressure. Am Rev Respir Dis 137:1159-1164

8.  Corbridge TC, Wood LDH, Crawford GP et al (1990) Adverse effects of large tidal volumes and low PEEP in canine acid aspiration. Am Rev Respir Dis 142:311-315

9.  Slutsky AS, Tremblay LN (1998) Multiple system organ failure: is mechanical ventilation a contributing factor? Am J Respir Crit Care Med 157:1721-1725

10.  Tomashefski JF Jr (2000) Pulmonary pathology of acute respiratory distress syndrome. Clin Chest Med 21:435-466

11.  Fein AM, Calalang-Colucci MG (2000) Acute lung injury and acute respiratory distress syndrome in sepsis and septic shock. Crit Care Clin 16:289-317

12.  Chesnutt AN, Matthay MA, Tibayan FA et al (1997) Early detection of type III procollagen peptide in acute lung injury. Pathogenic and prognostic significance. Am J Respir Crit Care Med 156:840-845

13.  Liebler JM, Qu Z, Buckner B et al (1998) Fibroproliferation and mast cells in the acute respiratory distress syndrome. Thorax 53:823-829

14.  Pugin J, Verghese G, Widmer MC et al (1999) The alveolar space is the site of intense inflammatory and profibrotic reactions in the early phase of acute respiratory distress syndrome. Crit Care Med 27:304-312

15.  Marshall RP, Bellingan G, Webb S et al (2000) Fibroproliferation occurs early in the acute respiratory distress syndrome and impacts on outcome. Am J Respir Crit Care Med 162:1783-1788

16.  Rocco PRM, Negri EM, Kurtz PM et al (2001) Lung tissue mechanics and extracellular matrix in acute lung injury. Am J Respir Crit Care Med 164:1067-1071

17.  Raghu G, Striker LJ, Hudson LD et al (1985) Extracellular matrix in normal and fibrotic human lungs. Am Rev Respir Dis 131:281-289

18.  Rocco PRM, Souza AB, Faffe DS et al (2003) Effect of corticosteroid on lung parenchyma remodelling at an early phase of acute lung injury. Am J Respir Crit Care Med 168:677-684

19.  Montgomery A, Stager M, Carrico C et al (1985) Causes of mortality in patients with the adult respiratory distress syndrome. Am Rev Respir Dis 132:485-489

20.  Meduri GM (1995) Pulmonary fibroproliferation and deaths in patients with late ARDS. Chest 107:5-6

21.  Martin C, Papazian L, Paya M-J et al (1995) Pulmonary fibrosis correlates with outcome in adult respiratory distress syndrome. A study in mechanically ventilated patients. Chest 107:196-200

22.  Grossman RF, Jones JG, Murray JF (1980) Effects of oleic acid-induced pulmonary edema on lung mechanics. J Appl Physiol 48:1045–1051

23.  Gregory TJ, Longmore WJ, Moxley MA et al (1991) Surfactant chemical composition and biophysical activity in acute respiratory distress syndrome. J Clin Invest 88:1976–1981

24.  Ingenito EP, Mark L, Davison B (1994) Effects of acute lung injury on dynamic tissue properties. J Appl Physiol 77:2689–2697

25.  Bachofen H (1968) Lung tissue resistance and pulmonary hysteresis. J Appl Physiol 24:296-301

26.  Hildebrandt J (1969) Dynamic properties of air-filled excised cat lung determined by liquid plethysmograph. J Appl Physiol 27:246-250

27.  Hildebrandt J (1970) Pressure-volume data of cat lung interpreted by a plastoelastic linear viscoelastic model. J Appl Physiol 28:365-372

28.  Ingenito EP, Davison B, Fredberg JJ (1993) Tissue resistance in the guinea pig at baseline and during metacholine constriction. J Appl Physiol 75:2541-2548

29.  Soubin SS, Fung YC, Tremer HM (1988) Collagen and elastin fibres in human alveolar walls. J Appl Physiol 64:1659-1675

30. Raghow R (1994) The role of extracellular matrix in postinflammatory wound healing and fibrosis. Faseb J 8:823-831

31. Yuan, H, Ingenito EP, Suki B (1997) Dynamic properties of lung parenchyma: mechanical contributions of fiber network and interstitial cells. J Appl Physiol 83:1420-1431

32. Fredberg JJ, Stamenovic D (1989) On the imperfect elasticity of lung tissue. J Appl Physiol 67:2408-2414

33. Yuan H, Kononov S, Cavalcante FSA et al (2000) Effects of collagenase and elastase on the mechanical properties of lung tissue strips. J Appl Physiol 89:3-14

34. Henke C, Marineili W, Jessurun J et al (1993) Macrophage production of basic fibroblast growth factor in the fibroproliferative disorder of alveolar fibrosis after lung injury. Am J Pathol 143:1189-1199

35. Krein PM, Sabatini PJB, Tinmouth W et al (2003) Localization of insulin-like growth factor-I in lung tissues of patients with fibroproliferative acute respiratory distress syndrome. Am J Respir Crit Care Med 167:83-90

36. Madtes DK, Rubenfeld G, Klima LD et al (1998) Elevated transforming growth factor-alpha levels in bronchoalveolar lavage fluid of patients with acute respiratory distress syndrome. Am J Respir Crit Care Med 158:424-430

37. Ward PA, Hunninghake GW (1998) Lung inflammation and fibrosis. Am J Respir Crit Care Med 157:S123-S129

38. Mercer RR, Crapo JD (1990) Spatial distribution of collagen and elastin fibres in the lungs. J Appl Physiol 69:756-765

39. Dubick MA, Rucker RB, Cross CE et al (1981) Elastin metabolism in rodent lung. Biochim Biophys Acta 672:303-306

40. Kida K, Yasui S, Utsuyama M et al (1984) Lung changes resulting from intraperitoneal injections of porcine pancreatic elastase in suckling rats. Am Rev Respir Dis 130:1111-1117

41. Fahrenbach WH, Sandberg LB, Cleary EG (1966) Ultrastructural studies on early elastogenesis. Anat Rec 155:563-568

42. Greenlee TK, Ross R, Hartman JL (1966) The fine structures of elastic fibers. J Cell Biol 30:59-71

43. Montes GS (1996) Structural biology of the fibres of the collagenous and elastic systems. Cell Biol Int 20:15-27

44. Pierce RA, Albertine KH, Starcher BC et al (1997) Chronic lung injury in preterm lambs: disordered pulmonary elastin deposition. Am J Physiol 273:L452-460

45. Raghow R, Lurie S, Seyer JM et al (1985) Profile of steady state levels of RNAs coding for type I procollagen, elastin, and fibronectin in hamster lungs undergoing bleomycin-induced interstitial pulmonary fibrosis. J Clin Invest 76:1733-1739

46. Moretto A, Dallaire M, Romero PV et al (1994) Effect of elastase on oscillation mechanics of lung parenchymal strips. J Appl Physiol 77:1623-1629

47. Rocco PRM, Leite-Junior JH, Souza AB et al (2002) Acute respiratory distress syndrome caused by pulmonary and extrapulmonary disease: effect of corticosteroid. Eur Respir J 20:36

48. Zin WA, Santos FB, Nagato LKS et al (2002) Temporal evolution of respiratory mechanics and pulmonary structural remodelling in Escherichia coli lipopolysaccharide-induced acute respiratory distress syndrome. Eur Respir J 20:36

49. Armstrong L, Thickett DR, Mansell JP et al (1999) Changes in collagen turnover in early acute respiratory distress syndrome. Am J Respir Crit Care Med 160:1910-1915

50. Murphy G, Docherty AJ (1992) The matrix metalloproteinases and their inhibitors. Am J Respir Cell Mol Biol 7:120-125

51. Shapiro SD, Senior RM (1999) Matrix metalloproteinases: matrix degradation and more. Am J Respir Cell Mol Biol 20:1100-1102

52. Lanchou J, Corbel M, Tanguy M et al (2003) Imbalance between matrix metalloproteinases (MMP-9 and MMP-2) and tissue inhibitors of metalloproteinases

(TIMP-1 and TIMP-2) in acute respiratory distress syndrome patients. Crit Care Med 31:536-542
53. Gurujeyalakshmi G, Giri SN (1995) Molecular mechanisms of anti-fibrotic effect of interferon gamma in bleomycin-mouse model of lung fibrosis: down regulation of TGF-beta and procollagen I and III gene expression. Exp Lung Res 21:791-808
54. Wilborn J, Crofford LJ, Burdick MD et al (1994) Cultured lung fibroblasts isolated from patients with idiopathic pulmonary fibrosis have diminished capacity to synthesis prostaglandin E2 and to express cyclooxygenase-2. J Clin Invest 95:1861-1868

# PERIOPERATIVE MEDICINE

# Chapter 8

# Pulmonary Diseases of Interest for Anaesthesiologists

F. CIANI

If one considers the most widespread pulmonary diseases, chronic obstructive pulmonary disease (COPD) deserves the first place on the list. COPD is worldwide the fourth most common cause of death and shows an increasing rate of incidence both in industrialized and in developing countries. Thus, for an anaesthesiologist an understanding of this disease is important now and probably in the future as well.

## Epidemiology of COPD

In 1990, COPD was 12th on the list of diseases with social impact but it is likely that in 2020 it will reach the 4th place. It has an overall 5% prevalence but is mostly concentrated in the middle to older age segment of the male population where it reaches a 20% of prevalence rate.

In Italy, the prevalence is higher in urban areas (Pisa) than in the country (Rovescala, Pavia), and more recent studies show an increasing incidence of COPD in the same urban area (see Fig. 1), whereas emphysema appears to be increasing only slightly [1].

Other interesting points of this study show that even in the range of 25-44 years of age, 11% of males and 6% of females show slight signs of bronchial obstruction and that the incidence of COPD is usually underestimated by the general practitioner.

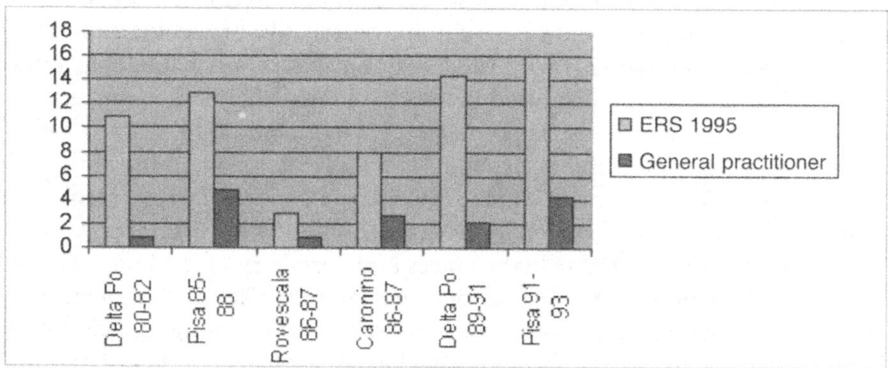


**Fig. 1.** European Respiratory Society (ERS)-based criteria and general-practitioner-based diagnosis of COPD in northern Italy

## Definition

COPD is defined by the American Thoracic Society (ATS) as a disorder characterized by abnormal forced expiratory air flow, of a structural or functional nature, that does not change markedly over several months. Clinicians use the term COPD to describe a group of clinical and pathologic findings that often produce disability of a chronic and unremitting nature and sometimes result in death. The diagnosis is usually based on the presence of chronic bronchitis associated with varying degrees of emphysema, with or without bronchospasm. More than 14 million Americans are afflicted with COPD [1]. Although chronic bronchitis is the most common component, most patients with COPD also have emphysematous involvement and may have episodes of bronchospasm. The incidence of chronic bronchitis has risen dramatically over the past 30 years, whereas emphysema appears to be increasing slightly in prevalence [1]. COPD and related conditions (e.g., asthma, bronchiectasis, hypersensitivity pneumonitis) rank as the fourth most frequent cause of death in the United States. In 1997, COPD accounted for 4.5% of all deaths (a total of 110,600), with an age-adjusted mortality rate of 21.4 per 100,000 people [2]. Of even greater significance is the chronic, progressive nature of the disease, which may result in severe, prolonged disability. As a consequence of the severe morbidity and mortality rate of COPD, its treatment and prevention have become an increasingly important public health issue. It is useful to address the three major components of the disease; chronic bronchitis, emphysema, and bronchospasm, because their manifestations, treatment requirements, and prognoses differ somewhat. The ATS defines chronic bronchitis as the persistence of cough and excessive mucus secretion on most days over a 3-month period for at least 2 successive years. The closest pathologic correlate to this syndrome is mucous gland hypertrophy, based on the "Reid Index," which is the ratio of the width of the mucous glands to the thickness of the bronchial walls. Most patients with chronic bronchitis do not have airflow obstruction; however, about 10-15% of smokers develop an abnormally rapid decline in airflow with aging, resulting in COPD [3]. Patients who do not develop airflow obstruction have simple chronic bronchitis; those who have a progressive decline in airflow have chronic obstructive bronchitis and constitute the majority of patients with COPD [3]. Emphysema is pathologic, rather than clinical, and can be diagnosed in vivo based on its clinical characteristics. The ATS defines emphysema as permanent enlargement of air spaces distal to the terminal bronchiole and destruction of the alveolar wall, in the absence of fibrosis. The classic subtype of emphysema associated with cigarette smoking is centrilobular emphysema, which involves destruction of the central portions of the acinus and affects primarily the apices and periphery of the lungs. Marked hyperinflation and airflow obstruction are characteristics of patients with advanced emphysema. They have abnormal values for diffusing capacity of the lung for carbon monoxide (DLCO), exhibit fixed obstruction, and respond poorly to bronchodilator therapy. Although marked variability of airflow obstruction is a characteristic of asthma rather than COPD, some patients with typical signs of chronic bronchitis (about 10% in one study) have significant changes in airflow after bronchodilator administration, comparable to those seen in patients with asthma. This reversible component of COPD represents the "opposite" of emphysema (i.e., reversible versus fixed obstruction) and has been labeled asthmatic bronchitis. In contrast to patients with emphysema, those with asthmatic bronchitis have little alteration of DLCO, exhibit wheezing on physical examination and eosinophils in the blood and sputum, and may have a family history of atopy. These patients appear to respond well to long-term therapy with bronchodilators and corticosteroids [4].

## Signs and Symptoms of COPD

COPD patients become aware of their disease late: the relationship between their symptoms and the underlying pulmonary function abnormality is poor so they refer to the physician when a large amount of their pulmonary function is lost. The most common symptoms are exertion dyspnoea and cough with or without sputum production.

Cough is an important physiologic defence mechanism for the lungs: it clears particulates, mucus, bacteria and viruses from the bronchial tree. Cough is present in about 50% of smokers after 10 years of smoking habit [5]. Chronic cough and sputum production are features of chronic bronchitis but they are not always related to bronchial obstruction: if a smoker quits smoking, cough disappears or reduces but bronchial obstruction persists [6].

Sputum is usual symptom in early stages of COPD: it is very difficult to evaluate the amount of smear since it is often swallowed by the patient; it is usually colourless, its daily amount is less than a cup of coffee and it may be a marker for future pulmonary complications [7].

Dyspnoea is certainly the most important symptom in COPD and is associated with the worst prognosis, the greatest functional impairment and the highest disability [8]. It can be defined as the awareness of an increased or inappropriate effort in breathing, but most COPD patients report it as a sensation of inspiratory difficulty [9]. The dynamic hyperinflation of the lung which occurs during exercise decreases the inspiratory reserve volume in COPD patients, who become aware of the increased effort of breathing [9]. Dyspnoea occurs after minimal exercise, when $FEV_1$ is less than 30% of the predicted value, and is a constant presence in the life of COPD patients. Dyspnoea may be better scored by means of different, simple, reproducible, non-specific scales, such as the Borg scale, visual analogical scale, MRC dyspnoea scale.

Wheezing is difficult to evaluate because it is intermittent: it is caused by a turbulent air flow in the large airways [10] but its role in COPD is still unclear.

Chest pain occurs often in COPD patients and is related to isometric contraction of the intercostal muscles. However, one must also consider that ischemic heart disease is often found in a population of heavy smokers. Chest pain may also occur because 40% of COPD patients also have oesophageal reflux [11].

In the advanced phase of COPD anorexia and weight loss due to increased total daily energy expenditure are markers of poor prognosis during acute exacerbations [12].

Among COPD patients, psychiatric disorders are common, partially because of the neurological effects of hypoxemia [13] and impaired sleep [14] .

## The Physical Examination of COPD Patients

The physical signs presented by COPD patients vary for many reasons: the degree of hyperinflation, the presence of disturbances in gas exchange and the severity of airflow obstruction. In mild to moderate COPD, physical examination is of poor sensitivity [15]. In the severe COPD patient, physical signs of the disease are always found.

In advanced COPD patients always show signs of respiratory distress. They sit leaning forward: this since breathing strategy allows the muscles that connect the limb girdle to the chest (i.e. latissimus dorsi) to act as inspiratory muscles.

Some COPD patients breath with pursed lips: the increase of intraluminal pressure in large airways reduces both deformation of the airways during expiration and the respiratory frequency, thereby minimizing the dynamic hyperinflation.

Pattern of breathing is a crucial sign. Most COPD patients show a breathing frequency > 16/min whereas patients with hypercapnia breath at a frequency > 25/min [16]. In the stable phase of COPD, sternocleidomastoid muscles do not take part in the respiration cycle; when this happens, one must consider it as a sign of impending respiratory failure [17]. Patients with severe COPD also show expiratory muscle activity, but its role is uncertain since downstream the flow-limited segments of the bronchial tree cannot be increased by their activation [18].

Barrel chest deformation has long been described as associated with pulmonary emphysema. It reflects diaphragmatic descent due to lung hyperinflation, but it may be illusive [19].

Lung hyperinflation also determines a lower position of the diaphragm and a reduction or, in the most severe cases, an inversion of the apposition zone. The contraction of the diaphragm pulls the lower ribs inward and the abdominal pressure becomes negative, causing the so-called paradoxical breath, which is not a sign of muscular fatigue but of diaphragm displacement. In this case, rib cage inspiratory muscles become important muscles of respiration [20].

Percussion of the chest is not very helpful in patients with COPD and evaluation of expansion of the thorax due to the altered chest wall configuration is misleading.

The auscultation of the thorax of patients with COPD is usually impaired because of adventitious sounds. Vesicular breath sound is decreased [21] by an amount proportional to the amount of bronchial obstruction. Wheezing is an important but non-specific sign of airflow limitation and is related to the severity of airflow limitation and to the response to bronchodilators [22]. Adventitious sounds, like inspiratory rales or crackles, are common findings and reflect sudden opening of the small airways and rapid equilibration of the pressures [23].

Heart sounds are difficult to hear in hyperinflated patients. Tachycardia and arrythmias are frequent.

## The Clinical Presentation of COPD Patients

The clinical presentation of COPD patient depends on the stage of the disease. In the late phases of the COPD, when $FEV_1$ falls below 30% of predicted or 1 l, patients tend to diverge into two main types: "pink and puffing" and "blue and bloated" (Table 1).

**Table 1.** Clinical and physiological feature of "pink and puffing" and "blue and bloated" patients

| Synonim | Type A (pink and puffing) | Type B (blue and bloated) |
| --- | --- | --- |
| Dyspnoea | At rest | Relatively less dyspnoeic |
| Weight | Thin<br>Hyperinflated | Obese<br>Oedematous |
| Gas exchange<br>Total lung capacity | Low/normal<br>Moderate increase | Normal<br>Small increase |
| Static lung compliance | Normal/high | Normal |
| Pulmonary artery pressure | Normal | Modest elevation |
| Red cell mass | Normal/low | High (smokers) |

There is indeed a broad spectrum of characteristics between these two types, but this model is useful to categorize most severe COPD patients.

Usually patients are identified when they seek help for cough, respiratory tract infections and dyspnoea. A minority of patients are recognized when they are hospitalized for an acute exacerbation.

## Investigations and Assessment of Severity of COPD

The main feature of COPD is airflow limitation. This is a slow, insidious process which begins in the peripheral parts of the bronchial tree (airways < 2 mm) and slowly advances in this functionally quiet zone (peripheral airways resistance represents only a tiny part, 25%, of the total airways resistance) to become clinically evident only at an irreversible stage of the disease [24]. The idea is to detect the onset of the disease in early stages in order to stop its progression and to improve its prognosis by the removal of risk factors. Disease onset can be detected using functional tests suitable to investigate small airways function: frequency dependence of dynamic compliance [25], nitrogen slope of the alveolar plateau [26], closing volume [27], maximal expiratory flow rates at low lung volume [28], density dependence of air flow [29]. However, these tests in many studies showed a link between their alteration and a subsequent decrease of $FEV_1$, but their abnormality could only partially explain the decline [30-32].

The reduction of $FEV_1$ in the course of the disease reflects well the progression of the obstruction but 3-5 years are required to assess an accurate rate of the decline. Values exceeding 50 ml/year suggest an accelerated progression of COPD [33]. The severity of airway obstruction has been differently graded by the ATS [34], the European Respiratory Society (ERS) [35], and the British Thoracic Society (BTS) [36] (Table 2).

**Table 2.** Grading of severity of airway obstruction in terms of $FEV_1$ (% of predicted)

| Society | Mild | Moderate | Severe |
| --- | --- | --- | --- |
| ATS | $\geq 50$ | 35-49 | $< 35$ |
| ERS | $\geq 70$ | 50-69 | $< 50$ |
| BTS | 60-79 | 40-59 | $< 40$ |

The response to bronchodilator in COPD is usually poor, not reaching minimal values of 200 ml and 12% [34] of increase from baseline, and this is one of the most important features that distinguish asthma from COPD.

In COPD, unlike asthma, the positive response to bronchial provocation test depends on baseline values [37].

Measurements of respiratory muscle function (i.e. maximum inspiratory or expiratory pressure) are indicated in malnutrition or steroid myopathy.

Single breath diffusion test has shown to be related to the extent of emphysema: if K CO (diffusion lung/alveolar volume) is normal, severe emphysema may be excluded but mild forms of COPD cannot be excluded [38].

There is a general relationship between reduction of $FEV_1$ and arterial oxygen tension ($PaO_2$); arterial carbon dioxide tension remains in the normal range until $FEV_1$ falls below 1.5-1.0 l.

Measurement of arterial blood gases in patients breathing room air is recommended in moderate to severe, stable COPD. In moderate COPD, an alternative approach is to measure oxygen saturation with an oximeter: if values < 94% are found, arterial gas sample must be obtained.

The relationship between semiquantitative assessment of macroscopic or microscopic emphysema and the degree of deterioration of functional tests is poor [39]. By contrast, loss of peribronchial alveolar attachments, which maintain airways shape, well correlate with the degree of airflow limitation [40].

Most COPD patients, even in the most advanced phase of the disease and even if they show an increase of arterial oxygen tension, have a normal or slightly increased minute ventilation [41]. Many studies suggest that the chemoceptor-mediated control of breathing is abnormally increased in COPD patients [42-43]. However, COPD patients show a reduced ventilatory response to hypoxia and hypercapnia, but it is not clear whether this represents an intrinsic reduction in respiratory chemosensitivity or is due to the increased mechanical load superimposed on the respiratory system in COPD, which limits the effects of the increased neural output.

Pulmonary arterial hypertension is a late finding in course of COPD, is associated with arterial hypoxemia ($PaO_2$ < 60 mmHg) and right ventricular hypertrophy and leads to a poor prognosis [44-45]. Factors that contribute to the onset of pulmonary artery hypertension are summarized in Table 3.

**Table 3.** Factors promoting the onset of pulmonary artery hypertension in COPD

1. Abnormal blood gas tensions
2. Disruption of pulmonary vascular bed
3. Abnormal pulmonary mechanics
4. Endothelial dysfunction
5. Increased cardiac output
6. Increased blood flow
7. Changes in blood volume

Increased pulmonary artery pressure in COPD is not related to the extent of emphysema, as measured by CT scans [46]. Endothelial dysfunction plays a major role in the development of pulmonary hypertension through a reduced nitric oxide synthesis. The potential role of nitric oxide in preventing excessive increases in pulmonary vascular tone due to hypoxemia may be lost in COPD patients.

Resting pulmonary function tests are not very accurate to predict exercise performance but maximum inspiratory pressure (MIP) and lung diffusion of CO (LD CO) are somehow related to maximum oxygen consumption and maximum ventilation [47-49]. Exertion dyspnoea may be measured using visual analogical scales, Borg scale, MRC scale. Exercise evaluation may be as simple as 6 min walking test, or shuttle walking test, or may include continuous measurements of many physiological parameters requiring complex instrumentation. These are useful in both planning and verifying the outcome of pulmonary rehabilitation programs.

Specific features of COPD on plain chest radiograph are signs of lung overinflation:

- Low diaphragms: the border of the diaphragm in the mid-clavicular line is at or below the anterior end of the sixth or seventh rib [50-51].
- Increase of retrosternal airspace: the horizontal distance of the posterior face of the sternum to the aorta exceeds 4.5 cm in lateral chest projection.
- An obtuse costophrenic angle.

- The inferior margin of the retrosternal space is $\leq$ 3 cm from the anterior aspect of the diaphragm.
- Reduction of size and number of pulmonary vessels.
- Vessel distortion.
- Areas of transradiency.

The accuracy of diagnosis of emphysema on plain chest radiograph increases with the increased severity of the disease. In early stages of emphysema, the plain chest radiograph may be normal.

## References


1. Adam PF, Benson V (1992) Current estimates from the national health interview survey. Vital Health Stat 184:1-232
2. Fletcher EC, Peto R (1997) The natural history of chronic airflow obstruction. Br Med J 1:1645-1648
3. Anthonisen NR, Wright EC (1986) IPPB Trial Group: Bronchodilator response in chronic obstructive pulmonary disease. Am Rev Respir Dis 133:814-819
4. Mandella LA, Manfreda J, Warren CPW, Anthonisen NR (1982) Steroid response in stable chronic obstructive pulmonary disease. Ann Intern Med 96:17-21
5. Anthonisen NR, Connett JE, Kiley JP et al (1994) Effects of smoking intervention and the use of an inhaled anticholinergic bronchodilator on the rate of decline of FEV1. The Lung Health Study. JAMA 272:1497-1505
6. Jamal K, Cooney TP, Fleetham JA et al (1984) Chronic bronchitis:correlation of morphologic findings to sputum production and flow rates. Am Rev Respir Dis 129:717-722
7. Vestbo J, Prescott E, Lange P (1996) Association of chronic mucus hypersecretion with FEV1 decline and chronic obstructive pulmonary disease morbidity. Copenhagen City Heart Study Group. Am J Respir Crit Care Med 153:1530-1535
8. Keatings VM, Collins PD, Scott DM et al (1996) Differences in interleukin-8 and tumor necrosis factor-alpha in induced sputum from patients with chronic obstructive pulmonary disease or asthma. Am J Respir Crit Care Med 153:530-534
9. O'Donnell DE, Bertley JC, Chau LK et al (1997) Qualitative aspects of exertional breathlessness in chronic airflow limitation: pathophysiologic mechanisms. Am J Respir Crit Care Med 155:109-115
10. Earis JE (1992) Lung sounds. Thorax 47:671-672
11. David P, Denis P, Nouvet G et al (1982) Lung function and gastro–oesophageal reflux during chronic bronchitis. Bull Eur Physiopat Respir 18:81-86
12. Baarends EM, Schols AM, Pannemans DL et al (1997) Total free living energy expenditure in patients with severe chronic obstructive pulmonary disease. Am J Respir Crit Care Med 155:549-554
13. Grant J, Heaton RK, McSweeny AJ et al (1982) Neuropsycologic findings in hypoxaemic chronic obstructive pulmonary disease. Arch Intern Med 142:1470-1476
14. Calverley PMA, Brezinova V, Douglas NJ et al (1982) The effect of oxygenation on sleep-quality in chronic bronchitis and emphysema. Am Rev Respir Dis 126:206-210
15. Badgett RC, Tanaka DV, Hunt DK et al (1993) Can moderate chronic obstructive pulmonary disease be diagnosed by historical and physical findings alone? Am J Med 94:188-196
16. Oliven A, Cherniak NS, Deal EC, Kelsen SG (1985) The effects of acute bronchoconstriction on respiratory activity in patients with chronic obstructive pulmonary disease. Am Rev Respir Dis 131:236-241
17. De Troyer A, Peche R, Yernault JC, Estenne M (1994) Neck muscle activity in

patients with severe chronic obstructive pulmonary disease. Am J Respir Crit Care Med 150:41-47

18. O'Donnel DF, Sanii R, Anthonisen NR, Younes M (1987) Effect of dynamic compression on breathing pattern and respiratory sensation in severe chronic obstructive pulmonary disease. Am Rev Respir Dis 135:912-918

19. Walsh JM, Webber CI, Fahej PJ et al (1992) Structural change of the thorax in chronic obstructive pulmonary disease. J Appl Physiol 72:1270-1278

20. Decramer M (1997) Hyperinflation and respiratory muscle interaction. Europ Respir J 10:934-941

21. Martinez FJ, Couser JI, Celli BR (1990) Factors influencing ventilatory muscle recruitment in patients with chronic airflow obstruction. Am Rev Respir Dis 142:276-282

22. Marini JJ, Pierson DJ, Hudson LD et al (1979) The significance of wheezing in chronic airflow obstruction. Am Rev Respir Dis 120:1069-1072

23. Nath AR, Capel LH (1974) Inspiratory crackles and mechanical events of breathing. Thorax 29:695-698

24. Macklem PT (1972) Obstruction in small airways. Acxhallenge to medicine. Am J Med 52:721-724

25. Woolcock AJ, Vincent NJ, Macklem PT (1969) Frequency dependence of compliance as a test for obstruction in the small airways. J Clin Invest 48:1097-1106

26. Buist SA, Ross BR (1973) Quantitative analysis of the alveolar plateau in the diagnosis of early airway obstruction. Am Rev Respir Dis 107:735-743

27. Dolfuss RE, Milic-Emili J, Bates DV (1967) Regional ventilation of the lung studied with boluses of xenon. Respir Physiol 2:234-246

28. Bouhuys A, Van de Woestijne KP (1970) Respiratory mechanics and dust exposure in byssinosis. J Clin Invest 49:106-118

29. Dosman J, Bode F, Urbanetti J et al (1975) The use of helium–oxygen mixture during maximum expiratory flow to demonstarte obstruction in small airways in smokers. J Clin Invest 55:1090-1099

30. Olofsson J, Svardsudd B, Skoog BE et al (1986) The single–breath N2 test predicts the rate of decline of FEV1. Eur J Respir Dis:69:46-56

31. Beaty TH, Menkes HA, Cochen BH et al (1984) Risk factors associated with longitudinal change in pulmonary function. Am Rev Respir Dis 129:660-667

32. Buist AS, Vollmer WM, Johnson LR et al (1988) Does the single-breath N2 test identify the smoker who will develop chronic airflow limitation? Am Rev Respir Dis 137:293-301

33. Burrows B, Lebowitz MD, Camilli AK et al (1986) Longitudinal changes in forced expiratory volume in one second in adults. Am Rev Respir Dis 133:974-980

34. (1991) American Thoracic Society: Lung function testing: selection of reference values and interpretative strategies Am Rev Respir Dis 144:1202-1228

35. Siafakas NM, Vermeire P, Pride NB et al (1995) Optimal assessment and management of chronic obstructive pulmonary disease. Eur Respir J 8:1398-1420

36. (1997) British Thoracic Society: Guidelines for the management of COPD. Thorax 52(Suppl):5-57

37. Ramsdale EH, Morris MM, Roberts RS et al (1994) Methacoline bronchiale responsiveness in chronic bronchitis; relationship to airflow obstruction and cold air responsiveness. Thorax 39:912-918

38. Burrows B, Fletcher CM, Heard BE et al (1966) The emphysematous and bronchial types of chronic airway obstruction. Lancet I:830-835

39. McLean A, Warren PM, Gillooly M et al (1992) Microscopic and macroscopic measurements of emphysema:relation to carbon monoxide gas transfer. Thorax 47:144-149

40. Lamb D, McLean A, Gillooly M et al (1993) The relationship between distal airspace size, bronchial attachments and lung function. Thorax 48:1012-1017

41. Sorli J, Grassino A, Lorange G et al (1978) Control of breathing in patients with chronic obstructive pulmonary disease. Clin Sci Mol Med 54:294-304

42. Fleetham JA, Bradley CA, Kryger MH et al (1980) The effect of low flow oxygen therapy on the chemical control of ventilation in patients with hypoxemia. Am Rev Respir Dis 122:833-840

43. Gribbin HR, Gardiner IT, Heinz GJ et al (1983) Role of impaired inspiratory muscle function in limiting the ventilatory response to carbon dioxide in chorinc airways obstruction. Clin Sci 64:487-495

44. MacNee W (1994) Pathophysiology of cor pulmonale in chronic obstructive pulmonary disease. Part One . Am J Respir Crit Care Med 150:833-852

45. MacNee W (1994) Pathophysiology of cor pulmonale in chronic obstructive pulmonary disease. Part two . Am J Respir Crit Care Med 150:1158-1168

46. Biernacki W, Gould GA, Whyte KF et al (1989) Pulmonary hemodynamics ,gas exchanges and the severity of emphysema as assessed by quantitative CT scan in chronic bronchitis and emphysema. Am Rev Respir Dis 139:1509-1515

47. Carter R, Peavler M, Zinkgraf S et al (1987) Predicting maximal exercise ventilation in patients with chronic obstructive pulmonary disease. Chest 92:253-259

48. Dilland TA, Piantadosi S, Rajagopal KR (1989) Determinants of maximum exercise capacity in patients with chronic airflow obstruction. Chest 96:267-271

49. Loiseau A, Dubreuil P, Loiseau P et al (1989) Exercise tolerance in chronic obstructive pulmonary disease: importance of active and passive components of the ventilatory system. Eur Respir J 2:522-527

50. Katsura S, Martin CJ (1967) The roentgenologic diagnosis of anatomic emphysema, Am Rev Respir Dis 96:700-706

51. Lennon EA, Simon G (1965) The height of the diaphragm in chest radiograph of normal adults. Br J Radiol 38:937-943

# Chapter 9

# Paediatric Respiratory Diseases

A. Sarti, C. Dell'Oste

## Introduction

Respiratory failure, the second most common cause of death in infants, accounts for around 50% of intensive care unit admission of infants and children [1]. This is due to the wide array and high incidence of respiratory diseases in the paediatric age group. It is also due to the fact that respiratory function is particularly at risk. The limited ability of the developing respiratory system to compensate for disease-induced mechanical abnormalities makes the child susceptible to respiratory failure, which is very often the cause or the main effect of most paediatric emergencies. Respiratory function is critical for all organ systems of infants and young children. Early recognition of respiratory insufficiency is critical to allowing quick treatment, before progression of the vicious cycle of asphyxia and haemodynamic deterioration, which may lead to cardiorespiratory arrest (Fig. 1).

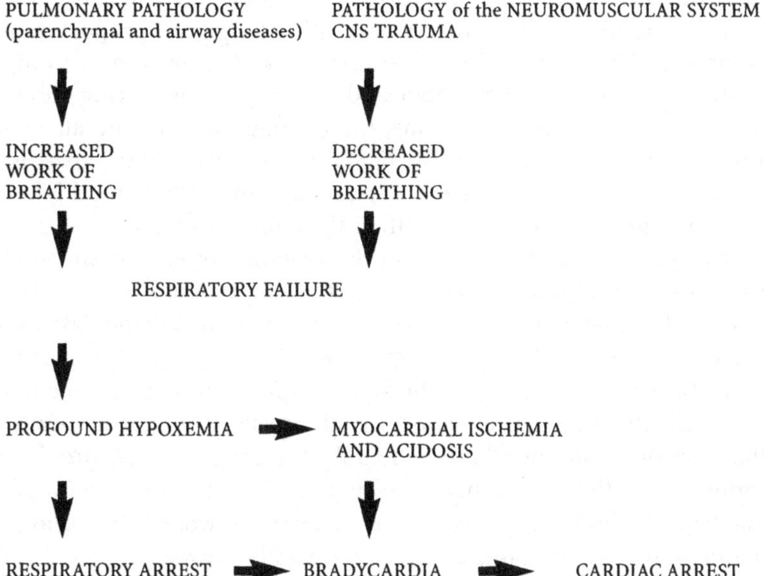


**Fig. 1.** Escalation of pulmonary disease emergencies

However, it must be appreciated that since many lung development changes occur in children up to at least 8 years of age, there is a great chance for spontaneous healing and improvement in respiratory function in the paediatric age, even after critical conditions. The understanding of the respiratory dysfunction depends  on the specific disease and also on the knowledge of the specific respiratory anatomy and physiology of the development stage of the single paediatric patient.

This paper reviewes some aspects of anatomy and physiology and the most frequent respiratory diseases the anaesthesiologist and the intensivist must face in the clinical practice beyond the neonatal age.

## Anatomy and Physiology

After birth, the development of the lung can be divided into two phases. During the first phase, from birth to the first 18 months of life, there is a brisk increase in the surface and volume of the bronchioalveolar spaces while  the capillary volume increases even more; the solid tissue grows more slowly. This process is very active in early infancy. Stimuli, such as hypoxemia and increased shear stress or tension in the vascular wall, can produce smooth-muscle hypertrophy and deposition of elastin and collagen, leading eventually to vasoconstriction and even obliteration of small pulmonary vessels. A failure to curtail this proliferative response is probably the origin of many cases of pulmonary hypertension complicating parenchymal lung diseases and right to left shunting in childhood.  In the second phase, all compartments of the lung grow proportionately to each other and the configuration of the air spaces becomes more complex because of the development of new septa, and because of lengthening and folding of the alveolar structures [2].  Thus, the configuration of the air spaces become progressively more complex. At birth, the alveolar surface area  is 2.8 $m^2$; it becomes 32 $m^2$ by 8 years of age and reaches 75 $m^2$ in adulthood [3].

The paediatric lung is less compliant than the adult lung because of the differences in the air space architecture and the amounts of elastin and surfactant. The amount of elastin increases over the first 18 years of life.

The airway enlarges in diameter and length with age. During the first 5 years of life, the growth of the distal airways lags behind that of the proximal airways; the narrow distal airway accounts for the high peripheral flow resistance in this age group. In infants and children, small distal airway resistance accounts for most of the work of breathing, whereas in adults the nasal passages provide the major proportion of flow resistance. The increased resistance to flow of the bronchi and bronchioles in the young results in increased work of breathing and increased vulnerability to diseases affecting the small airways.

Infants are described as obligate nasal breathers; thus, the obstruction caused by a naso-gastric probe may easily worsen the ventilation of a distressed child. The tongue is closer to the roof of the mouth and thus very easily obstructs the airway. Moreover, the infant's tongue is more likely to obstruct the view of the larynx during laryngoscopy. The infant's larynx is higher in the neck (C3-4) than is an adult's (C5) and it is "rostral" in the neck compared with that of the adult subject. The narrowest portion of the infant and small-child larynx is the cricoid cartilage. Thus, an endotracheal tube which easily goes through the glottis can stop at the cricoid level.

Resistance to flow is inversely related to the fourth power of the radius; therefore, a small decrement in the diameter of the airways in infants and small children, such as an inflammatory oedema at subglottic level, may lead to a dramatic increase in airways resistance. Cartilagenous support is essential for the stability of airway conduct. After birth, cartilaginous tissue increases and spreads up to the segmental bronchi. The weakness of this support in infants and small children accounts for dynamic compression of the trachea and bronchi in conditions associated with high air-flow rates, such as with bronchiolitis and asthma. A very common cause of upper airway obstruction in children is adenoidal and tonsillar hypertrophy due to frequent upper airway infections. Extrathoracic airway obstruction caused by croup, epiglottitis or a foreign body alters the airway dynamics. A more negative intrathoracic pressure leads to an increased tendency toward dynamic collapse below the level of the obstruction. Particularly at the extremes of transluminal pressure that occur when a child is crying, the tendency to collapse is increased [4]. Avoiding dynamic collapse is thus very important. It is common for children with respiratory diseases to breathe transiently at frequencies that depart from optimum. Agitation can in this manner reduce the efficiency of the respiratory system and precipitate respiratory failure. For this reason, it is imperative to keep the child with an airway obstruction as calm as possible, avoiding any unnecessary, frightening procedure. A brisk increase in the work of breathing may also occur with long endotracheal tubes of small diameter, or with a partially obstructed tube, because of thick, viscous secretions. An obstructed endotracheal tube may cause a respiratory distress very similar to that in a bronchospastic attack.

The chest wall of the infant is cartilagenous, soft and pliable. The infant's chest can behave much like a "flail" chest [5]. Since the chest wall is so compliant, the elastic recoil may lead to excessive reduction of the lung volume, increasing the risk of lung collapse. In fact, most tidal breathing in the infant and small child takes place in the range of closing capacity. The relationship between functional residual capacity (FRC) and closing capacity determines the matching of ventilation and perfusion and thus the $PaO_2$. This is crucial because most paediatric respiratory diseases show an alteration of closing capacity or functional residual capacity or both. FRC is also acutely decreased during anaesthesia, which can be reversed by the administration of PEEP [1]. Poorly ventilated areas of the lung have a parallel reduction in blood flow because of hypoxic pulmonary vasoconstriction. Thus, the oxygen-desaturated blood from areas with low ventilation-perfusion ratio mixes with oxygenated blood from well-ventilated areas. A potential disadvantage of all halogenated agents is their tendency to blunt hypoxic pulmonary vasoconstriction. Thus, any poorly ventilated area of the lung, e.g. an atelectasis, is well perfused and leads to desaturated and oxygenated blood mixing and hypoxemia. All injectable anaesthetics have no effect on hypoxic pulmonary vasoconstriction.

Units with high ventilation-perfusion ratios cause an increase of dead space ventilation, which can lead to a rise in arterial $CO_2$ if the child is unable to compensate with enough of an increase in minute ventilation.

The level of the pulmonary capillaries is the site of active exchange of water and solutes between the vascular space and the interstitium of the lung. This exchange is regulated across the endothelial cells by a balance of hydrostatic and oncotic forces. An increase of fluid filtration into the interstitial tissue and then into the alveoli may occur either when the microvascular pressure increases because of left ventricular failure or because of pulmonary vein obstruction or when the permeability of the endothelium is increased because of damage to the wall of the capillary vessels, which occurs in ARDS and in virtually any form of lung injury.

Oxygen demand is much higher per unit mass in infants than in adults. The higher oxygen consumption together with decreased oxygen supply in the lungs explains the inclination toward rapid hypoxemia and desaturation, with the appearance of cyanosis in infants and children during hypoventilation. This greater oxygen consumption accounts for the increased respiratory frequency, while tidal volume does not change much throughout age. In response to low oxygen, the newborn does not sustain an increase in ventilation. $CO_2$ response is also reduced in the young. Respiratory muscles seem to be more susceptible to fatigue in children than in adults. Thus, any condition that increases the work of breathing in children may easily fatigue the respiratory muscles and result in respiratory failure.

## Paediatric Respiratory Life Support [6,7]

Cardiopulmonary arrest in infants and children is rarely a sudden event and respiratory causes predominate. Current guidelines use the term "newly born" to refer to the neonate in the first minutes to hour after birth. The term "infant" includes the neonatal period and extends to one year of age. For the purposes of resuscitation, the term "child" refers to ages 1-8 years and the term "adult" applies to all victims beyond 8 years of age.

Because most paediatric arrests are secondary to progressive repiratory failure and/or shock and because ventricular fibrillation is uncommon, immediate cardiopulmonary resuscitation ("phone fast") is recommended for infants and children in the out-of-hospital setting rather than the adult approach, which is immediate activation of the emergency system before applying initial cardiopulmonary resuscitation ("phone first"). Opening the airway must be done with caution in infants, avoiding excessive head tilt, because it is easy to collapse the airway. Between 2 and 5 rescue breaths should be delivered initially to ensure that at least two effective ventilations are provided. Mouth-to-mouth-and-nose ventilation must be used for infants. A rescuer with a small mouth may have difficulty covering both the mouth and the nose of a large infant. Under these conditions, mouth-to-nose ventilation is applied. For children, mouth-to-mouth ventilation is suitable, like in adults. The volume of each rescue breath should be sufficient to rise the chest without causing gastric distention. Improper airway opening is by far the most common cause of inadequate ventilation during resuscitation. Gastric distention can be minimized by delivering the rescue breaths slowly. Gentle pressure on the cricoid cartilage during ventilation can help decreasing the amount of air driven to the stomach. Bag and mask ventilation in infants and children must be handled without difficulty by a professional rescuer. Paediatric-size ventilation bags (450-500 ml) should be used to ventilate term newly born infants, larger infants and children. The "E-C clamp" technique provides adequate sealing to the face of the mask if applied gently but firmly, avoiding excessive head tilt, particularly in infants. Two-rescuer bag-mask ventilation (four-hands technique) may be used by unskilled rescuers.

Ventilation via a tracheal tube is the most effective and reliable method of ventilation and airway control. A pillow to flex the neck  is not necessary for oral intubation of children < 2 years. For children older than one year, an estimate of tracheal tube size may be made using the following equation: tube size (mm) = (age/4) + 4.

The appropriate depth of insertion of a tracheal tube from the mouth may be estimated in children < 2 years of age using the following formula: depth (cm) = internal tube diameter (mm) x 3.

For children > 2 years of age the following equation must be used instead: depth (cm) = (age in years/2) + 12.

When it is impossible to oxygenate the child with bag-mask ventilation and when intubation cannot be accomplished, transtracheal ventilation may be attempted by needle-cannula cricothyrotomy.

## Physiology and Pathophysiology of the Lateral Decubitus Position

Gravity causes a vertical gradient for pulmonary blood flow in the lateral decubitus position. Gravity also causes a vertical gradient in pleural pressure in the dependent lung, which places it in a more favourable position on the compliance curve [5]. The abdominal content exerts more pressure on the dependent lung, resulting in doming and better contraction of the diaphgram during spontaneous ventilation. The induction of anaesthesia does not change the distribution of pulmonary blood flow. There is a loss of functional residual capacity in both lungs, which may be greater in the dependent lung because of the weight of the mediastinum and the abdomen. The upper, non-dependent lung moves to the more compliant portion of the pressure volume curve, whereas the lower lung becomes less compliant. Ventilation-perfusion matching is disturbed and a decreased $PaO_2$ easily develops. PEEP can restore ventilation to the lower lung. As the chest is opened, the ventilation-perfusion mismatch worsens and postive-pressure ventilation becomes mandatory.

An important difference exists between adults and children regarding the lateral decubitus position in the presence of unilateral lung disease. In adults, gas exchange is optimal when the "good" lung is dependent in the lower position [8]. By contrast, infants with unilateral lung disease show better oxygenation when the "good" lung is not dependent. Infants, both those breathing spontaneously and those receiving positive-pressure ventilation, distribute more ventilation to the upper, non-dependent lung [9]. This may be due to the unstable rib cage, which does not fully support the underlying lung [10]. In children, the best side must be found watching $SaO_2$ changes with both lateral positions.

## Respiratory Failure

Acute respiratory failure in paediatrics may be categorized into lung diseases of infants, in whom a single process involves only the lung, and those of older children, in whom pulmonary failure is often part of a multiple system dysfunction syndrome that is similar to that in adults with ARDS. Respiratory failure is defined as an alteration in arterial $PaO_2$ and $PaCO_2$. Respiratory failure caused by mechanical abnormalities ensues as the mechanisms that compensate for the increased work of breathing are not efficient enough to maintain normal or near-normal gas exchange. Mechanical abnormalities increase both the ventilatory requirement and the physical effort to fulfil these requirements. In addition to the increased work of breathing, many factors, such as malnutrition, electrolytes disorders and hypophosphatemia, increase the vulnerability of the ventilatory muscular pump. Even the increase of ventilatory demand caused by agitation or by an increase in temperature of the body may be sufficient to overcome the compensation mechanisms and precipitate significant hypoxemia and hypercarbia. An awake child with upper airway obstruction caused by croup or epiglottitis is much more stable in a mother's arms because the increased air flow generated by crying may easily precipitate respiratory failure. The clinical manifestations are the signs and symptoms of respiratory distress. Early recognition of respiratory distress is thus crucial to prevent escalation to respiratory failure.

By contrast, no distress is observed when respiratory failure is caused by neuromuscular or control abnormalities, and the only clinical clue is the observation of a decrease of the frequency and/or the depth of ventilation, which requires a very skilled eye and knowledge of the normal respiratory rate throughout infancy and childhood. Acute hypoxemia and hypercarbia are often associated with lethargy and confusion alternating with agitation and altered behaviour of the child.

Establishing a diagnosis and planning a therapy for children with respiratory diseases is aided by the clinician being able to distinguish between conditions that alter primarily the elastic (restrictive respiratory diseases) and the resistive (obstructive respiratory diseases) characteristics of the respiratory system [5].

Children with restrictive diseases breathe at fast rates, with shallow respiratory excursions. An expiratory grunt is common as the child attempts to raise the functional residual capacity by a partial closure of the glottis at the end of expiration. Lung percussion is usually dull and the auscultation reveals rales or crackles. Obstructive diseases are generally characterized by slower, deeper breaths. The pattern and the length of inspiration and expiration is very useful to diagnose the level of the obstruction: when the obstruction is extrathoracic from the nose up to the first half of the trachea, inspiration is more prolonged than expiration. With such conditions, an inspiratory stridor, can be easily heard. By contrast, expiration is more prolonged than inspiration when the obstruction is at the distal trachea, at the bronchi and at the level of the small airways. The child has to make use of the accessory muscles of the abdominal wall to eject the air out of the lungs. The auscultation reveals expiratory wheezes caused by turbulent flow in narrow airways.

Administration of supplemental oxygen is a safe and wise precaution for all children at risk of respiratory failure. Oxygen can be easily administered by nasal cannulas or hoods. Facial masks are not always well tolerated by infants and small children. The indication of ventilatory support is made on an individual basis considering the persistence or the worsening of gas exchange. Mechanical ventilation is life-saving, but can produce significant lung damage and adverse effects all over the body. Regardless of the underlying respiratory problem, the goal of the artificial ventilation is not to normalize arterial $PaO_2$ and $PaCO_2$, but rather to obtain adequate or acceptable gas exchange for the single patient, according to the underlying conditions. What can be considered adequate is very different at present from than it was some years ago. There is now a wide consensus among paediatric intensivists that some degree of hypercarbia and even some relative hypoxia is well tolerated and can reduce volutrauma and barotrauma. Permissive hypercapnia is considered an arterial $CO_2$ around 50-60 mmHg; its effects on pH are reduced by renal retention of bicarbonate. Moderate hypoxia, such as an arterial saturation around 85-90%, is also well tolerated if anaemia and insufficient cardiac output can be avoided. Lactate levels and mixed venous oxygen saturation may help in identifying the adequacy of cardiac output.

Inhaled nitric oxide may improve $PaO_2$ by reducing pulmonary vascular resistance.

## Upper Airway Obstruction

### The Child with a Runny Nose [11]

It is very common to evaluate a child scheduled for surgery, with symptoms and signs of a possible upper respiratory tract infection. There are many causes for a runny nose in children and each patient must be considered on an individual basis. It is very important to take a careful history and make an accurate diagnosis of the cause of the symptoms. Often, the parents state that their child always has a runny nose. The history may point to an acute onset of coryza. The examination of the mouth, nose and throat may help in identifying the amount and type of secretions and other evidence of an acute infection. An elevated temperature may suggest an infection, but a minor increase is seen frequently and may not be associated with infections. The problem is that there is an increased incidence of intraoperative and postoperative airway complications, such as episodes of desaturation and laryngospasm, in children with upper respiratory infections. The decision to postpone surgery is not without consequences for the child and the family because of many economic and emotional implications. However, it may be appropriate to be conservative, expecially if an endotracheal intubation is planned. The risks versus the benefits of proceeding with general anaesthesia should be discussed frankly with the parents and the surgeon.

## Congenital Larynx Abnormalities [12]

Congenital laryngeal webs and other anomalies of the larynx may be observed after birth. Stridor appearing in the first month of life is generally the result of laryngomalacia and tracheomalacia. The diagnosis is made by direct laryngoscopy. The symptoms of airway obstruction can be intermittent. Often they are worse when the infants lie on their backs and when an upper airway infection is superimposed on already narrowed airway. Stridor can also be caused by other malformations, such as cysts, haemangiomas and vascular anomalies. For this reason, a complete, accurate bronchoscopy is always indicated for these patients. Laryngomalacia usually resolves spontaneously during early infancy. Rarely, the infant must be intubated, and even more rarely, the patient requires a tracheostomy. Laryngeal abnormalities may require surgical intervention or laser treatment [13].

## Croup (Laryngotracheobronchitis) [14]

The term croup includes a group of acute, often infectious conditions characterized by a "croupy" cough. Inspiratory stridor, dyspnea, hoarseness and signs of respiratory distress, more or less pronounced, are always evident in the most severe cases. Symptoms are usually worse at night and increase quickly during the hours following onset. Agitation and crying aggravate the symptoms and may even hasten respiratory failure. The parainfluenza viruses account for 75% of cases. Occasionally, other viruses and bacteria may be involved. A radiograph of the upper airway shows very often the typical subglottic narrowing (steeple sign). Oxygen must always be administered in the hospital. Worsening hypoxemia and fatigue may ultimately lead to respiratory failure: the child is usually cyanotic, pale or obtunded. At this time, any manipulation of the pharynx may result in respiratory arrest. In a child showing signs of progressive fatigue, endotracheal intubation may become necessary (see "Epiglottitis"). A spasmodic type of croup occurs in children of 1-3 years of age and may be caused by viruses and other allergic or psychological factors. At laryngoscopy, a posterior laryngitis is usually seen, suggesting gastroesophageal reflux. It usually occurs in the evening or at night time and is characterized by a sudden onset, with no fever in most cases. The dyspnea is aggravated by excitement and agitation. Croup may recur several times.

## Epiglottitis [14]

This is an acute, life-threatening inflammation of the entire supraglottic region with a very rapid clinical course. It is now seen much less commonly since immunization against *H.influenzae* type B. The child, usually 2-7 years old, is well until the onset of high fever, severe sore throat, and inspiratory dyspnea. Prostration and fatigue ensue shortly thereafter. Within a few hours, the clinical course is complicated by progressive complete obstruction of the airway and death unless effective treatment is provided. Dysphagia is usually associated with drooling of saliva from the mouth. Painful or frightening procedures may result in sudden complete airway obstruction and cardiac arrest. If an epiglottitis is suspected, no attempts at stabilization, such as lying the child down, establishing an intravenous line or a forced visual inspection of the pharynx must be done. Oxygen is administered, avoiding constrained manoeuvres. The child must remain in the posture chosen, usually an upright position, stay together with the parents, and immediate transport to the hospital must be arranged. In the hospital, radiographs are performed to clarify the diagnosis only if the child is stable, and in the presence of a physician able to perform endotracheal intubation. As soon as possible, it is my practice to bring the patient to the operating room, trying to maintain a calm atmosphere. Anaesthesia is induced with sevoflurane in oxygen and a laryngoscopy is performed. The anatomy may be extremely distorted and sometimes it is even difficult to identify the glottic structures. The sight of air bubbles during exhalation may be the only clue to find the vocal cords. A small endotracheal tube is then inserted into the trachea. After some time a larger tube may be positioned in the trachea, as compression of the previous tube in the oedematous tissue enlarges the glottis passage. A tracheostomy is very rarely needed. After successful airway management, the child is sedated, treated with an antibiotic (ceftriaxone 100 mg/kg iv) and transferred to the pediatric intensive care unit for 48-72 h with assisted ventilation (CPAP). Acute pulmonary edema is not unusual after the relief of airway obstruction. Usually, this complication resolves within 24 h following appropriate treatment (oxygen, CPAP, diuretics).

## Lower Airway Obstruction

### Bronchiolitis [15]

This is an inflammatory obstruction of the small airways which occurs in the first two years of life, with a peak incidence at 6 months of age, mainly in winter and early spring. Respiratory syncytial virus is the aetiologic agent in more than

50% of all cases. The bronchial obstruction is due to edema and accumulation of cellular debris and viscous mucus. Since the resistance to flow is inversely related to the fourth power of the radius, the thinning of the bronchioli profoundly affects the air flow. Because the radius is even smaller in expiration, the ball-valve obstruction leads to air trapping and alveolar overinflation. The infant is usually tachypneic, in clear distress, with intercostal and subcostal retractions. Wheezings are often evident at auscultation. $SaO_2$ is reduced. The initial treatment is placing the patient in an atmosphere of warm humidified oxygen to relieve hypoxemia. Ribavirin is an antiviral agent which is currently used only for patients with bronchopulmonary dysplasia or cardiac abnormalities. Antibiotics are used if there is an associated pneumonia. Corticosteroids are used often to reduce inflammation. Some patients require endotracheal intubation and ventilatory assistance if $PaCO_2$ rises above 50 mmHg or severe hypoxemia persists despite oxygen therapy. Mechanical ventilation must consider the pathophysiologic basis of hyperinflation (see asthma).

## Asthma [16,17]

Asthma is the most common chronic disease of childhood. It is a leading cause of school absence and a common cause of hospital and intensive care admissions, too. The disease is intermittent and reversible and is characterized by narrowing of the airways due to inflammation, bronchospasm and accumulation of sticky mucus. The episodes may result in life-threatening respiratory failure. It is believed that allergy plays an important role in asthma. Airflow obstruction causes hyperinflation because of on expiratory ball-valve mechanism. Hypoxemia, hypocapnia and respiratory alkalosis are usually seen early in acute attacks. Ventilation/perfusion abnormalities result from non-uniform narrowing of the airway and changes in blood flow from the high intralveolar pressure, causing maldistributions in perfusion. Hypocapnia is due to hyperventilation. A normal level of $PaCO_2$ in the presence of respiratory distress means severe obstruction because of inadequate removal of $CO_2$. Elevated $PaCO_2$ occurs as the $FEV_{1.0}$ falls below 20% of the predicted value, and it indicates muscular exhaustion. Children with respiratory acidosis must be monitored closely in an intensive care unit. Intubation and mechanical ventilation must be considered when pharmacologic therapy [18] (beta-2-agonists, ipatropium, steroids, amynophilline) has failed to prevent fatigue and worsening hypercapnia. There are no absolute guidelines for initiating mechanical ventilation in status asthmaticus, except cardiopulmonary arrest; however, the following criteria are usually considered when deciding on an individual basis:
1. Coma or deterioration of mental status.
2. Progressive exhaustion.
3. Decreased wheezing associated with absence of breath sounds on auscultation.
4. Cyanosis or $SaO_2$ < 85-90 or $PaO_2$ < 55-60 mmHg, despite oxygen therapy.
5. Hypercapnia, $PaCO_2$ > 50 or rapidly increasing.

A suggested sequence for intubating an asthmatic child is as follows: pre-oxygenation with 100% oxygen, atropine 0.01 mg/kg iv, lidocaine 1-2 mg/kg iv, midazolam 0.2-0.3 mg/kg iv, ketamine 2-3 mg/kg iv, Sellick manoeuvre (cricoid compression) and an intravenous myorelaxant, such as suxametonium 1-2 mg/kg or rocuronium 1 mg/kg. Suxametonium is a better choice if a difficult intubation is suspected. However, it should be avoided if there is hyperkalemia, which is not unusual because of the beta-2 stimulation. Bag and mask ventilation with 100% oxygen prior to intubation may be difficult, but it becomes crucial to avoid dangerous hypoxemia after use of the drugs. Cricoid pressure may help in reducing gastric distention. Alternatively, halogenated agents, such as sevoflurane, may be used to induce anaesthesia during assisted ventilation. A chest radiography is always obtained after intubation to determine the position of the endotracheal tube and to get a "starting point" of x-ray assessment.

Mechanical ventilation must take account of the concept of limiting the risk of hyperinflation, barotrauma and volutrauma. Permissive hypercapnia is the recommended choice to be kept in mind in ventilating asthmatic children. Pressure-ventilation is often chosen to limit barotrauma. Expiration times must be long enough to allow air flow out of the obstructed bronchi, thus reducing air trapping. PEEP is generally not recommended, even if some centers use it, expecially during assisted spontaneous ventilation. Controlled ventilation is used initially. Then, pressure support may be chosen to facilitate weaning from the ventilator. Most chidren are ventilated for 36-72 h. The initial setting is usually as follows:

1. Peak pressure < 40 mmHg.
2. Tidal volume around 6-8 ml/kg.
3. Frequency around half the normal value for the age.
4. Inspiratory/expiratory ratio equal to 1/3 or 1/4.
5. No inspiratory pause.
6. PEEP: 0-3 cmH$_2$0
7. FIO$_2$ as needed to obtain SaO$_2$ 90%.

Subsequent adjustment should be done on the basis of clinical adequacy of ventilation and blood gases. PaCO$_2$ is maintained around 50-60 mmHg, with pH > 7.20. Monitoring includes pressure-volume curves, intrinsic PEEP (by means of end-expiratory breath hold) and plateau pressure (by means of end-inspiratory breath hold). Sedation and sometimes myorelaxation may be required to promote synchronization of the ventilator with breathing, which is favourable in reducing oxygen consumption and CO$_2$ production. Midazolam and ketamine (2-8 µg/kg/min) are the most frequent drugs used. Morphine is used with caution because of the possibility of worsening bronchospasm by morphine-induced histamine release. Drugs which cause hypotension are better avoided and it may become necessary to sustain cardiovascular function by inotropes.

Inhalational anaesthetics have been used in severe asthma. Isoflurane may be used in the ventilator circuit by progressive 0.1% increases, witholding all other sedatives until bronchospasm is reduced. Hypotension is the main concern. Intravenous fluids and/or vasoconstrictive agents may become necessary. The administration of magnesium sulfate 25-50 mg/kg iv, maximum 2 g, has gained interest in the treatment of asthma. Some improvements have been shown in recent studies. High doses of ketamine by continuous infusion, up to 40 µg/kg/min, may contribute to the succesful treatment of refractory bronchospasm.

## Foreign Bodies in the Respiratory Tract [6, 19, 20]

Most reported episodes of choking in children occur during play or eating, when parents or care providers are usually present. A foreign body which occludes the laryngeal inlet is an immediate threat to life. When a foreign body produces signs of complete airway obstruction, only a prompt relief may allow ventilation. Smaller objects or a piece of food may lodge in the main stem or lobar bronchus; the symptoms consist of coughing and sudden respiratory distress. After the initial symptoms, which may be forgotten, there is often a symptom-free period that may last hours, days, or even weeks.

If a responsive infant demonstrates signs of complete obstruction of the airway and spontaneous coughing is not successful to clear the airway, the rescuer must provide back blows and chest thrusts until the object is expelled or the victim becomes unresponsive. For the older child (1-8 years of age) a series of Heimlich abdominal thrusts are used to force air and the foreign body out of the airway. If the infant become unresponsive, the sequence of ABC of resuscitation is followed by the professional rescuer: open the victim's airway and attempt to provide rescue breaths. If the breaths are not effective, perform 5 back blows and 5 chest thrusts. This sequence is repeated until advanced life-support facilities are available. If the child becomes unresponsive, place the victim in the supine position, open the airway, and attempt to provide rescue breaths. If the repeated artificial breaths are not effective, the Heimlich manoeuvre is performed and the sequence is continued, alternating airway opening and inspection, rescue breaths and subdiaphragmatic thrusts.

Partial obstruction of the airway is more common if the object lies in the carena or the main bronchi. A non-obstructing, non-irritating foreign body may produce few symptoms. If there is a slight obstruction, a wheeze is produced. If the obstruction is severe, either overinflation or atelectasis may ensue. A ball-valve obstruction produces overinflation of the dependent area because air flow is interrupted in expiration, as the radius of the tube becomes smaller. Complete obstruction, by contrast, produces an atelectasis, as the air distal to the obstruction is reabsorbed. If the foreign body is a vegetable, such as a peanut, a severe bronchitis results, characterized by cough, mucus production, fever and worsening dyspnea. Chronic suppuration may occur if the vegetable remains in the airway for a long time. A chest X-ray may not reveal any change and it is always advisable trying to obtain films taken in deep inspiration and deep expiration. Early inspection of the airway and possible removal by rigid open-tube bronchoscopy is always indicated even if the presence of a foreign body is only suspected.

## Aspiration Pneumonia [21]

Children with gastroesophageal reflux or impaired consciousness and altered airway reflexes may regurgitate and aspirate food and vomitus. Hydrocloridric acid is the main determinant, but not the only one, of chemical lung injury. The child may show sudden distress just after the aspiration of a large amount of vomited food. Fever and tachypnea are usually present within 2 h after the episode. The chest X-ray reveals localized or, more often, bilateral infiltrates. Superimposed infection is very common. Immediate treatment consists of suctioning to reduce the chance of continuing aspiration. Oxygen is always used as needed. Endotracheal intubation and mechanical ventilation become necessary in severe cases. Clearing of infiltrates occurs within two weeks in most children. Hospitalized chronically ill children may become colonized and infected by gram-negative flora. Previously healthy children are often infected by mouth flora, predominantly anaerobes.

## ARDS [22-24]

Acute respiratory failure may occur after injury to the alveolar-capillary unit after a variety of insults in children with previous healthy lungs. It is often unclear whether the precipitating events are causative or merely associated phenomena. Shock, sepsis, aspiration pneumonia and diffuse infectious pneumonia are the most common causes in published pediatric series. The pathology and pathophysiology of the syndrome described in adults are not different than those in paediatric patients. The open lung approach, now much advocated in adult patients with ARDS, was first demonstrated in the young-animal lung lavage model of acute lung injury. It has been demonstrated that, in immature lambs, as few as six large tidal-volume breaths before the first spontaneous breath, a common scenario in the delivery suite, results in significant lung damage and blunts the effect of the exogenous administration of surfactant [25]. This concept was then applied using high-frequency oscillatory ventilation (HFOV) to treat premature infants. It is now clear that cyclic lung distention delivered by positive pressure ventilation can produce changes similar to those in ARDS in the lungs and damage to entire organ systems outside of the lungs. This damage may be mitigated by using small tidal volumes and high PEEP. Thus, oscillatory ventilation has a rationale to decrease lung damage during ventilation. If the clinician is to use HFOV, early intervention before the lung sustains significant damage is crucial. This has been demonstrated in a study in which premature infants were placed on HFOV in the delivery room [26]. If conventional ventilation is used in paediatric ARDS, a tidal volume as low as 5-6 ml/kg is associated with a reduction in mortality among patients with acute lung injury despite a significant degree of hypercapnia. Liquid ventilation is a very interesting concept in the treatment of ARDS, but the comparison of partial liquid ventilation with conventional ventilation in paediatric hypoxemic respiratory failure  did not show any advantage in using the liquid ventilation approach. There are data which show improvements in gas exchange in the prone position in paediatric patients [27, 28]. The role of extracorporeal membrane oxygenation (ECMO) in the treatment of children with pulmonary failure in this new era of lung-protection ventilation strategies remains to be determined. At present, when the facilities and experience with ECMO are limited, the value of this approach may only be judged on a case-by-case basis.

## Thoracic Trauma [29-31]

Trauma remains the single most common source of morbidity and mortality among children up to 14 years of age. Thoracic injuries may account for around 10% of admissions to trauma centres and they remain a substantial source of morbidity and mortality. The great flexibility of the thoracic cage in children allows the traumatic stress to propagate into the chest and thus pulmonary contusion is common, whereas rib fractures occur less frequently in children than in adults. Around 70% of chest injuries in children are the result of blunt trauma and very often there is not any external evidence of the trauma on the skin and the wall of the chest, such as rib fractures and brusing. If rib fractures are observed there is always a severe pulmonary contusion and other thoracic or abdominal organs may be involved. Chest radiographies are usually taken, but younger patients are more likely to have injuries without plain-film abnormalities. Chest computed tomography is very useful in the evaluation and management of thoracic injuries. Lung injury usually manifests as areas of consolidation. Pneumothorax may be missed by plain X-ray of the chest. Unilateral absence of breath sounds, tracheal deviation away from the affected site, jugular venous distention and hyper-resonance of the ipsilateral thorax indicate tension pneumothorax. The child with tension pneumothorax demonstrates severe respiratory distress and haemodynamic instability. The condition of the child may rapidly worsen as positive-pressure ventilation is started. Emergency treatment requires needle decompression, very often before obtaining a confirmatory chest X-ray. An over-the-needle catheter is inserted through the second intercostal space on the midclavicular line, just above the third rib. Injuries to the tracheobronchial tree are rare. They occur usually in the distal trachea or proximal bronchi. Most exhibit mediastinal air even if distal injuries may manifest as pneumothorax. Other findings include large air leak from the chest tube and cervical emphysema. Relevant hemothoraces occur in 15% of children sustaining blunt-force chest trauma. Prompt drainage of blood is necessary because pockets of blood are excellent culture media for bacteria. Antibiotic use for chest injury is controversial. However, circumstances of soft-tissue injury, pulmonary contusion with hemoptysis and need for operative intervention may well be indications for antibiotic prophylaxis.

# References


1.  Helfaer MA, Nichols DG, Rogers MC (1996) Developmental physiology of the respiratory system. In: Rogers MC, Nichols DG (eds) Textbook of Pediatric Intensive Care. Williams and Wilkings, Baltimore, pp 97-126
2.  Haddad GG, Fontan JJP (2000) Development of the respiratory system. In: Behrman RE, Kliegman RM, Jenson NB (eds) Nelson Textbook of Pediatrics, W.B Saunders Company, 16th edition, Philadelphia, pp 1235-1237
3.  Dunnil MS (2002) Postnatal growth of the lung. Thorax 17:329-344
4.  Wheeler M, Coté CJ, Todres ID (2001) Pediatric Airways. In: Coté CJ, Ryan JF, Todres ID, Goudsouzian NG (eds) Ice of Anesthesia for Infants and Children. W.B. Saunders Company, third edition, Philadelphia, pp 79-120
5.  Ulma G, Geiduschek JM, Zimmerman AA, Morray JP (2002) Anesthesia for thoracic surgery. In: Gregory GA (eds) Pediatric Anesthesia. Churchill Livingstone, New York, pp 423-464
6.  (2000) Pediatric basic life support Circulation 102: I-253
7.  (2000) Pediatric advanced life support Resuscitation 46:343-399
8.  Perez Fontan JJ, Haddad GG (2000) Respiratory pathophysiology. In: Behrman RE, Kliegman RM, Jenson NB (eds) Nelson Textbook of Pediatrics. W.B Saunders Company, 16th edition, Philadelphia pp 1240-1248
9.  Remolina C (1981) Positional hypoxemia in unilateral lung disease. N Engl J Med 304:523-526
10. Davies H, Kitchman R, Gordon I et al (1985) Regional ventilation in infancy. N Engl J Med 313:1626-1629
11. Steward DJ (2002) Preoperative evaluation and preparation for surgery. In: Gregory GA (ed) Pediatric Anesthesia. Churchill Livingstone, New York, pp 175-190
12. Stern RC (2000) Congenital anomalies. In: Behrman RE, Kliegman RM, Jenson NB (eds) Nelson Textbook of Pediatrics. W.B Saunders Company, 16th edition, Philadelphia, pp 1271-1274
13. Mancuso RF (1996) Stridor in neonates. Pediatr Clin North Am 6:1339-1348
14. Orenstein DM (2000) Acute inflammatory upper airway obstruction. In: Behrman RE, Kliegman RM, Jenson NB (eds) Nelson Textbook of Pediatrics. W.B Saunders Company, 16th edition, Philadelphia, pp 1322-1333
15. Orenstein DM (2000) Bronchiolitis. In: Behrman RE, Kliegman RM, Jenson NB (eds) Nelson Textbook of Pediatrics. W.B Saunders Company, 16th edition, Philadelphia, pp 1285-1278
16. Helfaer MA, Nichols DG, Rogers MC (1996) Lower airway disease: Bronchiolitis and asthma. In: Rogers MC, Nichols DG (eds) Textbook of Pediatric Intensive Care. Williams and Wilkings, Baltimore, pp 127-164
17. Smith SR, Strunk RC (1999) Acute asthma in the pediatric emergency department. Ped Clin North Am 46:1145-1165
18. Streetman DD, Bhatt-Metha V, Johnson CE (2002) Management of acute, severe asthma in children. Ann Pharmacother 36:1249-1260
19. Orenstein DM (2000) Foreign bodies in the larynx, trachea and bronchi. In: Behrman RE, Kliegman RM, Jenson NB (eds) Nelson Textbook of Pediatrics. W.B Saunders Company, 16th edition, Philadelphia, pp 1229-1236
20. Sarti A (2001) Recommendations on paediatric basic life support. In: Gullo A (ed) Anesthesia, Pain Intensive Care, Emergency. Springer Verlag, Milano, pp 607-620
21. Orenstein DM. Aspiration pneumonias and gastroesophageal reflux-related respiratory diseases. In: Behrman RE, Kliegman RM, Jenson NB (eds) Nelson Textbook of Pediatrics. W.B Saunders Company, 16th edition, Philadelphia, pp 1321-3136
22. Truman TL, Todres ID (1996) Acute respiratory distress syndrome. In: Todres ID, Fugate JH (eds) Critical care of infants and children. Little, Brown and Company, Boston, pp 147-154

23. Fackler JC, Arnold JH, Nichols DG, Rogers MC (1996) Acute Respiratory diostress syndrome. In: Rogers MC, Nichols DG (eds) Textbook of Pediatric Intensive Care. Williams and Wilkings, Baltimore, pp 197-233
24. Bohn D (2001) Lung salvage and protection ventilatory techniques. Pediatric Clin North Am 48:553-572
25. Bjorklund LJ (1997) Manual ventilation with a few large breaths at birth compromises the therapeutic effect of subsequent surfactant replacement in immature lambs. Pediatr Res 42:348-355
26. Rimensberger PC (2000) First intention high-frequency oscillation with early lung volume optimization improves pulmonary outcome in very low birth weight infants with respiratory distress syndrome. Pediatrics 105:1202-1208
27. Curley MA, Thompson JE (2000) The effects of early and repeated prone positioning in pediatric patients with acute lung injury. Chest 118:156-163
28. Korneki A, Frndova H (2001) A randomized trial of prolonged prone positioning in children with acute respiratory failure. Chest 119:211-218
29. Bliss D, Silen M (2002) Pedairtic thoracic trauma. Crit Care Med 30:S409-415
30. Cullen ML (2001) Pulmonary and respiratory complications of pediatric trauma. Respir Clin North Am 7:59-77
31. Cooper A (1995) Thoracic injuries. Semin Pediatr Surg 4:109-115

# Chapter 10

# Informed Consent: Origin, Controversies, Contradictions and Sociological Aspects

A. De Monte

If we refer to Oxford Advanced Learner's Dictionary [1], to *inform* means *to have* or *to show a lot of knowledge about a particular subject or situation: an informed critic; an informed choice / decision / guess / opinion. Consent* signifies *agreement, permission, permission to do something, especially given by somebody in authority. Children under 16 cannot give consent to medical treatment.* Literally that means the patient will  be taught in medical science and he will reach a level of knowledge allowing him to decide if the proposed therapy is right and safe for himself. But what is that level and how long does it take to be reached?

Obviously the above confirmation is deliberately provocative, just to underline that the term of *"informed consent"* already shows a list of problems that are quite often contradictory.

In this chapter, I will analyse various aspects involved and touched by the problem of *informed consent*. In particular, I will try to put in evidence the positive and negative aspects of informed consent with the goal of being able to use it as a tool of  participation and collaboration  that unites doctor and patient in a common choice of therapeutic strategy thereby of reducing mistrust and litigation between themselves.

I will try to clarify some aspects of difficult and equivocal interpretation that leave open doors to free interpretation of ethical, professional and legal matters. In particular, I will point out the risk of a real conflict of interest that the physician will incur upon providing information. This conflict can only remedied by a relationship of complicity, trust and intimacy with the patient that goes well beyond any bureaucratic formality [2-5].

## What Is Informed Consent

Firstly, why informed consent (IC) in medicine? What do we really mean by informed consent? And for whom do we need it?

From the patient's point of view, it should be both a defense and a guarantee; in the deontological field, the IC has an ethical meaning, in the insurance field it can assume economic aspects of great importance, as well as having legal implications.

Therefore, the consequences and motivations involved can be various.

At the moment the topic of IC is very *"trendy"* because it's often talked about it, and we frequently mention this subject out of context and, some times, without adequate knowledge and understanding of what we mean by IC.

One person identifies IC as a signature at the bottom of a clinical folder, another as a list of frightening information given to the patient, another as a legal medical shield to be used before performing any sort of treatment, some other as a moment of cultural growth for the patient.

But beyond the pure meaning of the word, what do we really mean by *informed consent*?

If we enter "informed consent" in the most common web search engine, *google.com*, we will find over 1150,000 entries (if we restrict the field of our search to Medline/Pub-Med of the National Library of Medicine of Bethesda, the number of entries will drop significantly to 24,000, still a great number).

Informed Consent has been defined as follows:

Informed consent is a process, not just a form. Information must be presented to enable persons to voluntarily decide whether or not to participate as a research subject. It is a fundamental mechanism to ensure respect for persons through provision of thoughtful consent for a voluntary act. The procedures used in obtaining informed consent should be designed to educate the subject population in terms that they can understand. Therefore, informed consent language and its documentation (especially explanation of the study's purpose, duration, experimental procedures, alternatives, risks, and benefits) must be written in "lay language", (i.e. understandable to the people being asked to participate). The written presentation of information is used to document the basis for consent and for the subjects' future reference. The consent document should be revised when deficiencies are noted or when additional information will improve the consent process[6].

Informed consent is the process by which a fully informed patient can participate in choices about his/her health care. It originates from the legal and ethical right the patient has to direct what happens to her body and from the ethical duty of the physician to involve the patient in her health care [7].

Finally, the Italian National Institute of Counselling defines *informed consent* as an opportunity and the absolute right for patients to be informed by their doctor, in the most clear, honest, real and consistent way on the treatments to which they will be submitted so that they should be able to agree with full conscience, in their interest and for their own good, to the treatments.

From the doctor point of view, the IC should be seen as the duty to inform the patient in all possible ways in order to allow the patient to make a fully aware and conscious decision [8].

It is clear from the above that the IC cannot be reduced to a simple signature on a form or even to a brief information. As reported by a study of bioethics of the National Society of Anaesthesia, ICU and Pain Therapy (SIAARTI), it will be more correct to speak of *information given* and *to consent to* [9].

With *information given* we have to include all processes of education and information mentioned in the above definitions. And with *"to consent to"* we formalize that the patient has fully understood the information given, he is satisfied and he agrees with the physician on the details of the treatments and gives permission to operate on and to act on his own body. Finally he enters into a contract to receive services both intellectual and physical from the doctor.

Nonetheless, major contradictions concern the drawing up of the informed consent.

## History

The origin of the informed consent in medicine and surgery, as the basis of a relationship between patient and doctor, goes back to the Calvinist spirit. This religious movement spread over France and Germany at the beginning of the XVI century [10], and it deeply impressed the development and evolution of modern society. The historical intellectual Max Weber dates the origin of modern capitalism (*protestant ethic and the capitalism spirit*) back to Calvinism [11]. The revolutionary essence of this movement is based on the doctrine of divine predestination to salvation or to damnation. Calvinism sustained, furthermore, that hard work in this world is devoted exclusively to create the reign of God on Earth, and success in terrene activities represents a tangible sign of predetermination to eternal salvation [12, 13].

Nothing could interfere with plans of achievement for the reign of God on Earth, not even illness could be of impediment to business success, and, when it comes to gamble on one's salvation, one could decide not to undergo treatment if that could compromise the good will of one's business.

From the XVI century to reach the modern terms and formulas of informed consent, many events have gone by, events that have not always put the defense and dignity of the sick person and of the human being as such in first place.

Wars, massacres and slavery have taken place, as integral, ongoing part of human history, in spite of social and cultural evolution.

Fundamental principles that have decreed the individual self-determination concept and the right of everyone to be arbitrator and owner of his own destiny have been formalized at international level by the Nürnberg Code (1946) and in the Helsinki declaration (1964). On these elements are based the modern foundations of IC.

As far as concerns the Italian situation, in recent times we must quote numbers of revisions of the Medical Deontological Code (1978, 1989, 1998) [9, 14]. In 1991, Italy acknowledged the new CEE directive n. 507 concerning the IC; while in 1992, the National Bioethical Committee issued an opinion on "informed consent in medicine".

In 1997, at Oviedo (Spain), Italy complied with the convention approved by the European Council of Human Rights and Biomedicine, a great part of which is dedicated to informed consent, deemed an element of necessity for all medical activities (therapeutic Art. 5) and scientific research and experimentation (Art. 15) [9].

In 1997, SIAARTI published a model form for IC in anaesthesia with the recommendation that it has to be filled out by every patient [1, 15].

Among the SIAARTI  members, there is a permanent study group dedicated to the anaesthesiology IC within the Bioethics Committee [1].

## Legislative Aspects

At the moment in Italy it does not exist a specific law requiring medical informed consent before proceeding with any diagnostic or therapeutic act.

The only exception is the transfusion of blood and blood products, where consent is compulsory and has to be obtained in advance.

Nevertheless we have a list of dispositions and laws which treat the matter of informed consent in a more or less explicit way.

*a)* Italian Constitution, Art. 13. *Personal freedom is inviolable. Any form of detention, inspection or personal perquisition, or other restriction of personal freedom is prohibited unless, for legal proceedings initiated by the Judicial Authority and only in those cases and manners provided for by law...* [16].

The following cases fall within the scope of medical activity: hospital admittance, medical visit, positioning patient on the operating table using complex systems, anaesthetic drug administration abolishing patient's will, etc. These can easily be configured as forms of *"...detention, inspection or personal perquisition, or other restriction of personal freedom...".*

*b)* Italian Constitution, Art. 32. *The State protects health as a fundamental right of the individual and of the community, guaranteeing free health care to the poorest.*

*None can be forced to receive a certain treatment if not by disposition of the law. The law cannot, in any case, violate limits imposed by respect for the human being* [16].

With this Article, the Constitution establishes that any medical treatment has to be performed on a voluntary basis of the individual, who makes himself available and agrees with the treatments proposed.

*c)* Criminal action, Art. 50. *An individual who has injured another individual or who has put him in a dangerous situation with his valid and aware consent is not punishable if it can be validly proved it* [17]. With this Article, the law recognises the absolute value and power of individual auto-determination, which allows a person to authorise another person to impose lesions on his own body. In other words: if we obtain the informed consent from the person who we are going to operate on, we are not liable to punishment even if we injured his physical integrity and put the patient at risk of death (for example: surgical intervention).

*d)* Criminal action, Art 54. *An individual who has committed an act which he was forced to perfom in order to save himself or others from real danger of immediate damage to the individual is not punishable.* This, in force of the law consents to intervene in case of an emergency even in the absence of informed consent. It is clear that the concept of emergency has to be used properly. A situation erroneously classified as an *emergency*, could constitute unskilfulness and negligence on the part of the doctor, who can be called to answer for liability of guilt [18].

These legislative directions do not necessarily expressly imply a need for patient consent, but they define what *cannot* be done without incurring a legal violation. They also indicate what we have to do and which actions are not punishable. (*I tell you what you can or cannot do, I do not tell you what you must do*).

It is clear that, based on this type of law, we have had a flourishing of the circumstances regarding jurisprudence, supported also by the Italian Corte di Cassazione (Supreme Court), which favours compulsory collection of informed consent [19].

This emerges only when a contentious situation is created by the offended part. In the absence of this element, nobody will investigate or verify the collection of IC.

Even if, in the first place, these sets of rules seem foggy and do not aid in assuming a well-defined position, they still are guarantors of the individual's freedom. It is enough to consider, for example, that in this way they guarantee the right of those who do not want to find out about the nature of their illness.

The physician must be aware that to have obtained IC does not mean that, in case of complication or lack of success, he is immune to any sanctions [10].

A negative result of a medical treatment can be impugned by a patient's complaint against the doctor. This contentious issue does not need to be necessarily heard in Criminal Court. On the contrary, the proceedings often take place in Civil Court, and end with a request by the patient for compensation for damages. In particular, Article n. 2236 of the Civil Code [20] shows that the doctor is responsible only for grave guilt and intent. This is applicable only when the service given was of particular difficulty. Whenever the service does not involve any particular problem, the doctor still has to answer for minor guilt.

It is useful to remember that complicated procedures for a general doctor or a specialist of a different field are not considered as such for a doctor expert in that field. For example, complications arising during epidural anaesthesia are handled under Article n. 1218 of the Civil Code, because we assume that for an anaesthesiologist an epidural puncture does not present technical problems or particular difficulties. Therefore, in this case, he is also liable [19, 20].

## Information

It has already been mentioned that IC is designed to educate the subject population in terms that they can understand [6]. This principal is in Article n. 30 of the Medical Deontological Code. *The doctor has to provide the most suitable information on diagnosis, prognosis, prospective and possible alternatives both diagnostic and therapeutic and also foresee consequences of such choices; the physician informing the patient has to take into consideration his capacity of comprehension in order to promote maximum collaboration in the diagnostic-therapeutic proposal* [14]. In these terms we locate the real problematic nature of informed consent: the dialogue between two people with different knowledge of such a very delicate field as individual health.

Based on what it has been said and written on informed consent, it is medical responsibility to inform and to make sure that the patient has correctly understood what has been transmitted by the doctor, and the patient must also have clearly understood all benefits of the procedure and also any possible risks [3-7, 21, 22].

From the doctor's point of view, he has to explain with clearness and objectivity all possible events, avoiding excessive *threatening information* or *superficiality.*

Correct information should consider four basic elements: risks, benefits, alternatives, and specific aspects of the procedure. In reality, we are far from satisfying all these conditions. In fact, Bottrell [23], in his recent analysis of 540 USA consent forms, found that only 26% of them included all four factors mentioned above.

Braddock [24] evaluated the informed consent acquisition in 1057 outpatients involving 65 surgeons. He found that a negligible number of informed consent to surgery was collected correctly.

In spite of a consolidated legal obligation to obtain informed consent prior to each medical treatment, the USA population show that the reading comprehension level of a consent form is quite low. It has been reported that in the 1970s less than half of the USA population understood common medical terms. In 1993, 40-44 million of USA citizens were almost illiterate, *defined as the inability to complete basic reading tasks required of a functioning member of society* [25]. Finally, Hopper [26] reports that, in 1998, only half of patients with a high school education were able to understand general hospital consent forms.

All these data evidence that informed consent is an educational process that requires several dozens of years before being completed and clearly accessible to the large majority of the population. As an example, Hopper [27, 28] found that more than 12 years were required to reach a massive comprehension of iodinated contrast media consent, and 15 years were required for general radiological procedures. Consent for surgical and anaesthesiological procedures is a much more complex decision to be explained to a *lay person*. Therefore, the length of time necessary to reach a fully aware and responsible attitude population is a lot longer.

As reported above, we understand clearly that information previous to consent, if it is to be exhaustive and thorough, needs a certain period of time well over that usuall time dedicated for a brief preoperative anaesthesiological evaluation.

Beyond the contents of the given information, there is an implicit meaning that has radically modified the role of the physician and of the patient. *The physician is not any longer authorised, in the name of a morality  that goes beyond that of the human being, to step over the will of the patient. For the same reasons, the patient may any delegate the doctor the responsibility to make a decision as to what is better for himself. This results in increased doubts and anxiety for the patient, who has to share with the doctor the weight of important decisions* [29].

The presence of anxiety and concerns during IC collection is supported by social studies that underline the great gap between the theoretical model and practical application. We have seen, in fact, that a patient tends to accept information in a partial and factious way; there could be also be an unconscious refusal to accept unpleasant news that causes concerns; for various cultural and social reasons patients quite often do not *dare* to ask for further explanation. The physician, on his part, orientates and heavily conditions patient choices, putting into discussion the autonomy of the decision itself.

Below are reported some ways in which the physician can influence the patient's decision (Fig. 1).

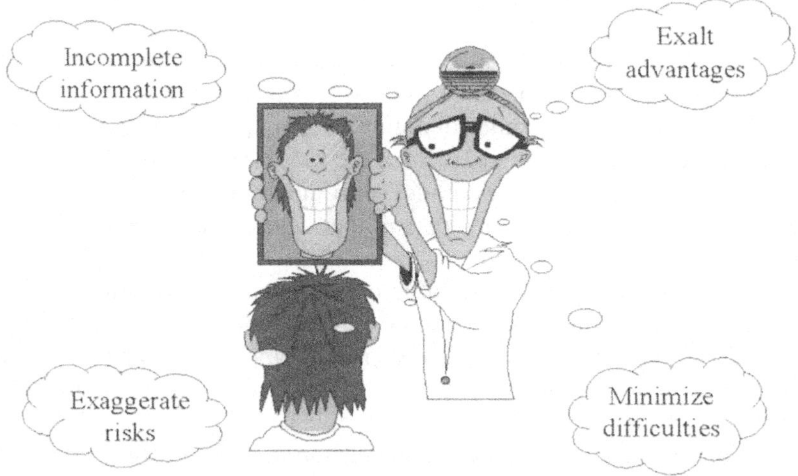


**Fig. 1.** Possible mechanisms of manipulation of information during medical evaluation

I) *To give incomplete information*: what is transmitted to the patient is a small surrogate of huge medical chapters that the doctor has learned after years of studies and experience; in this way, the information acknowledged by the patient is fragmentary and incomplete.

The ease of information flow does not depend only on the patient's characteristics but also on the humanity and sensibility of the physician to relate to the patient.

Also, the state of mind is important, to be able to understand and to introduce the problems. To place one self in a state of helpfulness and understanding, to be on familiar terms with the person in front of you, to use a language that is simple and understandable, it will raise a similar behaviour response by the patient a similar behaviour. All this makes for easy exchange of information between the people involved.

II) *To glorify the "pro"*: the physician can have some leaning toward a specific technique, as a consequence of different reasons, for example:
1. not being confident with local or regional anaesthesiology technique, he therefore suggests general anaesthesia;
2. lack of time due to previous engagements and therefore trying to convince the patient to accept the quickest technique,
3. long theater turnover time and the need to choose the least time-consuming anaesthesiological technique;
4. the wish of the anaesthesiologist to try new anaesthesiological techniques. In this case, the physician will suggest the technique, he wants to perform the safest and the most adaptable.

    Phrases such as: *"If you were my mother, If I were in your position…"* etc.,can have a greater persuasive effect than any other form of technical and formal information.

III) *To minimise the difficulties*: this strategy, in contrast to the previous one, can be used when the physician wishes to resort to therapies in which he is not particularly qualified or to methods of major complexity. In this case, we can detect a glossing over of information in which the risks are minimised despite a difficult technical approach, for example, continuous brachial plexus block compared to general anaesthesia in a patient that needs an arm operation.

IV) *Exaggerate risks*: this method of manipulation of information can be used, for example, when the anaesthesiologist does not want to do what the patient requires. It is an attitude to which we resort when we want to dissuade the patient from undergoing an operation because of the high risk he can incur (Fig. 1).
At this point it is right to ask who is the person that makes the final decision of consent. Sociologists Lidz and Meisel, in their studies, asserted that final decisions are not taken by the patient (or at least not only by the patient) but the choice is orientated and driven by the physician with a list of *recommendations*. Often it is the patient himself that gives up the responsibility of taking a decision and delegates everything to the doctor.

    Everyday practice is a proof of what we have said above. Which anaestheologist has not heard the common phrase: *"…you are the doctor…what do you suggest? …What would you choose?.."* We can assert that we commonly find that the patient, most of the time, is not aware of his pathology and knows even less about the remedies suggested; thus, what can we imagine when he comes to specific technical problems? Still, sociologists Liz and Meisel infer that : *consent doesn't exist, what we have found instead is: submission, absence of objection or, occasionally, a veto"*.

## Informed Consent: Conflict of Interest?

Within the National Health Service (NHS) in developed countries, the role of the patient has suffered radical transformation as a result of social evolution. In this process we can identify three major development phases which the NHS purchaser has gone through.

*Assist patient phase* (1945-1980). After World War II, NHSs were founded around Europe. Beyond all ideological criticisms of a central planned health program, the aim of the NHS was to build up a welfare model. The intention of this idea to improve the quality and productivity of labour will not be discussed in this chapter [30]. In such organisations, the individual is considered a common social resource. Employers and employees of NHSs have the goal to maintain the population in a healthy state for a common welfare. During this time, the individual was used to consider health assistance as something due, to him or her.

*Health consumer phase* (1980-2000). The scientific discoveries, biomedical industry developments and increased health expectations of the population over-ran NHS expenses. A more accurate and market-oriented health administration was required to run the limited economical resources. Therefore, a market-like mechanism was introduced (*quasi-market*) in which the individual became a *consumer* of NHS products, i.e. he assumes the consciousness to pay in exchange for a service.

*Customer phase* (1990s). In this phase, the individual acts as a customer who buys a product. Therefore, because he pays, he feels allowed to decide and to choose the one he wants, as well as the place and the doctor he prefers.

Above, I have schematically described three development phases through which the role of the patient has gone. Those changes had led to significant variations in both expectations and individual self-determination. It is clear that also the role of the doctor has changed due to changes of the patient's role. The physician has gone from a helping and sympathetic father to that of a specialist who supplies a highly qualified product.

The actual relation between *purchaser and provider,* is optimised by a negotiable exchange contract between the two plaintiffs involved.

According to the Oxford Advanced Learner's Dictionary, contract means: *an official written agreement.*

It is well known that each contract is drawn up with the signatures of the two plaintiffs involved. Therefore, in the contract of the physician-health demander, the doctor commits himself to supplying his competence and skill in exchange for renumeration and patient collaboration.

On the base of what has been analysed, it is clear that the contract between physician and patient presents some specific characteristics which distinguishes it from other forms of commercial contracts.

Let us analyse the dynamics that occur when we draw up a contract to buy a house. In this case, we have initially two plaintiffs, the buyer and the vendor (estate agent). The buyer formulates his request to the estate agent, specifying the main characteristics of the property he wants to buy. The vendor submits his proposal to the client. At this point, a third part comes on stage, the expert, who can be a relative, a friend or a surveyor engaged to defend one's interests. The buyer will ask him for advice to analyse the  advantages and disadvantages of the offer submitted, with the aim of deciding whether or not to buy the property. He can contact directly the estate agent or give this task to his consultant. But in the end, he remains the buyer and therefore he has to take on the responsibility of making the final decision of buying or not, taking into consideration his economic possibilities, his interest in the property, the surveyor's judgement, etc. (Fig. 2).

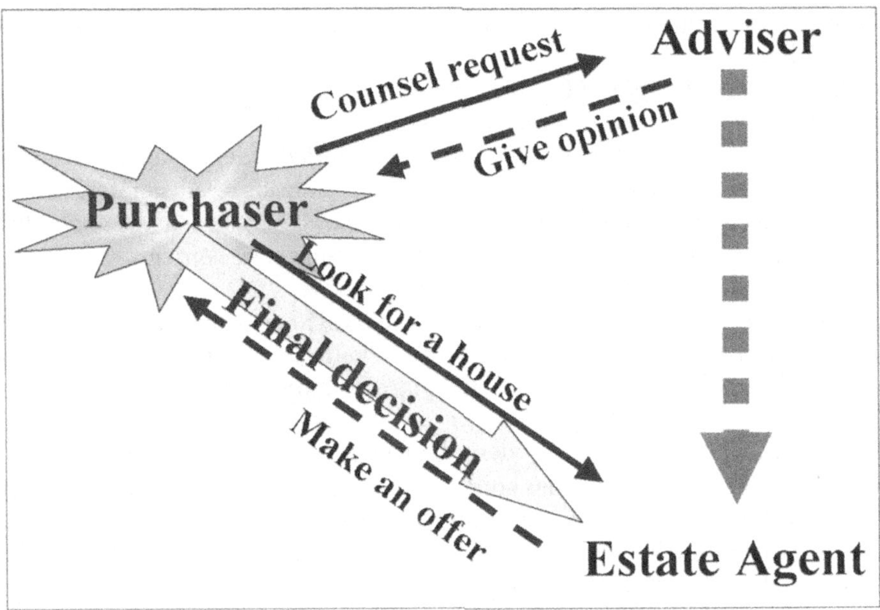


**Fig. 2.** Sequential actions of a house purchase. See text for details. ➡, purchaser action; --▶ estate agent and adviser action; ⇨ purchaser's final decision; ⋯▶ facultative counselling

Let us examine instead the dynamics that occur in the case of a contractual relation within the health field. In this case, too, the plaintiffs involved are two: physician and patient. The latter explains to the doctor his request, which ends up in a demand for health. The physician (similar to the estate agent) makes his diagnosis-therapeutic proposal.

At this point, the patient, if he is not a doctor himself, is confronted with two possible solutions: accepting the physician's proposal, therefore trusting him blindly to the point that the doctor acts as a consultant and a caregiver, or, alternatively, asking for a second opinion. In this case, the new doctor can support the proposal made by his colleague or suggest a different treatment, starting in this way a new contractual procedure.

A real conflict of interests occurs between the person that looks for health and the one who has to give it. Thus, the physician will cover both parts: the *hired person* and the *advising specialist* (Fig. 3).

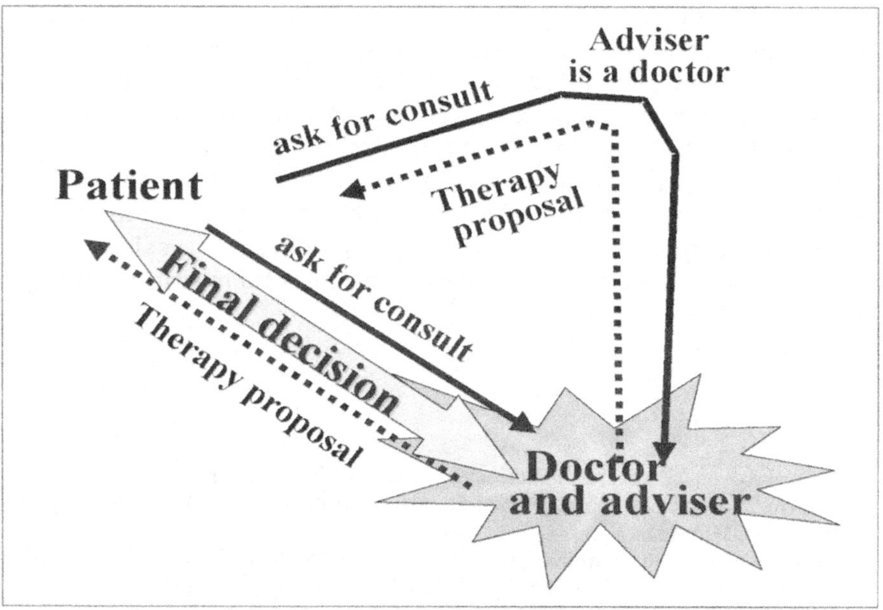


**Fig. 3.** Sequential actions of a medical consultation. See text for details. ➡ Patient action; --▶ doctor and advising doctor's action; ⟺ final decision taken by patient and doctor

It is therefore obvious, thus, that the physician has power in influencing, consciously or unconsciously, the patient's choice. It is up to the doctor and to his ability to relate to the patient to reach a relation of complicity and collaboration aimed to achieve the final goal, represented by the solution to the patient's problem.

Cannavò and Mulè [10] underlined that a bad relation between doctor and patient is not due to diagnostic or therapeutic error, but to:
- Inadequate information
- Poor attitude to listening
- Lack of interpersonal respect
- Inconsistent behaviour within the medical team
- Lack of participation in the diagnostic-therapeutic procedure
- Insufficient hospital comfort

## Conclusions

We have analysed the meaning, history, legal and sociological aspects of informed consent, or, better defined, *given information* and *acceptance of intervention*. The emerging picture is certainly one of very important topic, an emotional one but with undefined borders and strongly overlapping responsibilities

The need to educate the population and to level the different stages of information is one of the tasks that contributes to the several duties of the physician in his role not only as health provider but also as a member of society.

It is my opinion that we must be able to reach a relation of complicity and shared goals with the patient. We must be on the same wave-length as the patient, and we have to create a real alliance with the aim of solving the problem that afflicts the patient/health consumer/customer. If we can attain all these goals then the physician is better protected from any sort of legal actions, more so than provided by any simple signature collected in a rush during pre-operative medical evaluation.

## References


1. Oxford Advanced Learner's Dictionary (2000) Oxford University Press
2. Martinelli G (1999) Il problema del consenso informato in Anestesia e Terapia Intensiva. Min Anest 65:191-192
3. Kopp VJ (2002) Communication with patients before anesthesia and obtention of preanesthetic consent. Current opinion in Anaesthesiology 15:251-255
4. Dierdorf SF (2002) Anesthesia and informed consent. Current opinion in Anaesthesiology 15:349-350
5. Marchetti E (2002) Lo stato dell'arte sul consenso informato. Rischio Sanità 6:28-29
6. ohrp.osophs.dhhs.gov/humansubjects/guidance/ictips.htm
7. eduserv.hscer.washington.edu/bioethics/ topics/consent.html
8. www.therapeia.it/ConsensoInformato.html (counseling)
9. (2000) Gruppo di studio SIAARTI sul consenso all'anestesia La dichiarazione di avvenuta informazione e consenso all'anestesia. Min Anest 66:565-569
10. Cannavò G, Mulè D (2002) Valutazione del consenso informato prima dell'analgesia per il travaglio di parto. Rischio Sanità 5:20-25
11. Weber M (1905) The protestant ethic and the spiriti of capitalism. Penguin Twenty Century Classics
12. Lo sviluppo del Calvinismo e la tesi di Max Weber. http://www.cronologia.it/mondo41d.htm
13. Max Weber.http://www.carducci galilei.ap/rivoluzione/Economia/max_weber1.htm
14. (1998) Codice di Deontologia Medica Art. 30-37
15. (1997) Gruppo di studio SIAARTI per la sicurezza in Anestesia e Terapia Intensiva. Min Anest 63:271-273
16. (1947) Gazzetta Ufficiale della Repubblica Italiana. Edizione Speciale n. 298
17. Codice Penale. http://www.studiocelentano.it/codici/cp/index.htm
18. Marinello S (2001) Novità dalla cassazione in tema di consenso informato. RischioSanita 3:27-29
19. Rodriguez D, Picazio T, Pesaresi M (2002) Errore nella raccolta del consenso. In:

Responsabilità professionale del medico Anestesista Rianimatore pp 228-234
20. Codice Civile. http://www.studiocelentano.it/codici/cp/index.htm.
21. Mazzolo MG, Desinan L, De Monte A (2000) Il consenso informato in Day Surgery. Atti del XXXIII Congresso Nazionale SIMLA  1021-1040
22. Marinello S (2001) La difesa del medico dal reclamo  del paziente. Dal consenso informato alla cartella clinica. RischioSanità 2:25-27
23. Bottrell MM, Alpert H, Fischbach RL (2000) Hospital informed consent for procedure forms: facilitating quality patient-physician interaction. Arch Surg 135:26-33
24. Braddock CH, Edwards KA, Hasenberg NM (1999) Informed decision making in outpatient practice: time to get back to basics. JAMA  282:2313-2320
25. Kirsch I, Jungblut A, Jenkins L (1993) Adult literacy in America: a first look at the results of the national adult literacy survey. Washington, DC: National Center for Education, US Department of Education
26. Hopper KD, TenHave TR, Tully DA et al (1998) The readability of currently used surgical/procedure consent forms in the United States. Surgery 123:496-503
27. Hopper KD, TenHave TR, Hartzel J (1995) Informed consent forms for clinical and research imaging procedures: how much do patients understand? AJR Am J Roentgenol 164:493-496
28. Hopper KD, Zajdel M, Hulse SF et al (1994) Interactive method of informing patients of the risks of intravenous contrast media. Radiology 192:67-71
29. Lattuada L (2003) Il Consenso Informato: reportistica Aziendale 2002. Direzione Medica Ospedaliera ASS 3 Alto Friuli
30. Ranade W (1995) A future for the NHS? Longman Ed. London

# Chapter 11

# Total Intravenous Anesthesia and Respiratory System

A. Pasetto, L. Rinaldi

General anesthesia interferes with gas exchange even in patients with healthy lungs. This process is associated with alterations in the structure of chest-wall components such as the diaphragm. Almost 30 years have passed since Froese and Bryan [1] provided the first direct measurements of how anesthesia affects the shape and motion of the normal human diaphragm (Fig. 1). They described how the silhouette of the diaphragm created by fluoroscopy moved during breathing before and after the induction of anesthesia. Based on the interpretation of their results and subsequent studies by others [2], the following scenario evolved (and has been adopted by many anesthesia texts) (Fig. 2).

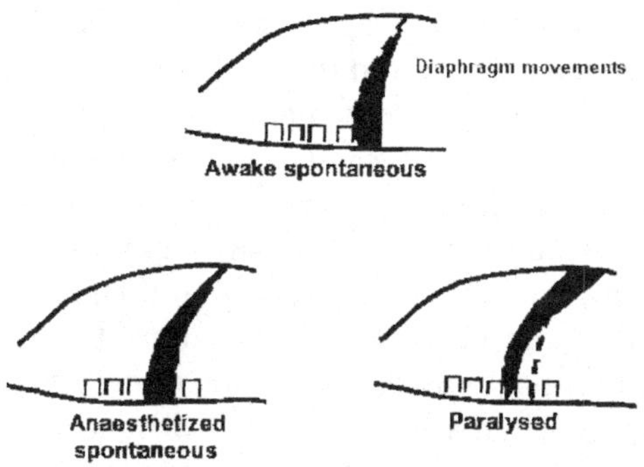


**Fig. 1.** Analysis of diaphragm movements during awake spontaneous breathing, sedation and mechanical ventilation with muscle paralysis. According to [1]

Anesthesia, with or without pharmacologic paralysis, produces a cephalad (headward) shift of the end-expiratory position of the diaphragm by reducing normal end-expiratory muscle tone. This shift in the diaphragm reduces the functional residual capacity (FRC) and compresses lung parenchyma in dependent regions, causing atelectasis. This atelectasis significantly contributes to intraoperative gas-exchange abnormalities by increasing shunt and may persist into the postoperative period [3] (especially after surgeries that invade the thorax or abdomen), perhaps leading to morbidity such as pneumonia. Some aspects of this scenario have been challenged by subsequent studies. In fact,

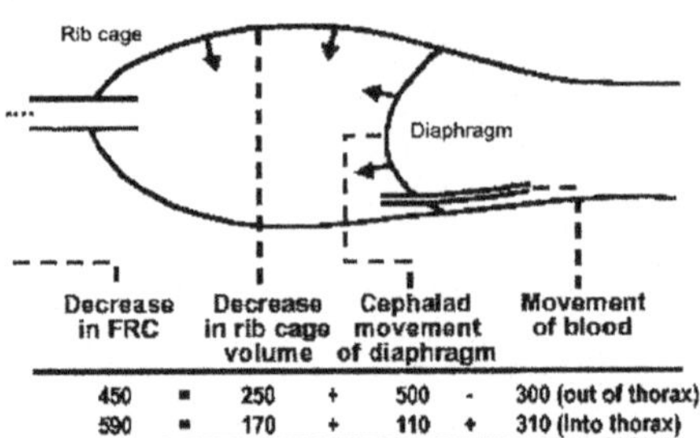


**Fig. 2.** Changes in FRC and thoracoabdominal dimensions according to Hedenstierna and Krayer. Data on changes in functional residual capacity (FRC) and thoracoabdominal dimensions adapted from [2, 34]

Froese and Bryan reported the end-expiratory position of the diaphragms of only two normal subjects, which in fact behaved somewhat differently. The most dependent (i.e., posterior in a supine subject) region of the diaphragm moved cephalad with the induction of anesthesia in both subjects. However, the nondependent region (i.e., anterior) actually moved in the opposite direction (caudad) in one subject, and cephalad in the other. Subsequent studies by several investigators have also found that, although anesthesia produces a consistent cephalad shift of dependent diaphragm regions, it causes either no change in position or an actual caudal shift of nondependent regions [4]. Kleinman *et al.* noted a similar pattern of results in their normal subjects, although none of the shifts were statistically significant because of considerable variation among subjects [5]. Thus, they confirmed that decreases in FRC produced by anesthesia in normal subjects cannot be attributed primarily to changes in diaphragm position. Furthermore, if atelectasis is caused by compression of lung parenchyma by a cephalad displacement of the dependent diaphragm, the greater the displacement, the greater should be the amount of atelectasis. Alas, there is no such correlation [6]. Thus, although there is little doubt that atelectasis is caused by anesthesia-induced changes in chest wall shape, the cause is not as simple as a cephalad shift of the diaphragm [7]. For example, anesthesia increases the curvature of the spine [8], which provides an anchor for all other chest-wall structures and thus may affect diaphragm and rib-cage configuration. Such secondary effects probably explain any changes in diaphragm shape produced by anesthesia, because there is currently little evidence that there is "normal" end-expiratory muscle tone in the diaphragm of awake subjects [9].

Besides, anesthesia produces ventilation/perfusion distribution changes. Pulmonary arteriolar pressure can be reduced, preventing the perfusion of non-dependent pulmonary regions. Mechanical ventilation, increasing alveolar pressure, interferes further on with upper regions of perfusion. While pulmonary perfusion is redistributed to dependent regions, ventilation of these dependent areas is reduced by atelectasis. This ventilation/perfusion mismatch contributes to gas-exchange impairment during anesthesia. Most effects of anesthesia on gas exchange can be observed already during spontaneus breathing, with little difference with muscle paralysis or mechanical ventilation [1].

Anesthetic drugs have two kinds of effects on the respiratory system: they cause alveolar hypoventilation and gas-exchange alteration.


## Alveolar Hypoventilation

Most intravenous induction agents produce dose-dependent respiratory depression characterized by a decrease in minute ventilation, related both to tidal volume or respiratory rate alteration, and a transient rightward shift in the $CO_2$ response curve [10, 11].

*Barbiturates* cause respiratory depression by enhancing the function of GABA-inhibitory synapses [12]. Induction apnea is frequent (40%) but transitory. In particular, thiopental depresses the rhythm and the depth of breathing [12, 13]. Tidal-volume depression is greater than respiratory-rate reduction in spontaneously breathing patients. Laryngeal and bronchial reflexes are attenuated only with high barbiturate doses [14].

By contrast, *benzodiazepines* (BDZ) usually cause less respiratory depression than barbiturates. However, they may produce greater respiratory depression in patients with COPD. BDZ present a slower onset and a longer time of action than the other class of intravenous anesthetic drugs [15, 16]. Moreover, they may enhance the respiratory effects of narcotics.

*Propofol* is now the most widely used induction agent. It is often the drug of choice in patients in whom a rapid and smooth recovery is required. In fact, it is characterized by the absence of a "hangover effect" and it produces a low incidence of postoperative nausea and vomiting [17]. However, the cardiovascular depressor effects produced by propofol appear to be more pronounced than those of thiopental [18]. An induction dose typically produces 30 s or more of apnea; its duration depends on propofol dose, injection rate and other drug administrations. Tidal volume decreases by about 60% and respiratory rate increases by about 40% [19]. Mechanical ventilation is mainly impaired in its abdominal component [20]. In healthy subjects, respiratory resistance and thoracic-abdominal compliance remain stable during propofol induction, compared to etomidate and thiopental anesthesia [21]. The same result was observed in patients with bronchial hyperreactivity, making propofol the preferred induction agent for asthmatic patients [22]. In addition, respiratory response to $CO_2$ and hypoxia is largly blunted [18], but hypoxic vasoconstriction is maintained with positive effects in thoracic surgery. Blood concentrations of 1 $\mu g.ml^{-1}$, which corresponds to clinical sedation without loss of consciousness, produce no significant respiratory parameter alterations.

*Etomidate* has minimal cardiovascular and respiratory-depressant effects and therefore is extremely useful in high-risk patients [23].

*Ketamine* anesthesia is associated with: 1) the maintenance of FRC, minute ventilation, and tidal volume; 2) an increase in rib-cage contribution to tidal breathing; and 3) an alteration of volume-motion relationships of the chest-wall compartments. In fact, ketamine presents a sparing effect on intercostal muscle activity, which may explain the maintenance of FRC [24].

*Opioids* produce a dose-related depression of the ventilatory response to $CO_2$ by a direct effect on respiratory centers in the medulla [25]; moreover, both the rate and the rhythm of breathing are affected. In fact, as the dose of opioids increases, the respiratory rate slows down, although this effect may be partially offset by an increase in tidal volume [25, 26]. Under opioids effect, the patient drive to breathe may be abnormal despite an apparently normal respiratory rate and state of consciousness [26]. Besides, opioids decrease the respiratory response to hypoxia and increase the duration of the respiratory pause [25]. These drugs have several side effects, since they produce muscle rigidity acting on mu receptors in the striatum, increase the rate of striated dopamine biosynthesis and inhibit the release of the inhibitory neurotransmitter GABA, decreasing the chest-wall compliance. In particular, fentanyl is a potent synthetic opioid. Its fat-soluble properties account for its rapid onset and relatively short duration [27]. The drug is extensively distributed throughout the body so its plasma levels decrease rapidly [27]. A large concentration gradient favors redistribution of fentanyl away from the central nervous system and this terminates its effect [26]. Another opioid largely used by anesthesiologists is remifentanil, which is an extremely short-acting opioid, since its metabolism depends on non-specific esterases. Patients given an infusion of remifentanil recover in 3-5 min after its infusion is stopped [26, 27].

## Gas Exchange Alterations

Gasses are exchanged between the atmosphere and the alveolar air, and gasses diffuse between the alveolar air and the blood flowing through the pulmonary capillaries. Oxygen is transported from the atmosphere, via the alveolar ventilation, and then carried by the pulmonary blood flow (equal to the cardiac output) into the cells and their mitochondria for metabolic purposes. Carbon dioxide, the final end-product of metabolism, migrates from the cells to the atmosphere.

The use of anesthetics drugs determines a gas-exchange impairment which is mirrored by an increase of the alveolar to arterial oxygen partial-pressure gradient (P(A-a)$O_2$). Two factors may contribute to this effect: a primary ventilation and perfusion mismatch and a decrease of the FRC.

The FRC is the gas volume that remains in the lungs at the end of exhalation after a normal breath; it is a static measure since it is obtained when there is no pressure difference between alveoli and atmosphere. Induction of general anesthesia is accompanied by a significant (18-20%) decrease in FRC, which usually causes a decrease in compliance [28, 29]. The maximum decrease in

FRC appears to occur within the first few minutes of anesthesia [28, 30] and in the absence of any other complicating factor, seems not to decrease besides during anesthesia. The FRC reduction remains during the postoperative period [31]. The possible causes of reduced FRC are:

- Supine position. Passing from the upright to the supine position, FRC decreases by 0,5-1 litres [31] because of a 4-cm cephalad diaphragm displacement by the abdominal viscera due to a change in thoracic-cage muscle tone. After induction of general anesthesia, there is a loss of muscle inspiratory tone and an appearance of end-expiratory tone in abdominal expiratory muscles at the end of exhalation. This expiratory muscles end-expiratory tone increases intra-abdominal pressure and forces the diaphgram cephalad, thus decreasing FRC [32, 33]. However, recent studies demonstrated that the dominant influence on diaphragm motion under anesthesia may be an anatomical difference between the crural and costal diaphragm regions rather than the abdominal hydrostatic pressure gradient [34].

- Surgical position. The Trendelemburg position allows the abdominal contents to push the diaphragm further cephalad, so that the diaphragm movement not only has to overcome the lungs' and thoracic-cage resistance, but also to lift the abdominal contents. The result is a predisposition to decreased FRC and atelectasis [35]. In the lateral decubitus position, the dependent lung experiences a moderate decrease in FRC [36]. The kidney and lithotomy positions also cause small decreases in FRC above that caused by the supine position.

The uniformity of distribution of ventilation and perfusion is decreased by anesthesia and the amount of this change is related to several factors, such as cardiac output (decreased by many anesthetic drugs), myocardial function and age [37]. An increase in alveolar dead-space is likely to be related to increased ventilation of lung gas-exchange units with high VA/Q [38]. Intrapulmonary shunting of mixed venous blood is increased in aneshesia by 10%. This effect is age related, and is minimal in the young [39]. The increased venous admixture during anesthesia is due partly to an increase of intrapulmonary true shunt and partly to increased perfusion of low V/Q regions (shunt effect). The latter component increases with age [39, 40].

Positive end-expiratory pressure (PEEP) reduces the shunt effect by increasing alveolar ventilation, but its positive effect on arterial $PO_2$ is offset by reduction of preload and cardiac output [40].

General anesthesia is usually administered with an increased inspired fraction of oxygen ($FiO_2$). When $FiO_2$ is > 0.5 it can produce denitrogenation atelectasis. When an enriched $O_2$ mixture is inspired, the alveolar oxygen partial pressure ($PAO_2$) rises, increasing the rate at which $O_2$ moves from alveolar gas to the capillary blood [41, 42]. The $O_2$ flux may increase so much that the net gas flow into the blood exceeds the inspired flow, and the lung unit will become progressively smaller [41, 43]. Collapse is most likely to occur if the $FiO_2$ is high, the V/Q is low, the time of exposure of the unit is long, and the $CvO_2$ is low [43, 44] (Table 1).

**Table 1.** Changes in factors influencing gas exchange after induction of anaesthesia. Adapted from Binslev L., Acta Anaesth. Scand 1981: 25:360

| | Awake | Anesthesia | | |
| --- | --- | --- | --- | --- |
| | | Spont. ventilation | IPPV | IPPV+PEEP |
| $FiO_2$ | 0.21 | 0.4 | 0.4 | 0.4 |
| Qs/Qt (%) | 1.6 | 6.2 | 8.6 | 4.1 |
| VD/VT (%) | 30 | 35 | 38 | 44 |
| Cardiac output (l/min) | 6.1 | 5.0 | 4.5 | 3.7 |
| $PaO_2$ (kPa) | 10.5 | 17.6 | 18.8 | 20.5 |
| V - mean V / Q | 0.81 | 1.30 | 2.20 | 3.03 |
| Q - mean V / Q | 0.47 | 0.51 | 0.83 | 0.55 |

The availability of intravenous sedatives, both hypnotics and opioids, with evanescent drug effects has promoted the advancement of total intravenous anesthesia (TIVA) techniques. These have some advantages compared to inhaled anesthesia:
- Smooth induction with minimal coughing or hiccuping (that is: high airways pressures) [45].
- Easier control of anesthetic depth [46].
- Ideal surgical conditions for brain surgery [4] with reduced cerebral flow [4, 5].
- Rapid, predictable anesthesia emergence with minimal hangover [46].
- Lower incidence of postoperative nausea and vomiting [45, 46].

Still few studies have investigated the effects of TIVA on the respiratory system compared to inhaled anesthesia. Speicher *et al.* studied postoperative pulmonary function after lung surgery. They found that pulmonary impairment after lung resection under propofol anesthesia was significantly smaller than under isoflurane anesthesia. TIVA with propofol is particularly suitable for this kind of operation [47]. Similarly, intrapulmonary shunt and alveolar-arterial oxygen tension difference did not show any significant variation during propofol anesthesia, while halothane produced a significant increase of these variables [48]. However, TIVA with propofol, alfentanil, and vecuronium is reported to depress mucociliary flow in patients with healthy lungs [49]. The possible disadvantage in patients with increased pulmonary risk (e.g. patients with chronic bronchitis and thoracic/abdominal surgery) should be clarified in further studies. In addition, Von Dossow *et al.* observed that thoracic epidural anesthesia in combination with general anesthesia with isoflurane does not impair arterial oxygenation to the same extent as TIVA, which might be a result of the major changes in cardiac output [50]. Also, no significant differences were observed in pulmonary mechanics between propofol TIVA and isoflurane anesthesia in patients with COPD [51]. Ventilation was also studied during ketamine anesthesia, because of its unique pattern of action [52], and comparing fentanyl and alfentanil TIVA [53], both of which caused an increase in total respiratory system and lung resistances, probably related to opioid-induced bronchoconstriction. Finally, TIVA has been studied for its respiratory effects during sedation with spontaneous breathing [54] and, dividing into two stages – the induction stage and the maintenance stage – the respiratory effect of propofol in TIVA, spontaneous ventilation appeared stable and adequate during maintenance of anesthesia [55].

# References


1. Froese AB, Bryan AC (1974) Effects of anesthesia and paralysis on diaphragmatic mechanics in man. Anesthesiology 41:242–255
2. Hedenstierna G, Strandberg A, Brismar B et al (1985) Functional residual capacity, thoracoabdominal dimensions, and central blood volume during general anesthesia with muscle paralysis and mechanical ventilation. A nesthesiology 62:247–254
3. Lindberg P, Gunnarsson L, Tokics L et al (1992) Atelectasis and lung function in the postoperative period. Acta Anaesthesiol Scand 36:546–553
4. Warner DO, Warner MA, Ritman EL (1996) Mechanical significance of respiratory muscle activity in humans during halothane anesthesia. Anesthesiology 84:309–321
5. Kleinman BS, Frey K, VanDrunen M et al (2002) Motion of the diaphragm in patients with chronic obstructive pulmonary disease (COPD) while spontaneously breathing versus during positive pressure breathing after anesthesia and neuromuscular blockade. Anesthesiology 97:298–305
6. Reber A, Nylund U, Hedenstierna G (1998) Position and shape of the diaphragm: implications for atelectasis formation. Anaesthesia 53:1054–1061
7. Spens HJ, Drummond GB, Wraith PK (1996) Changes in chest wall compartment volumes on induction of anaesthesia with eltanolone, propofol and thiopentone. Br J Anaesth Mar 76:369-373
8. Warner DO, Warner MA, Ritman EL (1995) Human chest wall function while awake and during halothane anesthesia. I. Quiet breathing. Anesthesiology 82:6–19
9. Druz WS, Sharp JT (1981) Activity of respiratory muscles in upright and recumbent humans. J Appl Physiol 51:1552–1561
10. Hickey RF, Severinghaus JW (1981) Regulation of breathing:drug effects. M Dekker. Lung biology in health and disease. Ed Hornbain T, New York, Vol 17 p 1251
11. Nunn JF (1993) Respiratory aspects of anaesthesia. Applied respiratory physiology. 4th Edition Butterworth-Heinemann, Oxford, p 384
12. Olsen RW (1988) Barbiturates. Int Anesthesiol Clin 26:262
13. Christensen JH, Andreasen F, Jansen JA (1982) Pharmacokinetics and pharmacodynamics of thiopentone a comparison between young and elderly patients. Anaesthesia 31:398
14. Chauvin M (1989) Tiopental EMC Roma-Parigi. Anestesia-Rianimazione 36304 A50,3
15. Haefely WE (1988) Benzodiazepines. Int Anesthesiol Clin 26:254
16. Forster A, Gardoz JP, Suter PM, Gemperle M (1998) Respiratory depression by midazolam and diazepam. Miller RD. Anesthesia 4th Edition. Vol I Churchill-Livingstone, NewYork, p 235
17. Cockshot ID (1985) Propofol pharmacokinetics and metabolism an overview, Postgrad Med J 61:45

18. Sebel PS, Lowdon JD (1989) Propofol: a new intravenous anesthetic. Anesthesiology 71:260
19. Blouin RT, Conard PF, Gross JB (1991) Time course of ventilatory depression following induction doses of propofol and thiopental. Anesthesiology 75:940-944
20. Fierobe L, Cantineau JP, Pandele G, Desmonts JM (1991) Effets respiratoires du propofol mesures par la spirometrie indirecte. Ann Fr Anesth Reanim 10:10-15
21. Eames WO, Rooke GA, Wu RS, Bishop MJ (1996) Comparison of the effects of etomidate, propofol and thiopental on respiratory resistance after tracheal intubation. Anesthesiology 84:1307-1311
22. Pizov R, Brown RH, Weiss YS et al (1995) Wheezing during induction of general anesthesia in patients with and without asthma. A randomized, blinded trial. Anesthesiology 82:1111-1116
23. Blouin RT, Conard PF, Gross JB (1991) Time course of ventilatory depression following induction doses of propofol and thiopental. Anesthesiology 75:940-944
24. Mankikian B, Cantineau JP, Sartene R et al (1986) Ventilatory pattern and chest wall mechanics during ketamine anesthesia in humans. Anesthesiology 65:492-499
25. Bodnar RJ et al (1988) Role of mu-opiate receptors in supraspinal opiate analgesia:a microinjection study. Brain Res 447:25
26. McClain DA, Hug CC Jr (1980) Intravenous fentanyl kinetics. Clin Pharmacol Ther 28:106
27. Dershwitz M et al (1995) Initial clinical experience with remifentanil a new opiod metabolized by esterases. Anesth Analg 81:619
28. Nunn JF (1987) Mechanism of pulmonary vetilation. Applied respiratory phisiology 3rd ed Butterworth London pp 64
29. Hedenstierna G (1990) Gas exchange during anesthesia Br.J Anaesth 64:507
30. Nunn JF (1987) Resistance to gas flow In: Applied respiratory physiology 3rd ed Butterworth, London pp 397
31. Craig DB, Wahba WM, Don HF (1971) Closing volume and its relationship to gas exchange in seated and supine positions. J Appl Physiol 31:717
32. Don HF, Craig DB, Wahbe WM (1971) the measurement of the gas trapped in the lungs at functional residual capacity and the effects of posture. Anesthesiology 35:582
33. Kayer S, Reheder K, Vattermann F (1989) Position and motion of the human diapharam during anaesthesia paralysis. Anesthesiology 70:891
34. Krayer S, Rehder K, Vettermann J et al (1989) Position and motion of the human diaphragm during anesthesia-paralysis. Anesthesiology 70:891-898
35. Strandberg A, Tokies I, Brismar B et al (1986) Atelectasis during anaesthesia and in the postoperative period. Acta Anesthesiol Scand 30:154
36. Tokics L, Hedenstierna G, Strandberg A et al (1987) Lung collapse and gas exchange during anesthesia effects of spontaneous breathing,muscle paralysis,and Peep. Anesthesiology 66:157
37. Fisherman AP (1963) Dynamics ofn the pulmonary circulation. In Hamilton WF (eds) Handbook of physiology-section 2-Circulation-vol II Williams and Wilkins, Baltimore pp 1667
38. West JB, Dollery CT, Neimark A (1964) Distribution of blood flow in isolated lung: relation to vascular and alveolar pressures. J Appl Physiol 19:713
39. West JB (1977) Ventilation/Blood flow and gas exchange 4th edBlackwell. Scientific Publications, Oxford
40. Zasslow MA, Beunmof JL, Transdale FR (1982) Hypoxic pulmonary vasoconstriction and the size of the hypoxic compartment. J Appl Physiol 53:626
41. Roberts JG (1990) The effects of hypoxic on the systemic circulation during anaesthesia In: Prys-Roberts (ed) The circulation in anaesthesia. Applied Physiology and pharmacology-Blackwell Scientific Publications, Oxford, pp 311
42. Nunn JF (1987) The minute volume of pulmonary ventilation. In: Applied respiratory physiology, 3rd ed. Butterworth, London, pp 65

43. Nunn JF (1982) Oxygen. In: Applied respiratory physiology 4th ed. Butterworth, London, pp 247
44. West JB (1977) Regional differences in the lung. Academic press, Orlando
45. Dundee JW, Wyant GM (1985) Intravenous anaesthesia 2th ed. Edimburgh and London, Churchill Livingstone
46. Blouin RT, Seifert HA, Babenco HD et al (1993) Propofol depresses the hypoxic ventilatory response during conscious sedation and isohypercapnia. Anesthesiology 79:1177
47. Speicher A, Jessberger J, Braun R et al (1995) Postoperative pulmonary function after lung surgery. Total intravenous anesthesia with propofol in comparison to balanced anesthesia with isoflurane. Anaesthesist Apr 44:265-273
48. Mendoza CU, Suarez M, Castaneda R et al (1992) Comparative study between the effects of total intravenous anesthesia with propofol and balanced anesthesia with halothane on the alveolar-arterial oxygen tension difference and on the pulmonary shunt. Arch Med Res Autumn 23:139-142
49. Konrad F, Schraag S, Marx T et al (1998) The effect of total intravenous anesthesia with propofol, alfentanil and vecuronium (TIVA) on bronchial mucosal transport. Anasthesiol Intensivmed Notfallmed Schmerzther Mar 33:171-176
50. Von Dossow V, Welte M, Zaune U et al (2001) Thoracic epidural anesthesia combined with general anesthesia: the preferred anesthetic technique for thoracic surgery. Anesth Analg 92:848-854
51. DeSouza G, deLisser EA, Turry P, Gold MI (1995) Comparison of propofol with isoflurane for maintenance of anesthesia in patients with chronic obstructive pulmonary disease: use of pulmonary mechanics, peak flow rates, and blood gases. J Cardiothorac Vasc Anesth 9:24-28
52. Mankikian B, Cantineau JP, Sartene R et al (1986) Ventilatory pattern and chest wall mechanics during ketamine anesthesia in humans. Anesthesiology 6:492-499
53. Joly LM, Benhamou D (1994) Ventilation during total intravenous anaesthesia with ketamine. Can J Anaesth 41:227-231
54. Ruiz Neto PP, Auler Junior JO (1992) Respiratory mechanical properties during fentanyl and alfentanil anaesthesia. Can J Anaesth 39:458-465
55. Luchini L, Marchesi P, Arcidiacono G et al (1990) Total intravenous anesthesia with spontaneous respiration, in minor general surgery. Minerva Anestesiol 56:827-830

# Determining a Rationale for the Choice of Neuromuscular Blocking Agents in Anaesthesia Practice

T. Pellis

Neuromuscular blocking agents (NMBAs) are used during anaesthesia to facilitate endotracheal intubation and provide surgically required muscle relaxation or paralysis; this allows a lighter plane of anaesthesia since NMBAs prevent patient movement. Using deeper planes of anaesthesia to keep patients still may produce unacceptable cardiovascular depression.

There is continuing development in the field of NMBAs with new products appearing at regular intervals. This suggests  that there may be inadequacies with existing agents. All new agents come at increased costs. The proportion of anaesthesia-related drug costs on a per patient basis are small. However, given the large number of anaesthetics administered over time, approximately 2 million per year in Italy alone, the total cost is significant.

The drug costs associated with anaesthesia vary from country to country but are a relatively small component of hospital drug budgets, accounting for no more than 12% [1]. As a group, NMBAs account for the largest portion of the anaesthesia drug budget, approximately one third [1]. These costs should be compared with surgical and patient admission costs. For example, prolonged block with succinylcholine or mivacurium may have significant pharmacoeconomic implications not only due to ventilatory costs and associated sedation and analgesia but also to the potential negative physical effects of prolonged ventilation and surgical procedure overruns and delays [2]. Appropriate selection of NMBAs can help not only to reduce biological costs secondary to complications but also to make surgical procedures proceed smoothly and without incident. Surgery is expensive and NMBAs are only a small part of the total expense.

The paucity of outcome studies in relation to anaesthetic drugs is not surprising given that anaesthesia is used to facilitate the provision of therapy rather than being therapeutic in its own right. Surgery with anaesthesia has a lower morbidity and mortality than surgery without anaesthesia. Aside from this basic finding, it is yet to be demonstrated that anaesthesia has any direct therapeutic effect; therefore the occurrence of side effects is poorly tolerated. Accordingly, the assessment of anaesthetic drugs has a different priority than that of therapeutic drugs. As anaesthetic drugs are 'non-therapeutic', it is also difficult to determine the best agent of choice. However, new NMBAs are marketed on the basis of improvements regarding the frequency of side effects, safety, reliability, duration, reversibility and undesirable haemodynamic effects.

A basic goal of modern day anaesthesia is to maintain normal physiological parameters. There are no studies to confirm this as best practice. It is based on the common-sense principle that the further a patient deviates from normal the more likely it is that he or she will suffer adverse events. NMBAs can cause significant physiological disturbance, for example, haemodynamic disturbance with vagolytic or vagomimetic effects and histamine release. They may also result in residual muscle paralysis and respiratory compromise, or allergy and anaphylaxis.

## Classification

NMBAs can be classified in two pharmacological groups – depolarising and non-depolarising. Non-depolarising NMBAs can also be classified according to their chemical structure in two major families as shown in Figure 1. They can be further classified depending on their duration of effect into short, intermediate and long-acting.

*Depolarising* NMBAs bind to postsynaptic cholinergic receptors on the skeletal muscle endplate of the neuromuscular junction, resulting in depolarisation. They also promote transient uncoordinated contraction of muscle fibres known as fasciculation. The endplate receptors remain refractory to depolarisation for a period of time, resulting in flaccid muscle paralysis. The only depolarising agent still in use is succinylcholine.

*Non-depolarising* NMBAs act as competitive antagonists for cholinergic receptors on the skeletal muscle endplate. By preventing the access of acetylcholine to these receptors, they induce flaccid muscle paralysis. The endplate is not depolarized and no fasciculations are produced.

*Very short-acting* agents have a duration of action of less than 12 min. *Short-acting* agents have a duration of less than 20 min, whereas *intermediate-acting* agents are effective 20-45 min. NMBAs with a duration of action greater than 45 min are generally considered to be *long-acting*. Residual weakness following attempted antagonism is more likely with long-acting than with intermediate-acting NMBAs [3].

The concurrent use of volatile general anaesthetic agents, such as isoflurane, potentiates neuromuscular blockade when these are administered in high concentrations. The influence of anaesthetic vapors on the effect of initial doses of NMBAs is minimal unless equilibration of anaesthetic agent is allowed to occur before administration of the NMBA [4]. More pronounced effects may be seen in the presence of sevoflurane and desflurane, which equilibrate more rapidly [5]. Depending on the requirement for muscle relaxation during surgery, further doses of NMBA may not be required after the intubating dose. The volatile agent alone may produce sufficient muscle relaxation.

NMBAs may also be used via continuous infusion. Infusions are typically employed for prolonged procedures or when patient movement might prove disastrous, e.g. during some neurosurgical procedures. Reliability of recovery

## Aminosteroids

**Pancuronium**   **Vecuronium**   **Rocuronium**

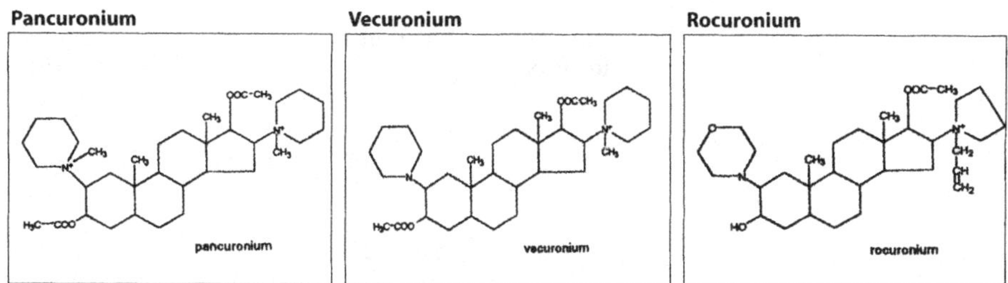

## Benzylisoquinolines

**Atracarium-Cisatracurium**   **Mivacurium**

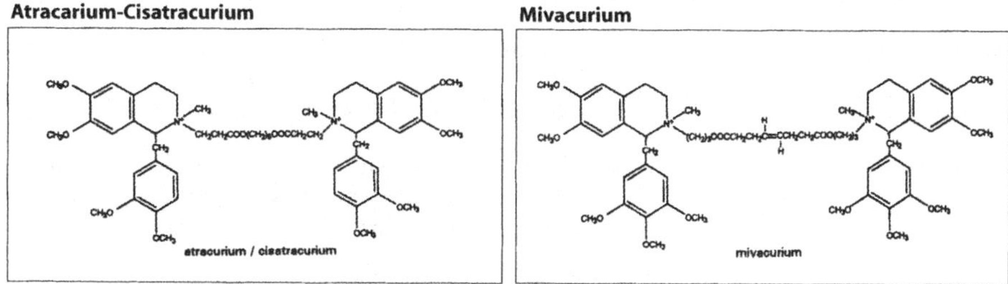

**Fig. 1** Classification of non-depolarizing NMBAs based on their chemical structure in Aminosetoids or Benzylisoquinolines

is critical with infusions in order to avoid prolonged block secondary to accumulation of NMBA. The use of infusions may be associated with increased wastage of NMBAs. Continuous infusion is not recommended for habitual use.

Ideally, neuromuscular function monitoring by peripheral nerve stimulation should be performed on all patients who receive NMBAs. In clinical practice this is often not the case. Monitoring is particularly indicated in patients undergoing long surgical procedures, in patients in whom blockade may be prolonged (neuromuscular diseases) or in whom reversal is intentionally avoided, and when drug interaction is suspected.

## Individual agents

The pharmacodynamic and pharmacokinetic features of clinically used NMBAs are summarized in the Table 1. *Succinylcholine* has a rapid onset and a very short action. It is chiefly used for rapid sequence induction, suspected difficult intubation, and, more rarely, in procedures in which only a brief period of relaxation is required. In spite of its numerous disadvantages, such as myalgia, malignant hyperthermia, hyperkalemia, myoglobinuria, masseter spasm, increased intraocular and intracranial pressure, vagal effects, prolonged blockade, and arrhythmias up to cardiac arrest, it is commonly used because of its unique properties of rapid, profound, and short-lived relaxation. It is of note

**Table 1.** Pharmacodynamic and pharmacokinetic properties of NMBAs. Adapted from [8]

| NMBAs | Onset | Clinical duration | Metabolism | Renal elimination | Hepatic elimin |
|---|---|---|---|---|---|
| Succinylcholine | 60-90 sec | 8-10 min | Pseudocholine-sterase 98-99% | < 2% | None = |
| Mivacurium | 2-3 min | 15-20 min | Pseudocholine-sterase 95-99% | < 5% | None = |
| Rocuronium | 1.5-2 min | 30-60 min | None | ~40% | ~60% |
| Vecuronium | 2-3 min | 60-75 min | Liver 30-40% | 40-50% | 50-60% |
| Pancuronium | 3-6 min | 60-100 min | Liver 10-20% | 85% | 15% |
| Atracurium | 2-3 min | 45-60 min | Hoffman elimination and ester hydrolysis | 10-40% | None = |
| *Cis*-atracurium | 2-3 min | 45-60 min | Hoffman elimination | ~15 | None = |

that in current day practice succinylcholine is the NMBA most commonly implicated in anaphylaxis [6].

Succinylcholine relies on pseudocholinesterase enzymes for metabolism. Reduced cholinesterase activity occurs congenitally, in pregnancy, extremes of age, burns, liver and renal dysfunction, chronic debilitation, carcinoma, collagen diseases, cardiac failure and with some drugs. Prolonged blockade ensues in patients with the inherited condition of plasma cholinesterase deficiency. In the mild forms of this condition, which affect 1/25 of the population, the patient is heterozygous for the normal gene (E1U) and one of three abnormal genes (E1A atypical, E1S silent or E1F fluoride-resistant). In these patients, block is prolonged by about 50% but this is unlikely to be a clinical problem. In the more severe forms, which affect about 1 in 2,500 people, the normal gene is absent and the patient is homozygous or heterozygous for one or more of the abnormal genes. In these patients, neuromuscular block may last from 2-4 h requiring treatment by sedation, or continuing anaesthesia, and controlled ventilation, with or without the administration of an anticholinesterase once there is a detectable twitch response. Once recovery has commenced, as shown by a response to peripheral nerve stimulation, it may be hastened by administering an anticholinesterase drug. Clearly the inconvenience caused by unexpected and prolonged neuromuscular block would be maximised in a busy day-case centre with no facilities for postoperative ventilation. When used in repeated or large doses, e.g. > 400 mg, it may produce a phase II block. This type of blockade resembles a non-depolarising block and is of uncertain duration.

*Mivacurium* is structurally similar to atracurium. It is a non-depolarising agent with a short duration of action but a slow onset. Mivacurium does not necessarily require reversal as it is metabolised by pseudocholinesterase enzymes at approximately 70-80% the rate of succinylcholine [7]. Mivacurium is marketed on the basis of its short duration of action, its suitability as an infusion and the fact that it does not require routine reversal. However, if twitch height has not returned to normal following neuromuscular blockade with mivacurium then reversal is recommended. Mivacurium does not have a rapid onset of action and, like other benzylisoquinolinium derivatives, causes release of histamine, which may cause significant hypotension, bronchospasm, erythema, and cutaneous flushing. It is recommended that the intubating dose be given over a minute. Mivacurium will not trigger malignant hyperthermia. Due to the risk of prolonged neuromuscular block in patients with pseudocholinesterase deficiency, the fact that a relatively short duration of block can be achieved by using smaller doses of alternative intermediate-acting agents, and the high cost of mivacurium, it is difficult to recommend this agent for routine use.

*Rocuronium* is an amino-steroidal non-depolarising muscle relaxant. It has the fastest onset of action of any of the existing non-depolarising NMBAs, with good to excellent intubating conditions at 60-90 s. At higher than $2xED_{95}$ dosage its onset of action approaches that of succinylcholine. The effective dose 95 $(ED_{95})$ is the mean dose required to produce 95% twitch depression (paralysis) at the adductor pollicis muscle. The standard intubating dose is taken to be $2xED_{95}$ to ensure paralysis of the diaphragm and airway musculature since these sites are relatively more resistant to neuromuscular block [9]. Rocuronium's other advantage is reduced formation of active metabolites when compared to vecuronium. Hepatic and renal dysfunction may prolong the effect of the block but less so than with pancuronium or vecuronium [10]. To avoid the potential complications of succinylcholine, many anaesthetists use rocuronium for rapid sequence induction when they are confident of intubating the airway. Rocuronium has an intermediate duration of action, comparable to vecuronium or *cis*-atracurium. There is no evidence of accumulation. It also has the major advantage of a very stable cardiovascular profile with no histamine release even at very high doses. Because of these advantages over vecuronium, it is slowly replacing the latter in clinical practice.

*Vecuronium* is an amino-steroidal non-depolarising NMBA. Since the 1980s it has achieved widespread popularity due to its reliability and haemodynamic stability. Vecuronium is an agent of intermediate duration and slow onset. Continuous infusion, as for rocuronium, is possible but no longer recommended given the production of active metabolites which may accumulate. The same metabolites may cause prolonged block in the presence of hepato-renal dysfunction, with prolonged infusion in intensive care units, in obesity, in the elderly and in neonates [11, 12]. Prolonged block from interaction with aminoglycoside antibiotics, magnesium, lithium and β-blockers have all been reported.

*Pancuronium* has a long duration of action and slow onset. Significant tachycardia and a rise in blood pressure are frequently reported following administration of pancuronium. Although it has not been demonstrated, it is widely believed that this vagolytic property has the potential to induce myocardial ischemia in patients with coronary artery disease. Pancuronium should only be used when prolonged relaxation is required, as the incidence of residual muscle paralysis in recovery is much higher with long-acting agents. Pancuronium has significant renal elimination and should be used with caution in patients who have renal impairment.

*Atracurium* is a benzylisoquinolinium non-depolarising NMBA. It has an intermediate duration of action with a slow onset. Atracurium's main advantage over other intermediate NMBAs is its organ-independent metabolism. Atracurium is metabolized by the Hoffmann reaction (nonenzymatic degradation at body temperature and pH) and ester hydrolysis, making it an excellent choice for patients with hepatic or renal failure. Laudanosine is produced as a non-active metabolite and subsequently renally excreted. Laudanosine is known to cause convulsions at high concentrations, thus caution must be used when utilising prolonged infusions of atracurium in patients with renal failure. The main limitation of this agent is histamine release, which appears to be dose-dependent and which accounts for haemodynamic instability and bronchospasm.

*Cis-atracurium* is one of the stereo-isomers of atracurium. It is a NMBA of intermediate duration and is clinically very similar to atracurium, although the onset time may be slightly slower. *Cis*-atracurium is also metabolised independently of renal and hepatic function, making it a good choice in patients with hepato-renal disease and for use in infusions. The Hoffmann elimination pathway accounts for 77% of total body clearance of *cis*-atracurium. Organ clearance is responsible for 23% of total body clearance, of which for more than half is kidney-dependent [13]. Approximately 16% of *cis*-atracurium is found unchanged in the urine; however, its clinical relevance in terms of prolonged recovery has not been clearly demonstrated. *Cis*-atracurium offers two advantages over atracurium: it releases less histamine and produces less laudanosine [14]. Being more potent than atracurium, less molecules are required to produce the same level of blockade, thus less laudanosine is produced. Histamine release starts at $5xED_{95}$ but becomes clinically relevant from $8xED_{95}$. Commonly used intubating doses of *cis*-atracurium range from 2 to 4x $ED_{95}$, offering a stable cardiovascular profile comparable to that of vecuronium.

## General Adverse Effects

All NMBAs can cause anaphylaxis and they are one of the most common drugs to do so among those used by anaesthetists. Malignant hyperthermia is a rare but serious disorder. Succinylcholine is a strong trigger for malignant hyperthermia whereas non-depolarising NMBAs are not considered triggers. Patients experiencing a major hyperthermic event have approximately a 5% mortality [15].

A major toxicity of NMBAs is ventilatory depression, especially in the recovery room. Residual post-anaesthetic neuromuscular blockade is associated with impaired hypoxic ventilatory control, increased incidence of pulmonary aspiration and reduced force of respiratory muscles, accounting for the increased morbidity. Intermediate- and short-acting NMBAs are less likely to result in post-operative residual curarisation than agents of long duration. Yet, given the severity of complications, administration of reversal agents and neuromuscular monitoring are strongly recommended.

## Specific Situations

*Routine Intubation.* Almost any NMBA can be used for routine intubation. Selection depends largely on the estimated duration of procedure, co-existing medical conditions (e.g. hepato-renal dysfunction), previous experience, the degree of tolerance to the side-effect profile, and the incidence of adverse effects associated with the particular NMBA chosen.

*Rapid Sequence Induction and Intubation.* If there is an increased risk of aspiration, a 'rapid sequence induction' is employed. Traditionally, this includes preoxygenation, an induction agent such as thiopentone followed by succinylcholine, cricoid pressure, and no positive-pressure ventilation. The ultimate goal of a 'rapid sequence induction' is to secure the airway as rapidly as possible. Rocuronium has an onset approaching that of succinylcholine, especially if used at greater than $2xED_{95}$ doses. Intubating conditions at 60 s after 1 mg/kg rocuronium are similar to those after 1 mg/kg succinylcholine [16]. Many anaesthetists prefer rocuronium over succinylcholine in order to avoid many of the numerous side effects of the latter. In addition, as succinylcholine is short-acting, another NMBA is needed to maintain neuromuscular blockade when the action of succinylcholine wears off. Using rocuronium avoids the need for another agent.

*Difficult Intubation.* There are many techniques for difficult intubation. Succinylcholine is used when there is uncertainty about the ability to successfully achieve endotracheal intubation. Its short duration of action allows the patient to breathe spontaneously again within 10 min.

*Hepato-renal Dysfunction.* For patients with hepatic and renal dysfunction, *cis*-atracurium is the drug of choice due to its independence from hepatic and renal metabolism. Clinically, however, there is little to separate *cis*-atracurium from rocuronium in this situation particularly in patients with renal dysfunction.

*Pregnancy.* NMBAs are very poorly lipid soluble and do not cross the placenta in clinically significant amounts. Traditional anaesthetic teaching would suggest that succinylcholine should be used to intubate the gravid patient. This should be followed by a non-depolarising NMBA. Pregnancy is associated with decreased levels of pseudocholinesterase enzyme.

*Pediatrics.* Neonates tend to be more susceptible to NMBAs than adults. Vecuronium has a more prolonged duration of action in neonates whereas the duration of action of *cis*-atracurium is similar in neonates as it is in children and adults [17]. Slightly older children display increased resistance to NMBAs especially succinylcholine where double the adult intubating dose may be required. Non-depolarising NMBAs may be used in a similar dose fashion as in adults. There is nothing particular in pediatric practice to favour one NMBA over another. Accordingly, the choice of the NMBA to use should rely on the same criteria that apply to adults.

## Cost

There are no good outcome studies to allow an informed opinion on the cost benefits of one NMBA over another. Costs of NMBAs may vary significantly from country to country. The absence of studies is due to the difficulty in differentiating NMBA costs from other factors, such as surgery time, the unpredictably of duration of the procedure, the low incidence of critical events and difficulties in calculating hidden costs and savings. In one study examining the effects of prescribing guidelines on the use of neuromuscular blocking agents reduced costs but increased adverse events by 2% [18]. The cost of these complications is likely to outweigh the increased costs of the new agents. Unfortunately, due to the absence of good studies, opinions on the pharmacoeconomics of NMBAs are founded to a large extent on speculation.

## References


1. DeMonaco HJ, Shah AS (1994) Economic considerations in the use of neuromuscular blocking drugs. J Clin Anesth 6:383-387
2. Armstrong DK, Crisp CB (1994) Pharmacoeconomic issues of sedation, analgesia and neuromuscular blockade in critical care. New Horizons 2:85-93
3. Bevan DR, Donati F, Kopman AF (1988) Reversal of neuromuscular blockade. Anesthesiology 69:272-276
4. Wulf H, Kahl M, Ledowski T (1998) Augmentation of neuromuscular blocking effects of cisatracurium during desflurane, sevoflurane, isoflurane and i.v. anaesthesia. Br J Anaesth 80:308
5. Wulf H, Ledowski T, Linstedt U et al (1998) Neuromuscular blocking effects of rocuronium during desflurane, isoflurane, and sevoflurane anesthesia. Can J Anaesth 45:526
6. Hunter JM (1987) Adverse effects of neuromuscular blocking drugs. Br J Anaesth 59:46-60
7. Savarese JJ, Ali HH, Basta SJ et al (1988) The clinical neuromuscular pharmacology of mivacurium chloride (BW 1090U), a short acting non-depolarising ester neuromuscular blocking drug. Anesthesiology 68:723-732
8. Savarese JJ, Caldwell GE, Lien CA, Miller RD (2000) Pharmacology. In: Miller RD (ed) Anaesthesia, 5th ed. Curdelli Livingstone, Philadelphia, pp 412-490
9. Brull SJ, Silverman DG (1993) Intraoperative use of muscle relaxants. Advances in the use of muscle relaxants. Anesthesiology Clinics of North America 11

10. Khuenl-Brady KS, Sparr H (1996) Clinical pharmacokinetics of rocuronium bromide. Clinical Pharmacokinetics 31:174-183
11. Brull SJ, Silverman DG (1993) Intraoperative use of muscle relaxants. Advances in the use of muscle relaxants. Anesthesiology Clinics of North America 11
12. Sanders KA, Aucker R (1996) Early recognition of risk factors for persistent effects of vecuronium. Southern Medical Journal 89:411-414
13. Kisor DF, Scmith VD (1999) Clinical pharmacokinetics of cisatracurium besilate. Clinical Pharmacokinetics 36:27-40
14. Savarese JJ, Mogensen J, Reich D et al (1996) The haemodynamic profile of cisatracurium. Current Opinion in Anesthesiology 9:S36-S41
15. Ording H (1985) Incidence of malignant hyperthermia in Denmark. Anesth Analg 64:700
16. Andrews JL, Kumar N, Van der Brom RHG et al (1999) A large sample randomized trial of rocuronium versus succinylcholine in rapid-sequence induction of anesthesia along with propofol. Acta Anaesthesiol Scand 43:4
17. Meretjo OA (1990) Neuromuscular blocking agents in paediatric patients: influence of age on the response. Anaesth Intensive Care 18:440-448
18. Gora-harper Ml, Hessel E, Shadick D (1995) Effect of prescribing guidelines on the use of neuromuscular blocking agents. Am J Health Syst Pharm 52

# Chapter 13

# Recovery Room

Y. LEYKIN

## Introduction

The *recovery room* (RR) is defined, according to the Society of Anaesthesiology of Great Britain and Ireland, as "the place where the patient coming from the *operating theatre* stays till recovery of *consciousness* and *haemodynamic* and *respiratory* steady-state" [1]. The RR was created to make a smooth passage from the operating theatre to the ward, since correct *perioperative management* improves the outcome of surgery. As a matter of fact, emergence from the drug induced coma necessary during operation is the most critical phase, 50% of perioperative deaths occur during the first perioperative hours [2]. Moreover, technical and pharmacological improvements in the surgical and anaesthesiological fields have allow elderly patients and patients with ASA III and IV pathologies to be operated on. These patients need highly intensive levels of *monitoring* in the immediate post-operative period. Therefore the RR has gained ever greater importance nowadays.

The first RR in GB was described in 1801; in the USA, the first RR was opened in 1873, at the Massachusetts General Hospital in Boston [3]. During World War II, the RR became more important, and specifically trained staff was devoted to this special ward. In the late 1980s, the need for a RR increased as "day hospital" procedures became more popular.

At the beginning of the 1990s, most Anaesthesiological Societies provided guidelines on the postoperative management of the patient.

## Guidelines

The *Anaesthesiological Societies* of most countries regulate the activities of the RR. In France, the Société Française d'Anesthésie et de Réanimation published, in 1990 and 1994 guidelines regarding the surveillance and post-anaesthetic care of the patient. These guidelines were the basis for a law in 1994 [4]. In 1990, the American Society of Anesthesiology indicated the "standards" for *post-operative monitoring*, which are the following [5]:
- All patients undergoing anaesthesia of any kind need adequate post-operative monitoring.
- *Medical responsibility* for the RR is in the hands of the anaesthesiology department.

- Clinical conditions of the patients should be recorded upon their admission to the RR and monitored periodically.
- Patients should be accompanied to the RR by the *anaesthesiologist* along with adequate clinical and instrumental monitoring.
- The RR staff should receive adequate information about the patient.
- The anaesthesiologist is responsible for discharge or transfer of the patient from the RR.

The *Italian Guidelines* were written by the Commission on Safety in Anaesthesiology and Intensive Care of the Società Italiana di Anestesia, Analgesia, Rianimazione e Terapia Intensiva (SIAARTI) [6, 7]. These are *recommendations* on optimisation of post-operative care in an equipped area. This document takes into account that the Italian situation is inhomogeneous, as far as the medical and nursing staff, and the location and the equipment are concerned. The recommendations should therefore be a goal to achieve. All recommendations are presented as possibilities, leaving each department free to choose its own way.

SIAARTI guidelines differ from those of other countries:
- Post-operative surveillance may take place in the operating room area or in a dedicated room.
- It is not specified whether the anaesthesiologist accompanies the patient to the RR.
- The surveillance is performed by highly trained nurses.
- The anaesthesiologist gives information to the nurses on the post-anaesthetic requirements.
- The anaesthesiologist is responsible for discharge or transfer of the patient to the ward.
- No specific RR record is foreseen.
- Instrumental monitoring is divided into suggested and optional equipment.
- There is no RR indication for day surgery.

## Objectives

The patient's stay in the RR has the following objectives:
- Recovery from *anaesthetic drugs'* effect.
- Stabilisation of *vital signs* (circulation and ventilation).
- Stabilisation of *body temperature.*
- Control of *hydro-electrolyte balance.*
- Intensive care support in case of *acute complications.*
- Definition of adequate *post-operative analgesia.*
- Recovery of *motor activity* after locoregional anaesthesia.

## Organisation (Location, Equipment, Staff)

The RR should be *close* to the operating theatre, and the laboratory and radiology should be of rapid and easy access. The number of bays of the RR should be *1.5 per theatre*, but if the throughput is rapid, as in day-surgery units, more will be needed. Temperature should be 21-22 °C and relative humidity 38-45% [8].

The bays should be surrounded by a large area (standard floor area is about 9 m², but as large as 18 m² may be useful for patients needing a higher level of monitoring or mechanical support) to guarantee easy access to the head of the patient and the positioning of transport carts, ECGraphs, echographs, medication carts, etc.

An efficient RR should be equipped with a patient trolley or bed having the following characteristics [1]:
- Oxygen cylinder with key, gauge, flowmeter, tubing, suitable oxygen masks.
- Rapid availability of head-down tilt operated from the head end.
- Mounting sites for infusion poles.

Every recovery bay should be equipped with:
- Oxygen supply with a set of facial masks and ventilation bags.
- Suction device.
- ECG, pulseoxymeter, invasive and non-invasive blood pressure monitor.

Cardiorespiratory equipment:
- Respiratory device with adequate monitoring (capnography).

The personnel working in the RR should be *highly professionally trained*. The nurses should be able to promptly recognise any sign of impaired vital signs and provide adequate support to the patients until the anaesthesiologist arrives. There should be one nurse every two patients. An anaesthesiologist should always be available [7].

## Reception of the Patient

When the patient arrives, both the anaesthesiologist and the nurse who accompany him give a full *report* to the colleagues in charge in the RR. It should include:
- Patient's name and age.
- Surgical procedure performed.
- Anaesthetic technique used and its duration.
- Blood loss and fluid balance.
- Final monitoring record.
- Any complication encountered during anaesthesia.
- Number and type of drains and catheters.
- Post-anaesthetic requirements for: positioning, oxygen therapy, intravenous fluid, drug therapy and analgesia.

The patient should be immediately monitored and routinely *observed* at least every 15 min, recording:
- Skin colour.
- Respiratory function.
- Cardiovascular function.
- Consciousness.
- Bleeding.
- Pain.
- Body temperature, if below 36 °C at admission.
- Motor block, if locoregional anaesthesia.

## Normal Recovery from General Anaesthesia

The *physiologic recovery* from general anaesthesia is not completed in the operating theatre, nor in the recovery room. It can be subdivided into three steps [2]:
- Phase 1, early recovery: from the end of administration of anaesthetic drugs until the recovery of reflexes and conscience. This takes minutes.
- Phase 2, intermediate recovery: recovery of movement and thinking ability. This takes hours.
- Phase 3, late recovery: complete recovery of psychomotor ability. This takes days.

The duration of these three phases actually depends on the elimination time of all given medications.

The volatile agents are excreted unmodified by the lungs. Their elimination half-life is proportional to their solubility. Sevoflurane and desflurane have a faster elimination than isoflurane. The rate of metabolism of the gases used at present is very low.

The intravenous ipnotic drugs more used are propofol, thiopentone and ketamine. The rate of elimination of these drugs is faster for propofol and longer than for thiopentone and ketamine.

Muscle relaxants have very different times of action, but all non-depolarising muscle relaxants are reversed by anticholinesterase (neostigmine). Their duration can be prolonged by low body temperature. Succinilcholine is metabolised by pseudocholinesterase, a lack of which results in a slower metabolism in the liver. This may last several hours.

At the end of the anaesthesia a good analgesic level should be present, to allow a faster recovery of the patient. This is important especially when using fast-metabolised opioids.

## Normal Recovery from Locoregional Anaesthesia

Patients are generally admitted to the RR after combined epidural and general anaesthesia or after complications encountered during locoregional procedures. They all recover from motor block and start post-operative analgesia.

The recovery from locoregional anaesthesia is completed by the following steps (Table 1) [9]:
– Cardiovascular stabilisation.
– Sensitivity recovery.
– Motor block disappearance.

**Table 1.** Bromage scoring system

| Score | Block | Residual movement |
|---|---|---|
| IV | None | Complete knee and foot flexion |
| III | Partial | Knee flexion still possible |
| II | Almost complete | Foot flexion still possible |
| I | Complete | Knee and foot immobile |

## Complications

The complications in the perioperative period are described below:

### Respiratory

*Upper airway obstruction* is frequently due to reduced muscular tone and falling of the tongue in the hypopharynx. It may also complicate rhyno-laryngoiatric operation (blood, foreign bodies).

*Inadequate ventilation* in the immediate postoperative period is provoked by:
1. Drugs depressing the *ventilatory drive*, administered either intravenously or intrathecally (opioids, sedatives, hypnotics).
2. Incomplete recovery after administration of *muscle relaxants*.
3. Impaired ventilation because of operation on upper abdomen or thorax.

*Hypoxemia.* An *oxygen saturation* lower than 90% frequently occurs in the postoperative period. Pulse-oximetry is therefore mandatory while transferring the patient from the operating theatre to the RR until the patient will be discharged. Hypoxemia is caused by perfusion-ventilation mismatch, pulmonary shunt, hypoventilation; predisposing factors are obesity, bronchopneumopathies, abdominal surgery [10, 11].

*Laryngospasm* is a prolonged closure of the vocal chords as a defence reflex against any foreign body or blood in the hypopharynx.

*Aspiration of gastric content* is seldom observed in the RR. Higher risk is given by *full stomach* or increased abdominal pressure (obesity, pregnancy, bowel obstruction), associated with a reduced protection reflex of the airway [12].

### Cardiovascular

Most frequent cardiovascular complications are as described in [13-15]:

*Hypertension* (blood pressure values 20% higher than preoperative) is frequently caused by:

1. Pain.
2. Bladder distension.
3. Respiratory distress with hypercarbia.
4. Excessive fluid administration.
5. Cardiovascular surgery.
6. Perioperative drugs.
7. Concomitant diseases (pheochromocytoma, hyperthyroidism, increase of intracranial pressure, preeclampsia).

*Hypotension* (blood pressure values 20% lower than preoperative) is the complication occurring most frequently. It can depend on:

1. Pre-load reduction, due to hypovolemia or venous vasodilatation.
2. Myocardial impairment of contractility, may be a consequence of anaesthetic drugs, cardiac failure, myocardial infarction, pulmonary thromboembolism, cardiac tamponade or tense pneumothorax.
3. Post-load reduction, peripheral resistance reduction, due to neuroaxial blocks, septicaemia or anaphylaxis.

*Tachycardia* can be caused by pain, anxiety, anticholinergic drugs. If it persists, it may be a sign of hypovolemia, anaemia or respiratory distress.

*Bradycardia* in the postoperative period can be due to anticholinesterase, opioids, hypothermia or vagal stimuli.

*Dysrhythmias.* The presence of an irregular pulse in the postoperative period may be caused by the residual effects of anaesthetic gases sensitising the myocardium. Premature atrial contractions need no treatment. Premature ventricular contractions may be caused by hypoxia, hypercarbia, hypokalemia, acidosis, digitalis overdose, hyperthyroidism. Treatment is required if the ectopic beats occur frequently and cause hypotension. It consists of lidocaine bolus (1 mg/kg) followed by an infusion of 1-4 mg/min, or ß-blocker (propranolol or esmolol). Atrial fibrillation needs treatment if the ventricular response is rapid and causes hypotension. It consists of electrical cardioversion or digitalisation.

*Myocardial ischemia.* Perioperative *myocardial infarction* is the most common cause of death in non-cardiac surgical patients [2]. Myocardial ischemia during operation or in the immediate perioperative period puts the patient at risk of arrhythmias, ischemic episodes or cardiac failure in the first postoperative week [16]. Most postoperative infarcts occur on the second or third postoperative day [17]. The mechanism of myocardial ischemia is a reduction of *oxygen supply* or an increased oxygen demand.

## Restlessness, Excitement and Confusion

The most important causes of these abnormal recoveries from anaesthesia are [18, 19]:
– Hypoxaemia.
– Hypercapnia.
– Gastric overdistension.
– Bladder overdistension.

## Post-operative Nausea and Vomiting (PONV)

PONV complicates 20-30% of all operations [13]. Concomitant conditions which facilitate PONV are: age (children), gender (women), obesity, kinetosis, anxiety, gastroparesis, type and duration of the surgical procedure (laparoscopy, eye surgery for strabismus, ear surgery). The choice of drugs used for anaesthesia is also important [20]. *Prophylaxis* for PONV is challenging: droperidol, metoclopramide and ondansetron [21] have all been used with poor success. A good management of post-operative pain, on the other hand, reduces PONV, elicited by visceral reflexes.

## Hypothermia

Intraoperative mild hypothermia (body temperature between 33 and 36.4 °C) is a consequence of a temporary impairment of the *thermoregulatory centre* and of vasodilatation induced by anaesthetic drugs [1]. Postoperative hypothermia causes:
- Discomfort to the patient.
- Delayed recovery from general anaesthesia, as it slows down enzyme activity and drug metabolism, as well as neurologic activity of the patients.
- Shivering. In the post-operative period the patient's temperature increases by shivering. Oxygen consumption is increased 3 to 4 -fold. Intraocular and intracranial pressures increase as well. It is therefore dangerous in patients with reduced oxygen transport [22], in eye surgery or with eye pathologies, after head surgery or trauma. Hypothermia can be abolished by petidine (20-30 mg i.v.) or doxapram, clonidine, ketanserin.
- Haemocoagulative alterations: modified platelet activity, prolonged coagulation time [23].

Postoperative hypothermia should be prevented in the operating theatre and corrected in the RR using *warmed fluids* and *warming blankets*.

## Hyperthermia

In the postoperative period, hyperthermia is rarely encountered [13]. It can be caused by *transfusion reactions*, infections, adverse reaction to drugs, thyroid storm, malignant hyperthermia [1].

## Seizures

These can be a consequence of *drug overdose* (teophilline, lidocaine, amphetamine), abstinence from some substances (ethanol, benzodiazepine, barbiturates, opioids), infections (meningoencephalitis, brain-abscess), brain-enlarging lesions (tumour or haemorrhage) or metabolic impairment (hepatic or ureic encephalopathy). The treatment is symptomatic.

## Blood Transfusion Reactions

These reactions are *immunologic* (fever, shivering, urticaria, haemolysis, fatal haemolysis, anaphylaxis) or infectious (viral or bacterial contamination). Acute haemolytic reactions follow immediately the transfusion of mismatched blood. Transfusion should be stopped immediately, because the haemolysis is quantity dependent, and circulation should be maintained with fluid and inotropic agents. Febrile non-haemolytic reactions are caused by the presence of anti-leukocyte antibodies against donor blood. It appears 1-6 h after the transfusion. Skin rash and anaphylaxis are a consequence of sensitisation to blood proteins.

## Haemorrhage

*Post-operative bleeding* in the operation field is often caused by insufficient haemostasis and may require immediate surgical evaluation. Other causes for bleeding are inborn or acquired modification of coagulation. The latter may be preoperative (coagulation deficiencies, anticoagulation therapy, drugs interfering with platelet activity, liver failure) or intraoperative (massive transfusion, surgery of the liver, administration of heparin in major vascular surgery).

Postoperative haemorrhage should be assumed in the presence of signs of hypovolemia (anxiety, agitation, dyspnoea, tachycardia, paleness, oliguria, even if blood pressure values are normal), hypotension, excessive bleeding from drainage or dressings. The clinical consequences depend on the site, quantity and velocity of bleeding [24].

## Discharge Criteria

The patient can be discharged to a ward or to the intensive care unit, or in case of day surgery he can return home.

Before the patient is discharged, the recovery staff must be sure that:
- The patient is *fully conscious* and reflexes have returned so he can protect his airway.
- Breathing is adequate and blood saturation is satisfactory.
- Cardiovascular system is stable.
- Pain is well controlled.
- No blood loss is ongoing.
  If the patient is returning home he should:
- Be able to dress.
- Have no *nausea* or *vomiting*.
- Have been able to void.
  Also:
- His wound should have been inspected and the dressing changed.
- He should have written and verbal instructions on follow-up, and a telephone number to call in case of any complications.
- He should be accompanied by a responsible person [25].

Patients who are inappropriately or prematurely discharged are more likely to have *post-operative complications* or to suffer injuries due to psychomotor impairment. By contrast, an inappropriate delayed discharge may occupy beds useful for other patients.

To help decide timely discharge, many *scoring systems* have been adopted. One of the earliest was *Aldrete's* [26]. It mimics the Apgar scoring system and is useful for evaluating recovery of patients transferred to a ward (Table 2). It is not appropriate for ambulatory patients.

**Table 2.** Aldrete scoring system

| Parameter | Score |
| --- | --- |
| Motility (voluntar or on command) | |
|   ☐  4 limbs | 2 |
|   ☐  2 limbs | 1 |
|   ☐  none | 0 |
| Respiration | |
|   ☐  Deep breathing and active cough | 2 |
|   ☐  Dispnoea, superficial breathing | 1 |
|   ☐  Apnoea | 0 |
| Circulation (systolic blood pressure) | |
|   ☐  – 20% than pre-anaesthetic value | 2 |
|   ☐  – 20-50% than pre-anaesthetic value | 1 |
|   ☐  – 50% than pre-anaesthetic value | 0 |
| Conscience | |
|   ☐  Awake | 2 |
|   ☐  Awakable on calling | 1 |
|   ☐  Not awakable | 0 |
| Colour | |
|   ☐  Normal | 2 |
|   ☐  Pale | 1 |
|   ☐  Cyanotic | 0 |

To specifically address the intermediate recovery phase of the ambulatory patient, the *Post-anaesthesia Discharge Scoring System (PADSS)* was developed. It assesses: vital signs, activity and mental status, pain, nausea, vomiting, surgical bleeding, intake and output (Table 3) [27].

PADS allows patients to be discharged significantly earlier than those based on clinical criteria alone, and gives medico-legal documentation as well.

Since intake and voiding were not accepted as universal criteria, PADS was modified and these two requirements deleted (Table 4) [28, 29].

Patients whose recovery from anaesthesia is prolonged or complicated should be transferred to the intensive care unit directly from the operating theatre or after admission to the RR.

**Table 3.** Post-anaesthesia discharge scoring system

| | |
|---|---|
| **Vital signs** | |
| ☐   Within 20% of preoperative value | 2 |
| ☐   20-40% of preoperative value | 1 |
| ☐   40% of preoperative value | 0 |
| **Ambulation and mental status** | |
| ☐   Oriented x3 and has a steady gait | 2 |
| ☐   Oriented x3 or has a steady gait | 1 |
| ☐   Neither | 0 |
| **Pain or nausea and vomiting** | |
| ☐   Minimal | 2 |
| ☐   Moderate | 1 |
| ☐   Severe | 0 |
| **Surgical bleeding** | |
| ☐   Minimal | 2 |
| ☐   Moderate | 1 |
| ☐   Severe | 0 |
| **Intake and output** | |
| ☐   Has had oral fluid and has voided | 2 |
| ☐   Has had oral fluid or has voided | 1 |
| ☐   Neither | 0 |

Maximum score is 10; patients scoring 9 or 10 are considered fit for discharge home, "x3" means that the patient is oriented sufficiently to know his name, his location and the time

**Table 4.** Modified Postanaesthesia Discharge Scoring System. Maximum score is 10; patients scoring 9 or 10 are considered fit for discharge home

| | |
|---|---|
| **Vital signs** | |
| ☐   Within 20% of preoperative value | 2 |
| ☐   20-40% of preoperative value | 1 |
| ☐   40% of preoperative value | 0 |
| **Ambulation and mental status** | |
| ☐   Steady gait/no dizziness | 2 |
| ☐   With assistance | 1 |
| ☐   No ambulatory or dizziness | 0 |
| **Nausea and vomiting** | |
| ☐   Minimal | 2 |
| ☐   Moderate | 1 |
| ☐   Severe | 0 |
| **Pain** | |
| ☐   Minimal | 2 |
| ☐   Moderate | 1 |
| ☐   Severe | 0 |
| **Surgical bleeding** | |
| ☐   Minimal | 2 |
| ☐   Moderate | 1 |
| ☐   Severe | 0 |

# References


1. Eltringham R, Casey W, Durkin M (1998) Post-operative recovery and pain relief. Springer, London
2. Hatfield A, Tronson M (2001) The complete recovery room book. The Oxford University Press, Oxford
3. Zuck D (1995) Anaesthetic and postoperative recovery rooms. Anaesthesia 50:435-438
4. Dècret n°94-1050 du Décèmbre
5. (1990) A.S.A. Standards for Postanesthesia Care. Approved by House of Delegates on October 12, 1988 and last amended on October 23
6. Torri G (2000) Ruolo della PACU nel postoperatorio. Atti del congresso S.I.A.A.R.T.I Napoli 25-28 Ottobre
7. (1994) S.I.A.A.R.T.I. Raccomandazioni per la sorveglianza Post-anestesiologica
8. (1999) Virtual Congress of the Royal Australians College of Surgeons. www.virtual-congress.racs.edu.au/open/index.htm
9. Gauthier-Lafaye P, Muller A (1998) Anestesia locoregionale e trattamento del dolore. Masson, Milano, p 246
10. Rose DK, Cohen MM, Wigglesworth DF (1994) Critical respiratory events in the postanaesthesia care unit. Anesthesiology 81:410-418
11. Moller JT, Wittruo M, Johansen SH (1990) Hypoxemia in the Postanestesia Care Unit: an observer study. Anesthesiology 73:890
12. Warner MA, Warner ME, Weber JG (1993) Clinical significance of pulmonary aspiration during the perioperative period. Anaesthesiology 78:56
13. Hines R, Barash PG, Watrous G (1992) Complications Occurring in the Postanesthesia Care Unit: A Survey. Anesthesia Analgesia 74:503-509
14. Peskett MJ (1999) Clinical indicators and other complications in the Recovery Room or Post Anaesthetic Care Unit. Anaesthesia 54:1143-1149
15. Rose DK, Cohen MM, DeBoer DP (1996) Cardiovascular events in the Postanaesthesia Care Unit. Anesthesiology 84:772-781
16. Roy WL, Edelist G, Gilbert B (1979) Myocardial ischemia during non-cardiac surgical procedures in patients with coronary-artery disease. Anesthesiology 51:393-397
17. Ashton CM, Petersen NJ, Wray NP (1993) The incidence of perioperative myocardial infarction in men undergoing noncardiac surgery. Annals of Internal Medicine 118:504-510
18. Parr SM, Robinson BI, Glover PW, Galletly DC (1993) Level of consciouness on arrival in the recovery room and the development of early respiratory morbidity. Anest Analg 19:369
19. Parik SS, Chung F (1995) Postoperative delirium in the elderly. Anesth Analg 80:1223
20. Whatcha MF, White PF (1992) Postoperative nausea and vomiting. Its etiology, treatment and prevention. Anesthesiology 77:162
21. Tramer MR, Philips C (1999) Cost-Effectiveness of Ondansetron for postoperative nausea and vomiting. Anaesthesia 54:226-234
22. Frank SM, Fleisher LA, Breslow MJ (1997) Perioperative maintenance of normothermia reduces the incidence of morbid cardiac events. A randomised data. JAMA 277:1127-1134
23. Schmeid H, Kurz A, Sessler DI (1996) Mild hypotermia increases blood loss and trasfusion requirements during total hip arthroplasty. Lancet 347:289-292
24. Paul L (2001) Marino Terapia Intensiva. Masson, Milano
25. Brown M, Brown EM (1997) Comprehensive Postanesthesia Care Williams & Wilkins, Baltimore, Maryland, USA pp 477-479
26. Aldrete JA, Droulik D (1970) A postoperative recovery score. Anesth Analg 49:924
27. Chung F (1995) Discharge criteria a new trend. Can J Anaesth 42:1056-1058

28. Chung F (1995) Are discharge criteria changing. J Clin Anesth (Suppl 1):645-685
29. Leykin Y, Costa N, Gullo A (2001) Recovery Room. Aspetti clinici ed organizzativi. Minerva anestesiologica 67:539-544

# Chapter 14

# Post-operative Respiratory Complications

Y. Leykin, S. Milesi

## Introduction

The positive outcome of any surgical procedure depends on the correct management of the pre-, intra- and post-operative periods. Actually, it is not possible to consider the last as a separate entity even if it has its own properties, it is also the direct evolution of the two preceding periods. Therefore, these periods should be better identified as perioperative medicine [1].

The recovery from anaesthesia can be divided into three phases:
– Phase 1, early recovery: from the end of administration of anaesthetic drugs until the recovery of reflexes and consciousness.
– Phase 2, intermediate recovery: recovery of movement and thinking ability.
– Phase 3, late recovery: complete recovery of psychomotor ability, which can take days and weeks.

The anaesthesiologist is involved in the treatment of the patient in the first and second phases, but the effects will be seen in the following period.

It is important to state what is meant by complication. In fact, in the literature there is not a homogeneous utilization of this word. Some Authors define "complication" as any deviation from a normal course. Other Authors consider complication only an event causing a different outcome (prolonged hospital stay or increased use of antibiotics).

## Effects of General Anaesthesia on the Respiratory System

### Healthy People

The vital capacity (VC) is the lung volume at the end of a maximal inspiration: the VC is composed of the tidal volume ($V_T$), inspiratory reserve and expiratory reserve. It is reduced during anesthesia, with the patient breathing spontaneously and is reduced by 75% after upper abdominal procedures and by 50% after lower abdominal or thoracic operations [2]. Recovery of normal pulmonary function may take several weeks [3].

The functional residual capacity (FRC) is the volume of gas in the lungs at the end of tidal expiration, when the gas flow is zero and the alveolar pressure equals ambient pressure. It is related to the overall respiratory reserve. General anesthesia and the supine position decrease FRC, and atelectatic plaques form in dependent portions of the lungs [4], while positive pressure ventilation and positive end expiratory pressure (PEEP) can minimize this effect.

The closing capacity (CC) is the lung volume above the residual volume at which airways in dependent lung zones begin to close. In most patients, CC is less than FRC. When tidal breathing occurs within the CC range of lung volume, pulmonary blood flow is directed to areas of low ventilation, leading to increased shunt and hypoxemia.

Ventilation/perfusion (V/Q) mismatch is increased due to alveolar hypoventilation and increased closing capacity. During positive pressure ventilation, non-dependent portions of the lung receive a greater proportion of ventilation than do dependent portions. The distribution of pulmonary blood flow is determined by gravity, since blood flow tends to be increased in dependent portions of the lung. Moreover, the hypoxic pulmonary vasoconstriction is impaired. The end result is a variable increase in both physiologic dead space and shunt as compared with spontaneous ventilation.

The respiration mechanics are also modified. In the supine position, the diaphragm is displaced cephalad by abdominal pressure. General anesthesia, muscle paralysis and positive-pressure ventilation profoundly change the pattern of respiratory-muscle use and chest-wall motion.

The ventilatory response to hypercarbia is reduced by inhalation anesthetics, barbiturates and opioids. Carbon dioxide tension ($PaCO_2$) is elevated with spontaneous ventilation during general anesthesia, as is the apneic threshold, that is the $PaCO_2$ at which patients who have had hyperventilation to apnea resume spontaneous ventilation.

The effect on ciliary function is impaired by general anesthesia, especially with high, cold, unhumidified gas flow, which dries secretions and can easily damage respiratory epithelium. Thickened secretions and reduction of ciliary function decrease the patient's resistance to infections.

Biological effects can also be caused by general anesthesia. It decreases the number and the activity of alveolar macrophages, increases the alveolar-capillary permeability, inhibits the release of surfactant, increases the activity of pulmonary nitric oxide synthetase and enhances the sensitivity of the pulmonary vasculature to $\alpha$-adrenergic agonists.

## Elderly Patients

Older age per se is no longer considered a risk factor [5], but the physiological modifications of ageing have to be taken into account when elderly people undergo surgery. Closing capacity increases with age and the forced expiratory volume in 1 s ($FEV_1$) declines by 8-10% each decade because of the decrease of compliance of the pulmonary system and of muscle power [6]. Arterial blood oxygen tension decreases progressively with age-induced ventilation/perfusion mismatch, diffusion, block and anatomical shunt.

Preoperative clinical predictors of adverse pulmonary outcomes are: site of surgery, duration and type of anesthesia, COPD, asthma, preoperative hypersecretion of mucus, and chest deformation. Chronic smoking within 1 month preoperatively increases risk approximately sixfold [5].

## Children

Similar to the adult, also in the normal infant or child, general anesthetics depress respiration, decreasing FRC, vital capacity, and tidal volume; they increase  dead volume/tidal volume ratio, respiratory rate, and ventilation/perfusion mismatch. Pulmonary function, inspiratory muscle tone, and $CO_2/O_2$ ventilation response curve are all depressed. The neonate is particularly susceptible to respiratory depression because of increased $O_2$ requirements (higher metabolic rate). The oxyhaemoglobin dissociation curve for neonates is shifted to the left. This shift represents the increased affinity for oxygen of fetal haemoglobin. A low concentration of 2,3 diphosphoglycerate is responsible for this increased affinity. As a result of the leftward shift of the curve, neonates require a higher haemoglobin level to maintain $O_2$ delivery to the tissue [2].

## Effects of Surgery and Anaesthesia

The effect of anaesthesia, which is of short duration, cannot easily be disjuncted from the effect of surgery (much longer in duration). For example, Rock [4] reported a reduction in FRC for 1-2 weeks after operation, a V/Q mismatch and a reflex effect of the surgical incision on the phrenic nerve.

Operations longer than 4 h have a higher incidence of respiratory complications, together with emergency, thoracic and abdominal surgery [7].

## Post-operative Monitoring

As a consequence of the physio-pathological modifications induced by operation described above it is evident that the patient should be accurately monitored in the immediate post-operative period. The first evaluation is performed upon exit from the OR, and should consider:
- A, Airway (airway not obstructed).
- B, Breathing (thorax movements, colour of the skin).
- C, Circulation (pulse, blood pressure, peripheral perfusion).
- D, Drugs (drugs, infusion, drainage, paddings).
- E, Extras (specific evaluation depending on the operation).
- The following monitoring should be performed at fixed time intervals:
- Consciousness (reflexes, reactivity, answer capability).
- Oxygenation (skin colour, pulse-oxymetry).
- Ventilation (respiratory rate, capnography, blood gas analysis).
- Circulation (perfusion, pulse, blood pressure, ECG, central venous pressure, diuresis).
- Pain.
- Body temperature.
- Hydro-electrolytic balance.

The best location where the patients can be monitored and treated in the post-operative period is the recovery room (RR) and in case of complication the intensive care unit.

## Recovery Room

The RR should be close to the operating theatre, and the laboratory and radiology should be of rapid and easy access.

The number of bays of the RR should be 1.5 per theatre, but if the throughput is rapid, as in day-surgery units, more will be needed.

Temperature should be 21-22 °C and relative humidity 38-45%.

The bays should be surrounded by a large area (standard floor area is about 9 m², but as large as 18 m² may be useful for patients needing a higher level of monitoring or mechanical support) to guarantee an easy access to the head of the patient and the positioning of transport carts, ECGraphs, echographs, medication carts, etc.

An efficient RR should be equipped with all devices needed to deal with all possible postoperative complications. In the RR there should be:

1. A patient trolley or bed, which should have the following characteristics:
   oxygen cylinder with key, gauge, flowmeter, tubing, suitable oxygen masks;
   rapid availability of head-down tilt operated from the head end;
   mounting sites for infusion poles.
2. Every recovery bay should be equipped with: oxygen supply with a set of facial masks and ventilation bags; suction device; ECG, pulse-oxymeter, invasive and non-invasive blood pressure monitor.
3. Cardiorespiratory equipment:
   Appropriate ventilator with disconnecting alarms
   Respiratory device with adequate monitoring (capnography)
   Infusion sets and intravenous cannulae
   Intravenous fluids, both colloids and cristalloids
   Cardiac defibrillator.
   The following should be stored in a "difficult-intubation" trolley:
   Oral and nasopharyngeal airways
   Laryngeal mask airways
   Endotracheal tubes and intubation equipment
   Crico-thyroid puncture set
   Bronchoscopes
   Jet ventilator
   Wright's respirometer.
4. Pediatric equipment.
5. Miscellaneous.
6. Drugs and fluids.

The personnel working in the RR should be highly professionally trained. The nurses should be able to promptly recognise any sign of impairment of the vital signs and provide adequate support to the patients until the anaesthesiologist arrives. There should be one nurse for every two patients.

The anaesthesiologist in charge of the RR can either be in the RR or working in the OR and called for help when needed [8].

## Complications

The definition of complication and the limits of time in which they arise can differ widely, according to the various Authors. Jin and Chung [9] consider mortality associated with anaesthesia and surgery as the death rate within 30 days of operation. Overall mortality in the general population is 1.2% [10]. It becomes higher with ageing: in patients age 60-69 years it is 2.2%, 2.9% in those 70-79 years, 5.8-6.2% in patients over 80 years and 8.9% in those older than 90 years. Abdominal emergency operation on patients older than 80 has a mortality rate of 9.7%. Thoracotomy in patients older than 70 has a mortality rate of 17%. Finally, any type of major surgery performed on patients older than 90 has the highest mortality rate: 19.8%.

The respiratory complications usually include atelectasis, pneumonia, bronchitis, bronchospasm, hypoxemia, respiratory failure and hypoventilation [4, 9]. Hypoxemia and hypoventilation cannot probably be considered complication by themselves, but they may be better considered as symptoms.

In the immediate postoperative period we can usually identify early complications (atelectasis, pneumothorax, aspiration, upper airway obstruction) and symptoms. The most frequent respiratory symptoms are hypoxemia, tachypnoea, dispnoea, bronchospasm, and hypoventilation. It is important to recognize these symptoms early and treat them immediately, because they can lead to complications. Vaughan [11] showed 9.5% (over 1005 patients) with respiratory complication; Abdy [12] reported 2.8% (over 1000 patients), 13 of whom needing reintubation. In the days after surgery, episodic or sustained arterial desaturation may play a role in the development of other complications. In fact, if postoperative hypoxemia develops, tachycardia and hypertension will ensue at a time when anemia decreases arterial oxygen content. This may induce myocardial ischemia in patients with coronary artery stenoses. A recent study showed that postoperative oxygen therapy decreased heart rate and increased arterial oxygen saturation several days after abdominal surgery. Perioperative supplemental oxygen also has been shown to decrease both postoperative nausea and vomiting and surgical wound infections by approximately 50%. Oxygen therapy may be beneficial even if administered for only several hours after surgery, especially in patients who have undergone major abdominal surgery [13, 14].

Regional anesthesia confers a significantly lower risk of postoperative hypoxemia. Epidural analgesia may reduce the incidence of postoperative atelectasis and pulmonary infection especially in older patients.

Postoperatively, the residual effects of anesthetic agents, the prolonged effect of neuromuscular relaxants and post-surgical pain can contribute to pulmonary complications. Respiratory depression is recognised as the most common cause of postoperative death and coma attributable to anesthesia [9].

The high frequency of respiratory "complications" in the first hours after general anesthesia suggests close monitoring of these patients, especially after a long-lasting procedure, when preoperative risk factors are present, and when thoracic, abdominal or emergency surgery was performed.

## Signs of Respiratory Complications

Since the function of the respiratory system is to deliver $O_2$ to the tissues and to eliminate $CO_2$ from the periphery, any respiratory complication will lead to hypoxemia and/or hypercarbia. The signs of a respiratory complication can be erroneously ascribed to other systems, since they can present as alteration of the cardiovascular, neurologic, or gastro-intestinal system. On the other hand, alterations occurring in other systems can reflect on the respiratory system.

Signs of hypoxemia are:
- Cyanosis. Central cyanosis, a bluish colouration of lips, tongue and mucous membrane is a sign of sever hypoxemia. Peripheral cyanosis, blue hands, feet and finger-nail beds, is always present with a central cyanosis, but it may present alone. In this case it may indicate that the patient is cold, has venous congestion or is shocked. This may be difficult to detect in the presence of anemia or poor peripheral perfusion. Cyanosis is detectable when deoxy-haemoglobin is higher than 3 g and it corresponds to $PaO_2$ less than 50 mmHg (6.6 kPa) and oxygen saturation of 85%. Also methylene blue and prylocaine can cause central cyanosis.
- Restlessness and confusion indicate impaired cerebral saturation.
- Tachycardia followed by bradycardia is also a sign of hypoxemia.
Signs of hypercarbia are:
- Tachycardia.
- Hypertension.
- Sweating.
- Irregular pulse, especially bigeminism.
- Flushed skin (vasodilation).
- Clouding of consciousness.

These clinical signs should be confirmed by an arterial blood analysis.

At the beginning of the use of pulse-oxymetry, an interesting study showed that clinical signs of hypoxemia could easily be unrecognized. In a post-anaesthesia care unit, 200 patients were studied: 55% had one or more mild hypoxemic episodes ($SpO_2$ < 90%), 28% showed one or more episodes with $SpO_2$ < 85% and 13% had severe hypoxemia ($SpO_2$ < 80%), recorded by the pulse-oxymeter. These episodes occurred even when supplemental oxygen was administered (in 55% of the episodes, corresponding to 32% of the patients). Of these episodes, 95% were clinically unrecognized by the staff. This study suggested that hypoxemia is more common and severe than previously assumed and it can be detected by the pulse-oxymeter; however, the Authors did not find any correlation between hypoxemia and post-operative complications [15]. By contrast, Greif [13, 14] demonstrated in recent studies that oxygen administration reduced post-operativer wound infection, nausea and vomiting.

The causes that may lead to the previously cited signs are as follows:

*(a) Upper Airway Obstruction*

A partial obstruction of the upper airway is characterised by stertorous breathing, use of the accessory muscle to breathe, external paradoxical respiration (movements of abdomen and thorax not synchronous, but in different phases). A complete obstruction is characterised by no movement of air detectable at the airway, no breath sounds, signs of hypoxia and hypercarbia.

The causes are:

1. The tongue may fall back and obstruct the pharynx in the unconscious patient.
2. Foreign materials in the pharynx (mucus or saliva, gastric content from vomiting, blood, teeth, etc.).
3. Laryngospasm, due to stimulation of the larynx during emergence from anesthesia (foreign body, suction extubation).
4. Laryngeal oedema, due to trauma, intubation or infection. It is especially dangerous in children, in whom a small amount of reactive oedema will rapidly occlude the narrow lumen of the larynx.
5. External pressure on the trachea due to enlarging haematoma following neck surgery (thyroidectomy, carotid surgery) or jugular cannulation;
6. Paralysis of vocal cords following lesion of recurrent laryngeal nerve during total thyroidectomy or as a complication of intubation.
7. Tracheal collapse following thyroidectomy.

*Management*

- Extend the neck.
- Lift the jaw forward.
- Insert oral or nasal airway.
- Turn the patient on lateral decubitus.
- Trendelemburg position to facilitate the elimination of foreign materials.
- Apply suction to the pharynx.
- Should these manouvers be unsuccessful, then laryngoscopy is needed to clear the pharynx under vision.
- If the cords are in spasm, give oxygen by anaesthetic face mask. Apply gentle pressure to the reservoir bag to overcome the spasm.
- If unsuccessful, give succinylcholine to relax the cords and ventilate the lung. Endotracheal intubation may be necessary.
- If the cause of upper airway obstruction is laryngeal oedema, the management should be as follows:

- Sitting position to improve venous drainage.
- Steroids.
- Humidification.
- Diuretics.
- Inhalation of racemic epinephrine.
- If no other solution is possible to solve the obstruction, emergency cricothyrotomy should be performed.

## (b) Hypoventilation

Hypoventilation is a reduced alveolar ventilation resulting in an increased arterial carbon dioxide tension ($PaCO_2$). In the postoperative period it can be due to reduced respiratory drive, reduced muscle function or as the direct result of acute or chronic lung disease and to conditions affecting the mechanics of respiration.

1. Depression of respiratory drive occurs with any anaesthetic agent. Opiates, barbiturates and inhalation agents all depress the respiratory centre. Opiates effects can be reversed by use of small doses of antagonists, without eliminating the analgesic effect. But the effect of an antagonist may be of shorter duration than that of opiates. A low $PaCO_2$ following hyperventilation during anesthesia and the loss of hypoxic drive following administration of high oxygen concentration mixture to patients suffering from chronic lung disease are also causes of the depression of respiratory drive.
   *Management*
   - Administration of naloxone 0.1-0.4 mg i.v. (administered 0.1 mg every 2-3 min  titrated to effect). The onset of action is in 1-2 min and the duration of action of 0.4 mg is about 45 min in an adult of 70 kg. The reported half-life is 60-90 min in adults and 3 h in neonates [16].

2. Muscle function is impaired after surgery, and vital capacity is reduced in nearly all patients to the greatest extent on the day of surgery. The impairment of diaphragmatic function results in reduced carbon dioxide elimination and oxygenation. Inadequate ventilation may also result from residual muscle paralysis due to the use of neuromuscular blocking agents or from neuromuscular disease.
   *Management*
   The treatment will depend on whether the residual paralysis is due to depolarising (phase I) or non-depolarising (phase II) block. The record of anesthetic will usually clarify the type of block, but if doubt remains two tests may add information.
   - Peripheral nerve stimulation. If a train of 4 supramaximal stimuli at a frequency of 2 Hz is applied to the ulnar nerve, contraction of the hand muscles will result. A fade with successive stimuli indicates a non-depolarising (phase II) block. Significant paralysis is present if the ratio of the fourth to the first response is 50%.

- Edrophonium test. Intravenous administration of this short-acting anti-cholinesterase drug will increase muscle strength if a non-depolarising (phase II) block is present. It is advisable not to use the longer-acting neostigmine as it will exacerbate a depolarising block.

*Phase I block.* If succinylcholine is not metabolised in 5-10 min, the following should be suspected:

(a)   Abnormal cholinesterase (rare inherited condition).
(b)   Reduced amounts of cholinesterase (liver disease or malnutrition).
(c)   Concurrent administration of anti-cholinesterase (e.g. ecothiophate used in the treatment of glaucoma).

The recovery can be facilitated administering cholinesterase with fresh frozen plasma. The blood of the patient should then be checked for cholinesterase and dibucaine (pathologic if lower than 80%).

*Phase II block* may be due to:

(a)   Excessive administration of muscle relaxants.
(b)   Sensitivity to relaxants (myasthenia gravis).
(c)   Potentiation of relaxants (hypokalemia, acidosis, large quantities of antibiotics, hypocalcemia).
(d)   Impaired excretion or metabolism of relaxants.
(e)   Excessive administration of depolarising relaxants.

The treatment consists of ventilation control, administration of neostigmine, correction of acidosis or electrolyte imbalance.

3. Bronchospasm is a cause of hypoventilation. Pre-existing asthma or chronic obstructive pulmonary disease can lead to bronchospasm after surgery, but also pulmonary oedema and aspiration can present with bronchospasm. Therefore it is of greatest importance to find the etiology before starting the treatment.
   *Management*
   - Oxygen, bronchodilators, steroids, in case of asthma.
   - Diuretics, vasodilators, inotropic agents in case of pulmonary oedema.

4. Conditions affecting the mechanics of respiration can be:
   (a)   Pain from a high abdominal or thoracic incision.
   (b)   Obesity.
   (c)   Tight abdominal or thoracic strapping.
   (d)   Pneumothorax or haemothorax.
   *Management*
   - Oxygen.
   - Sitting position.
   - Analgesia.
   - Physiotherapy.
   - X-ray to verify lung expansion and drainage of pneumothorax or haemothorax.

## Our Experience

In the years 2000-2002, in our Medical Centre 22,634 surgical procedures requiring anaesthesia were performed. Immediately after surgery, the patients were treated either in the operating theatre or, those who needed more than 1 h observation or who had developed any anomalous symptoms, in the recovery room. All patients were administered $O_2$ supplementation.

A total of 3,125 patients were admitted to the RR. There were no deaths. The overall rate of anomalous symptoms or complications was 2.5% and 2.9% in the first and second year, respectively. Of the patients admitted to the RR, 0.02% developed respiratory symptoms (Table 1).

**Table 1.** Respiratory complications in recovery room

|  | 1st year | 2nd year | Total |
|---|---|---|---|
| Number of operations | 11,626 | 11,008 | 22,634 |
| Patients admitted to the RR | 1,047 | 985 | 2,032 |
| Hypoxemia | 26 | 4 | 30 |
| Dispnoea | 3 | 3 | 6 |
| Tachypnoea | 5 | 2 | 7 |
| Bronchospasm | 3 | 3 | 6 |
| Total of symptoms | 37 | 12 | 49 |

## How To Prevent or Reduce the Risk of Complications

Reducing complications is a primary medical goal. A first step is to identify any patient with a possible pre-existing pathology which if treated before surgery could improve the surgical outcome. Asthma, chronic obstructive pulmonary disease and obstructive sleep apnoea will be briefly discussed below.

In the history of the patient it is also very important to check for any sign of dyspnoea, coughing and wheezing, or smoking [9].

*Asthma.* Risk factors include recent asthma symptoms, recent use of anti-asthma drugs or therapy for asthma symptoms in a medical facility, and history for tracheal intubation for asthma [4]. Usually the airway hyperreactivity persists for several weeks after an acute episode of asthma. Improvement in asthma symptoms does not exclude the development of bronchospasm in response to various stimuli.

*Management*
- Steroids 24-48 h before surgery; these can be discontinued after surgery without tapering, in the absence of bronchospasm.
- $\beta_2$-adrenergic agents for patients with wheezing.
- Use of laryngeal mask airway, which is associated with fewer airway reactions.

*Chronic obstructive pulmonary disease (COPD).* Patients with COPD are at high risk for the development of complications.

*Management*
- Stop smoking: cessation 24-48 h before surgery decreases carboxyhaemoglobin levels to normal, abolishes the stimulant effects of nicotine on the cardiovascular system, and improves respiratory ciliary beating. More than 4-6 weeks are required to improve lung function [4].
- Respiratory infections should be treated with antibiotics.
- If bronchospasm is present, it should be treated.
- Patients may have chronically fatigued respiratory muscles. Impaired nutrition, electrolyte and endocrine disorders can contribute to respiratory muscle weakness and should be corrected before surgery. Pulmonary rehabilitation before surgery is helpful in reducing complications.

*Obstructive sleep apnoea (OSA).* This is a breathing disorder characterized by repeated collapse of the upper airway during the rapid eye movement phase of sleep, with cessation of breathing. It is most common in men, obese and elderly patients. Almost all patients with OSA have a history of snoring. Associated conditions are hypertension, arrhythmias, congestive heart failure, coronary artery disease, and stroke. These patients are likely to have worsening of their disease process after anaesthesia and may be at postoperative risk for development of more episodes of apnea and more severe episodes of hypoxemia.

*Management*
- Judicious use of sedatives.
- Difficult-airway precautions are appropriate, including availability of laryngeal mask airway, fiberoptic bronchoscope, and a tracheotomy kit.
- Short-acting agents are preferred.
- Non-invasive ventilatory devices such as BiPAP should be available postoperatively.
- Postoperative narcotic analgesia should be avoided.

To minimize complications after general anesthesia [4, 9], remember that:
1. In elderly people, the opioid perioperative requirements are lower than in younger patients.
2. Short- or intermediate-acting neuromuscular relaxants have to be used and antagonists should be given to reverse their residual effects.
3. Supplemental oxygen should be administered by facemask during awakening from anesthesia and for several days to prevent late nocturnal hypoxemia.

## References


1. Leykin Y, Zannier G (2002) Focus sulla recovery room: aspetti organizzativi. Minerva anestesiologica 68 (Suppl 1)9:221
2. Bell C, Kain ZN (eds) (1997) The pediatric anesthesia handbook Yale University St. Louis, Missouri, USA
3. Sheperd KE (1997) Specific considerations with pulmonary disease pp35-46. In: WE Hurford, MT Bailin, JK Davison, KL Haspel and C Rosow (eds) Clinical Anesthesia procedures of the Massachusetts General Hospital, Lippincott Williams & Wilkins, Philadelphia, PA, USA
4. Rock P (2002) Evaluation and perioperative management of the patient with respiratory disease. American Society of Anesthesiologists Annual Meeting Refresher Course Lectures 253, pp 1-7 Orlando, Florida October 12-16
5. Smetana GW (1999) Preoperative pulmonary evaluation. N Engl J Med 340:937-944
6. Knudson RJ, Lebowitz MD, Holberg CJ, Burrows B (1983) Changes in the normal maximal expiratory flow-volume curve with growth and ageing. Am Rev Respir Dis 127:725-734
7. Klotz HP, Candinas D, Platz A et al (1996) Preoperative risk assessment in elective general surgery. Br J Surg 83:1788-1791
8. Eltringham R, Casey W and Durkin M (1998) Post-operative recovery and pain relief. Springer-Verlag London
9. Jin F, Chung F (2001) Minimizing perioperative adverse events in the elderly. Br J Anaesth 87:608-624
10. Pedersen T, Eliasen K, Henriksen E (1990) A prospective study of mortality associated with anaesthesia and surgery: risk indicators of mortality in hospital. Acta Anaesthesiol Scand 34:176-182
11. Vaughan RS (1997) Airway management in the recovery room. Anaesthesia 52:617-618
12. Abdy S (1999) An audit of airway problems in the recovery room. Anaesthesia 54:372-392
13. Greif R (1999) Supplemental oxygen reduces the incidence of postoperative nausea and vomiting. Anesthesiology 91:1246-1252
14. Greif R (2000) Supplemental perioperative to reduce the incidence of surgical wound infection. N Engl J Med 342:167-167
15. Moller JT, Wittrup M, Johansen SH (1990) Hypoxemia in the postanaesthesia care unit: an observer study. Anesthesiology 73:890-895
16. Stern RJ (1997) Drugs, diseases and anesthesia. Lippincott-Raven Publishers Philadelphia PA USA

# INTENSIVE CARE

# Debate on Cardiac Resynchronisation Therapy

M. ZECCHIN, G. SINAGRA

Intraventricular delay, especially left bundle branch block (LBBB), is present in up to 20% of patients with heart failure due to left ventricular (LV) dysfunction and can be considered a marker of disease. Although LBBB has been always considered a consequence rather than a cause of LV impairment, the delayed movement of the lateral wall towards the interventricular septum leads to a waste of energy and a reduced efficacy of LV contraction.

In 1990, experimental studies on animals suggested that a simultaneous stimulation of both ventricles has "a favourable effect on systolic function and on diastolic relaxation" [1]. The first human trials were carried out in 1996 on a few patients with advanced heart failure, extremely severe LV dysfunction and very long QRS interval. The good results of these initial studies led to the first cross-over study, the PATH-CHF [2]. Forty-two patients with class III-IV heart failure and QRS duration > 120 ms underwent implantation of two pacemakers (one traditionally stimulating the right ventricle, the other stimulating the left ventricle through a pericardial electrode and triggered by right ventricle stimulation). The study showed a clear improvement of patients during biventricular pacing and worsening of heart failure when the stimulation was switched off. In addition, hospitalization for heart failure was greatly reduced in the year following implantation.

Subsequently, the MUSTIC [3], but especially the MIRACLE [4] trials clearly confirmed the role of biventricular stimulation in improving signs and symptoms of heart failure, quality of life, exercise duration and LV performance. Benefits with respect to survival are also likely, but controlled data are still lacking and the results of ongoing or recently completed studies with mortality as a primary end-point are awaited. In the COMPANION [5] study, 1520 patients with heart failure (III or IV NYHA class), LV ejection fraction $\geq$ 35%, LV end-diastolic diameter $\geq$ 60 mm and QRS duration $\geq$ 120 on optimal medical treatment (including beta-blockers) were randomized to conventional treatment, conventional treatment+biventricular stimulation (RCT), or conventional treatment+implantable defibrillator with biventricular stimulation (RCT+ICD). The results showed a 36% reduction in total mortality in the RCT+ICD group vs. the conventional treatment group. The RCT group had an intermediate effect, with a nearly significant 23% reduction of mortality (P = 0.059).

Since then, many studies on cardiac resynchronization therapy (CRT) have been published (Table 1) and many others are ongoing (Table 2).

**Table 1.** Studies on long-term effects of cardiac resynchronization therapy (CRT)

| | End of study | Patients (n) | Randomized | Inclusion criteria | Follow-up (months) | Effect of CRT |
|---|---|---|---|---|---|---|
| French Pilot [21] | 1998 | 50 | No | III/IV cl. | 15 | -1.5 NYHA, +40% $VO_2$ peak |
| InSync [22] | 1998 | 103 | No | III/IV cl. | 12 | -1.2 NYHA, +40% QOL, +60% in 6 min WT |
| InSync Italian Registry [23] | 2000 | 190 | No | II/IV cl. | 10 | +31% in 6 min WT, +60% QOL |
| PATH-CHF [2] | 1998 | 42 | No | III/IV cl., QRS > 120 ms | 3 | +22% in 6 min WT, +43% QOL, +20% $VO_2$ peak |
| MUSTIC SR [3] | 1999 | 67 | Yes | III cl., EF < 35%, EDD > 60 mm, QRS > 150 ms | 3 | +23% in 6 min WT, +32% QOL, +8% $VO_2$ peak |
| MUSTIC AF [18] | 1999 | 43 | Yes | III cl., EF < 35%, EDD > 60 mm, AF | 3 | +9% in 6 min WT, +13% $VO_2$ peak |
| MIRACLE [12] | 2000 | 453 | Yes | III/IV cl., EF ≤ 35%, EDD ≥ 55 mm, QRS ≥ 130 ms, 6 min WT ≤ 450 s | 6 | +13% in 6 min WT, +13% QOL |
| COMPANION* [5] | 2002 | 1520 | Yes | III/IV cl., EF ≤ 35%, EDD ≥ 60 mm, QRS ≥ 120 ms | 12 | *-24% in mortality; -19% deaths/hospitalization[a] |

* Effect of *CRT* only (*CRT*+defibrillator excluded)
*Cl*, NYHA functional class; *AF*, atrial fibrillation; *EF*, left ventricular ejection fraction; *EDD*, left ventricular end-diastolic diameter; *QOL*, Quality of life; *SR*, sinus rhythm; *WT*, walking test

**Table 2.** Ongoing studies [23] on CRT

| Study | Inclusion criteria | Follow-up | Primary end-point |
|---|---|---|---|
| CARE-HF | III/IV cl., EF < 35%, QRS > 150 ms (or > 120 ms + dissynchrony at echo) | 1.5 years | Death/cardiovascular, hospitalization |
| PACMAN | III/IV cl., EF < 35%, QRS > 150 ms | 6 months crossover | 6 min WT |
| PATH-CHF II | II/IV cl., EF < 35%, QRS > 120 ms | 6 months crossover | 6 min WT and $VO_2$ |
| Ventak | II/IV cl., EF < 35%, QRS > 120 ms | 3 months crossover | $VO_2$ |
| VECTOR | II/IV cl., EF < 35%, QRS > 140 ms | 6 months crossover | 6 min WT and QOL |
| PAVE | AV node ablation/chronic AF | 6 months | 6 min WT and QOL |
| BELIEVE | II/IV cl., EF < 35%, QRS > 130 ms | 1 year | Echo parameters |
| Insync III | III/IV cl., EF < 35%, QRS > 130 ms | 6 months | 6 min WT and QOL |
| MIRACLE ICD | II/IV cl., EF < 35%, QRS > 130 ms | 6 months crossover | 6 min WT and QOL |
| OPTISITE | AV node ablation/chronic AF | 6 months | 6 min WT and QOL |

For abbreviations, see Table 1.

## Mechanisms

In patients with LBBB, fibers in the posterolateral wall of the left ventricle shorten in a very late phase of the cardiac cycle, when the interventricular septum has already begun its relaxation. The delayed contraction of some LV segments, in patients with LBBB (representing mechanical LV asynchrony) not only reflects a loss of systolic force, but also causes inappropriate energy consumption and increased LV wall stress in early diastole. This would presumably interfere with regional myocardial perfusion that could, in turn, further reduce LV systolic performance and aggravate remodeling. Moreover, since cardiac resynchronization therapy (CRT) reduces the number of segments displaying delayed contraction, pacing not only improves systolic function by recruiting this contractile reserve, but also facilitates diastolic filling of the left ventricle [6].

Finally, the delayed contraction of the posterolateral wall impairs the efficiency of posterior papillary muscle, favoring mitral regurgitation. It is well known that the presence of functional mitral regurgitation in heart failure is strongly dependent on alterations in LV shape, as the tethering forces that act on the mitral leaflets are higher in dilated, more spherical ventricles [7]. However, ventricular asynchrony might, independently from LV geometry, alter the leaflet-tethering forces and aggravate functional mitral regurgitation. As experimental studies convincingly demonstrate, it is not isolated papillary muscle dysfunction per se that causes functional mitral regurgitation, but altered papillary displacement by dysfunction and remodeling of the underlying myocardium. Thus, asynchronous activation of the medial and lateral segments supporting the papillary muscles might independently contribute to functional mitral regurgitation severity in heart failure [8]. CRT in selected patients with advanced heart failure and electrical conduction delay acutely reduces the severity of mitral regurgitation by decreasing the effective orifice area. This effect is directly related to an improvement in LV systolic function, causing an accelerated rise in the transmitral pressure gradient, which effectively counteracts the increased tethering forces that impair mitral valve competence.

CRT improves LV function without increasing global LV oxidative metabolism; it actually reduces oxygen consumption (unlike inotropic stimulation) [9] resulting in improved myocardial efficiency. Oxidative metabolism of the interventricular septum increases relative to the lateral wall [6]. As a consequence, there is also a significant decrease in catecholaminergic activation [10], so that RCT can be included in the group of therapies acting on neuro-hormonal activation (e.g. ACE-inhibitors, beta-blockers and potassium-sparing diuretics) and is not only a "mechanical" treatment.

## Identification of Responders

Not all patients with heart failure, LV dysfunction and LBBB have the same benefit from RCT. About 20-30% of subjects treated do not show any improvement.

Thus, considering the cost and technical difficulties of implantation, a correct selection of patients is mandatory.

An important issue in patient selection is the etiology of heart failure. Patients with ischemic heart disease, and in particular those with previous myocardial infarction, may benefit less from RCT [11]. It is possible that, in the presence of ischemic/necrotic tissue (for example, an akinetic interventricular septum), an earlier contraction of the posterolateral wall makes little contribution to LV performance. It is also possible that the pacing lead may not be placed at the optimal site with regard to ischemic areas. Today, the relation between the pacing site and ischemic areas needs to be better defined in order to decrease the proportion of nonresponder patients, potentially due to a rather detrimental pacing site for cardiac function [11]. However, the benefit in terms of death or hospitalization was similar in ischemic and non-ischemic patients in the COMPANION Study [5].

As discussed earlier, intraventricular delay may in some patients lead to functional mitral regurgitation. As a consequence, in these patients there is consistent benefit from RCT, as mitral regurgitation can dramatically decrease just after implantation. Moreover, many studies [11, 12] have confirmed that mitral regurgitation significantly improves in patients treated with CRT.

One of the first parameters evaluated in predicting CRT results was the QRS duration before implantation and the reduction of QRS after biventricular stimulation. The longer the QRS the greater the desynchronization, and the greater the QRS reduction the more physiological the LV contraction. Actually, there is some association between QRS duration and septal to posterolateral wall delay, as well as a significant correlation between QRS duration and acute response in term of $dP/dT$. In addition, a large reduction of the QRS interval (i.e. > 25%) is usually accompanied by a long-term improvement [11]. However, there is an increasing awareness that QRS duration and QRS reduction after stimulation have little importance in predicting long-term results. Responders and nonresponders presented with a similar QRS duration before pacemaker implantation [11], and CRT resulted in a similar degree of QRS narrowing in both groups. Improvement was evident also in patients with narrow (120-150 ms) QRS [13]. This is not surprising because it has been shown that electro-mechanical resynchronization may not be apparent on the surface electrocardiogram. Indeed, LV pacing alone may provide short-term clinical improvement in patients with heart failure, even when the paced QRS complex is wider than in sinus rhythm. LBBB may be the result of abnormalities that do not necessarily cause late contraction of the left free wall (e.g. peripheral conduction defect or global LV dysfunction), and the same QRS morphology and duration can lead to different patterns of LV contraction and different responses to CRT. Thus, the detection of mechanical, rather than electrical, asynchrony with imaging (especially echo-Doppler) techniques is the best way to select patients who can benefit from CRT. The interventricular delay (measured evaluating the interval between opening of the pulmonary and aortic valves) is of little value; more important is the delay between different LV segments, especially between the septum and the posterolateral wall. This can be evaluated, for example, with M-mode echo measuring the difference between the maximum systolic excursion of the interventricular septum and the maximum systolic excursion of the LV posterior wall [14]. Tissue Doppler imaging (TDI) is a relatively new technique for measuring direction and velocity of a tissue (i.e. ventricular wall). More complex TDI modalities allow visualization of the longitudinal motion amplitude in each myocardial segment during systole and determination of whether this motion represents contraction or is merely passive. Pre-implantation TDI screening may improve the selection of candidates likely to benefit from CRT [15]. This hypothesis is currently being tested in a substudy in the Cardiac Resynchronization in Heart Failure study (CARE-HF) [16]. However, there are many technical problems (for example, M-mode evaluation of maximum systolic displacement in patients with very poor systolic function, or obtaining good images of TDI in some patients), and a clear standardization of methods is still lacking.

## Right Bundle Branch Block

Although most of information on CRT was acquired in patients with LBBB, the largest trials did not exclude patients with intraventricular delay due to right bundle branch block (RBBB). The delayed contraction of the right ventricle can hide a "reversed" desynchronization of the LV walls, as the septum can be activated later than the LV posterolateral wall. As a matter of fact, in some patients, but not in all, this interval can be consistent. Garrigue *et al.* showed [17] that a large interval between setpal and LV lateral wall activation and a significant reduction of this interval were associated with significant clinical and functional improvement in patients with RBBB, while a reduction of interventicular activation (measured by the time difference between the electromechanical delay of the right ventricular (RV) free wall and that of the LV septal wall) again was of little value. Therefore, an accurate echocardiographic evaluation can identify also patients with RBBB who may benefit from RCT.

## Atrial Fibrillation

To avoid spontaneous beats or inconstant stimulation, patients in atrial fibrillation (AF) who are candidates for RCT must be pacemaker-dependent (because of advanced spontaneous AV block or AV junction ablation). The first published clinical trial on RCT excluded patients with AF, but recent studies have shown a clear benefit also in these patients. In the MUSTIC trial, the peak $VO_2$ increase, the reduction in the Minnesota score, the NYHA class improvement, and the mitral regurgitation reduction at 12 months were similar in patients with sinus rhythm and those with AF [18]. The effect was not due merely to the regularization of cardiac rhythm, as biventricular stimulation was superior to RV stimulation alone in patients with AF and AV junctional ablation [19].

## Conclusions

Despite the recent introduction into clinical practice and technical difficulties due to catheter positioning, CRT can no longer be considered an investigational treatment. It has been already included as IIa indication (weight of opinion is in favor of usefulness) for treatment of patients with dilated cardiomyopathy, NYHA class III heart failure and QRS duration $\geq$ 130 ms in the ACC/AHA/NASPE 2002 Guideline Update for Implantation of Cardiac Pacemakers and Antiarrhythmia Devices [20]. Many clinical trials have demonstrated that CRT can improve heart failure symptoms and LV function in selected patients. However, some issues are not resolved yet. First, it is not well understood why and which patients do not improve with CRT: with respect to an "electrical" stratification of patients, when QRS duration and its reduction should be considered. We therefore apply a "mechanically based" identification, with echocardiographic techniques, of patients who are more likely to benefit from this novel therapy. Second, the benefit of CRT in terms of life expectancy remains to be clarified. Although some preliminary data show favorable results on cardiac mortality (MIRACLE, COMPANION) and possibly on sudden death (probably due to neuro-hormonal effects), the results of ongoing or recently completed studies must be awaited in order to have a definitive answer.

## References


1. Mower MM (1990) Preliminary animal studies on biventricular pacing. Clin Res 38:822A
2. Stellbrink C, Breithardt OA, Franke A et al (2001) PATH-CHF (PAcing THerapies in Congestive Heart Failure) Investigators; CPI Guidant Congestive Heart Failure Research Group: Impact of cardiac resynchronization therapy using hemodynamically optimized pacing on left ventricular remodeling in patients with congestive heart failure and ventricular conduction disturbances. J Am Coll Cardiol 38:1957-1965
3. Cazeau S, Leclercq C, Lavergne T et al (2001) for the Multisite Stimulation in Cardiomyopathy. Effects of multisite biventricular pacing in patients with heart failure and intraventricular conduction delay. N Engl J Med 12:873-880
4. Abraham W, Fisher WG, Smith AL et al (2001) The Multicenter InSync Randomised ClinicaL Evaluation (MIRACLE)—results of a double blind controlled trial to assess resynchronisation therapy in heart failure patients. J Am Coll Cardiol 38:604-605
5. Bristow MR, Saxon LA et al (2004) Cardiac-resynchronization therapy with or without an implantable defibrillator in advanced chronic heart failure. N Engl J Med 350:2140-2150
6. Ukkonen H, Beanlands RSB, Burwash IG et al (2003) Effect of Cardiac Resynchronization on Myocardial Efficiency and Regional Oxidative Metabolism. Circulation 107:28-31
7. Kono T, Sabbah HN, Stein PD et al (1991) Left ventricular shape as a determinant of functional mitral regurgitation in patients with severe heart failure secondary to either coronary artery disease or idiopathic dilated cardiomyopathy. Am J Cardiol 68:355-359
8. Breithardt OA, Sinha AM, Schwammenthal E et al (2003) Acute Effects of Cardiac Resynchronization Therapy on Functional Mitral Regurgitation in Advanced Systolic Heart Failure. J Am Coll Cardiol 41:765-770

9.  Nelson GS, Berger RD, Fetics BJ et al (2000) Left ventricular or biventricular pacing improves cardiac function at diminished energy cost in patients with dilated cardiomyopathy and left bundle branch block. Circulation 102:3053–3059

10. Hamdan MH, Zagrodzky JD, Joglar JA et al (2000) Biventricular Pacing Decreases Sympathetic Activity Compared With Right Ventricular Pacing in Patients With Depressed Ejection Fraction. Circulation 102:1027-1032

11. Reuter S, Garrigue S, Barolo SS et al (2002) Comparison of Characteristics in Responders Versus Nonresponders With Biventricular Pacing for Drug-Resistant Congestive Heart Failure. Am J Cardiol 89:346-350

12. Sutton MGJ, Plappert T, Abraham WT et al for the Multicenter InSync Randomized Clinical Evaluation (MIRACLE) Study Group (2003) Effect of Cardiac Resynchronization Therapy on Left Ventricular Size and Function in Chronic Heart Failure. Circulation 107:1985-1990

13. Gasparini M, Mantica M, Galimberti P et al (2003) Beneficial effects of biventricular pacing in patients with a "narrow" QRS. PACE 26:169-174

14. Pitzalis MV, Iacovello M, Romito R et al (2002) Cardiac resynchronization therapy tailored by echocardiographic evaluation of ventricular asynchrony. J Am Coll Cardiol 9:1615-1622

15. Søgaard P, Egeblad H, Kim WY et al (2002) Tissue Doppler Imaging Predicts Improved Systolic Performance and Reversed Left Ventricular Remodeling During Long-Term Cardiac Resynchronization Therapy. J Am Coll Cardiol 40:723–730

16. Cleland JGF, Daubert JC, Erdmann E et al (2001) The CARE-HF study: rationale, design and end-points. Eur J Heart Fail 3:481–489

17. Garrigue S, Reuter S, Labeque JN et al (2001) Usefulness of biventricular pacing in patients with congestive heart failure and right bundle branch block. Am J Cardiol 88:1436-1441

18. Linde C, Leclercq C, Rex S et al (2002) Long-Term Benefits of Biventricular Pacing in Congestive Heart Failure: Results from the MUltisite STimulation in cardiomyopathy (MUSTIC) study. J Am Coll Cardiol 40:111–118

19. Leon AR, Greenberg JM, Kanuru N et al (2002) Cardiac Resynchronization in Patients With Congestive Heart Failure and Chronic Atrial Fibrillation. Effect of Upgrading to Biventricular Pacing After Chronic Right Ventricular Pacing. J Am Coll Cardiol 39:1258–1263

20. ACC/AHA/NASPE (2002) Guideline Update for Implantation of Cardiac Pacemakers and Antiarrhythmia Devices: Summary Article Circulation 106:2145-2161

21. Leclercq C, Cazeau S et al (2000) A pilot experience with permanent biventricular pacing to treat advanced heart failure. Am Heart J 140:862-870

22. Gras D, Mabo P, Tang T et al (1998) Multisite pacing as a supplemental treatment of congestive heart failure: preliminary results of the Medtronic Inc. InSync Study Pacing Clin Electrophysiol 21:2249-2255

23. Leclercq C, Kass DA (2002) Retiming the failing heart: principles and current clinical status of cardiac resynchronization. J Am Coll Cardiol 39:194-201

# Chapter 16

# Acute Pulmonary Embolism: Hemodynamic Aspects and Treatment

G. DELLA ROCCA, C. COCCIA, I. REFFO

Pulmonary embolism (PE) is a major international health problem, with an annual estimated incidence of over 100,000 cases in France, 65,000 cases among hospitalized patients in England and Wales, and at least 60,000 new cases per year in Italy. The diagnosis is often untreated, difficult to obtain and is frequently missed [1]. Mortality in the untreated is approximately 30%, but with adequate treatment this can be reduced to 2-8%. Numerous cases go unrecognized and hence untreated, with poor outcomes. Indeed the prevalence of PE at autopsy (approximately 12-15% in hospitalized patients) has not changed over three decades [2].

PE may occur as a single event or in the form of successive episodes. The prognosis may be influenced in the acute and post-acute phases. In the acute phase, a first attack may cause death, produce mild or severe clinical consequences or no symptoms at all. In general, anatomically large emboli pose a greater threat than small ones. In rare cases, however, embolization of the peripheral branches of the pulmonary arteries, leaving the main branches free, may produce symptoms of marked severity and even cause sudden and unexpected death [3]. There is a considerable risk of recurrent PE, especially during the first 4-6 weeks [4, 5]. The risk is greatly increased in the absence of anticoagulant therapy [6]. Hence, the short-term outcome of patients who survive an initial PE episode is influenced greatly by whether or not therapy is instituted. This action, in turn, is obviously determined by whether or not a timely diagnosis is made [6, 7]. Right ventricular afterload stress, detected by echocardiography, is a major determinant of short-term prognosis when PE is clinically suspected [8, 9] and detection of a patent foramen is a significant predictor of an ischemic and morbidity in patients with major PE [10]. The onset of massive PE may be preceded by a number of smaller PEs, which often escape the attention of clinicians. Multiples PEs and infarcts of different age (recent, organizing and organized) are found at necroscopy in 15-60% of cases [4]. This finding is important, since it means that these patients suffered from successive emboli and that death might have been prevented if an early diagnosis had been made.

Both the magnitude of embolization and the absence or presence of pre-existing cardiopulmonary disease [11, 12] are responsible for the hemodynamic consequences of acute PE, in terms of pulmonary artery and systemic pressure, right atrial pressure, cardiac output, pulmonary vascular resistance and input impedance, and coronary blood flow.

For clinical purposes, the Task Force on Pulmonary Embolism, European Society of Cardiology [1], has classified PE into two main groups: massive and non-massive. Massive PE consists of shock and/or hypotension (defined as a systolic blood pressure < 90 mmHg or a pressure drop of ≥ 40 mmHg for major > 15 min if not caused by new-onset arrhythmia, hypovolemia or sepsis). Otherwise, non-massive can be diagnosed. A subgroup of patients with non-massive PE may be identified by echocardiographic signs of right ventricular (RV) hypokinesis. The Task Force proposes that this subgroup be called sub-massive, because there is growing evidence that the prognosis of this patients group may be different from those with non-massive PE and normal right ventricular function.

The *pathophysiology* of circulatory failure due to PE is primarly caused by a reduced cross-sectional area of the pulmonary vascular bed and by pre-existing cardiac or pulmonary disease [12, 13]. This occurs because of the mechanical effect of the embolus itself, as well as secondary effects, including hypoxic/acidotic vasoconstriction and release of vasoactive substances. The resultant increase in pulmonary arterial pressure leads to increased RV afterload, myocardial wall tension and oxygen consumption [12].

In PE, the acute increase in pulmonary arterial pressure causes an increase in RV afterload and in right ventricular end-diastolic pressure. The consequent depression in RV performance and the RV distension depends on the extent of thromboembolism and on cardiopulmonary compensatory mechanisms. It is likely that the sequence of events that follows is more profound in acute PE, because the right ventricle is not hypertrophied and thus less able to overcome the initial increase in afterload. The increase in RV afterload and the RV dilation lead to an increase in RV myocardial work and oxygen consumption [14]. RV failure results in reduced LV preload whereas the increase in RV-end-diastolic pressure reverses the diastolic trans-septal pressure gradient [15]. The leftward shift of the interventricular septum and the pericardial constraint in the face of RV dilatation results in diastolic ventricular interdependence, decreased LV end diastolic volume and consequent decrease of LV output [16, 17]. The impaired LV diastolic function contributes to low cardiac index and systemic hypotension that reduces RV coronary pressure and myocardial blood flow [12]. As the systemic pressure ultimately falls and the RV pressure increases, the pressure gradient between the aorta and the RV narrows. Unlike the left ventricle, the RV under normal conditions has high compliance and can be perfused throughout the cardiac cycle. However, when pulmonary hypertension causes increased RV intracavitary pressure, right coronary blood flow in systole can become dependent on the pressure gradient between the aorta and RV. The resulting RV ischemia has been confirmed at autopsy in patients who had acute massive PE by an increase in creatinine kinase MB isoenzyme, troponin I or T or even right ventricular infarction, despite normal coronary arteries [18-20].

Indeed RV failure may be defined as the point at which cardiac output (CO) and systemic blood pressure fall despite increased right ventricular end-diastolic pressure. The reduced CO amplifiers the aterial desaturation caused by

**Table 1.** Hemodynamic consequences of PE [1]

| | | |
|---|---|---|
| (A) | *Changes of pulmonary hemodynamics* | |
| | Precapillary hypertension | Reduced vascular bed<br>Bronchoconstriction<br>Arteriolar vasoconstriction |
| | Development of collateral vessels | Broncho-pulmonary arterial<br>anastomoses |
| | Blood-flow changes | Pulmonary arterio-venous shunts<br>Flow redistribution<br>Flow resumption (lysis, etc.) |
| (B) | *Changes of systemic circulation and cardiac function* | |
| | Arterial hypotension<br>Tachycardia<br>RV overload and dilation<br>Increased central venous pressure<br>LV geometrical changes | |
| (C) | *Changes of coronary circulation* | |
| | Reduced transcoronary pressure gradient | Aortic hypotension<br>Right atrial hypertension |
| | Reduced flow per myocardial unit<br>Relative hypoperfusion of RV subendocardium | |

ventilation-perfusion mismatch in PE [21], in turn worsening myocardial oxygenation and performance (Table 1, Fig. 1).

A typical echocardiography picture of haemodynamically significant PE includes dilated, hypokinetic RV, an increased RV/LV ratio caused by interventricular septal bulging into the LV, dilated proximal pulmonary arteries, increased velocity of the jet of tricuspid regurgitation (usually in the range of 3-3,5 mj s$^{-1}$), and disturbed flow velocity pattern in the RV outflow tract. Furthermore, the inferior vena cava does not collapse on inspiration [12, 16]. Recently, RV regional systolic wall motion abnormalities were suggested as a more specific diagnostic sign of acute PE [1, 22].

PE is generally associated with hypoxaemia, but up to 20% of patients with PE have normal arterial oxygen pressure ($PaO_2$). Since most are also hypocapnic, it was hoped that the oxygen alveolo-arterial difference ($A\text{-}aDO_2$) would be more sensitive to PE than $PaO_2$ but critical trials were disappointing [23] revealing that 15-20% of patients with proven PE also have normal $A\text{-}aDO_2$. In acute PE, particularly in massive PE, hypoxaemia may be due to: (a) ventilation/perfusion mismatching: the V/Q ratio, which is increased in the hypoperfused areas, may be reduced in some relatively over-perfused zones, or in atelectatic areas; (b) shunting within the lung or the heart due to either the opening of pre-existing pulmonary arterial-venous anstomoses or to a patent

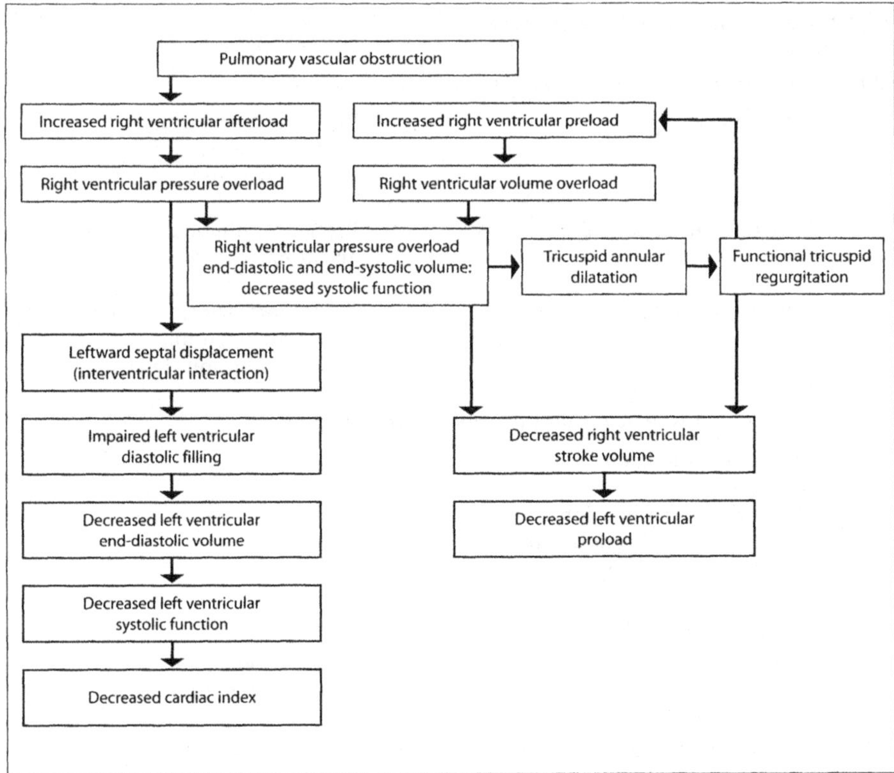


**Fig. 1.** Pathophysiology of right and left heart failure [16]

foramen ovale; (c) reduced mixed venous oxygen saturation, secondary to a decreased cardiac output; (d) altered diffusion component [1] (Table 2).

The goals of *treatment* are to support cardiocirculatory and respiratory function reversing right ventricular failure and systemic hemodynamic impairment, prevent further extension of clots and/or further embolization, reduce recurrencies at long term, minimize long-term morbidity by preventing the development of pulmonary hypertension.

During the post-acute phase of PE, the prognosis is largely dependent on adequate clot resolution and revascularization of the pulmonary arterial and deep venous systems. This is influenced by a range of factors, such as the presence of congenital thrombophilia, the adequacy of anticoagulant therapy and the presence of permanent risk factors. Even when patients survive their initial episode of PE, the long-term prognosis is largely determined by underlying conditions. Factors associated with higher mortality are advanced age, cancer, stroke and cardiopulmonary disease.

Deep vein thrombosis (DVT) and PE are both part of one entity: venous thromboembolism (VTE). A correlation between thrombosis location and the incidence and severity of PE has been demonstrated by a prospective clinical study [24]. The incidence of PE was 46% if DVT was confined to the calf,

**Table 2.** Respiratory consequences of PE [1]

| (A) | *Changes of respiratory dynamics* | |
|---|---|---|
| | Hyperventilation | Pulmonary arterial hypertension |
| | | Reduced compliance |
| | | Atelectasis |
| | Increased airway resistance | Local hypocapnia |
| | | Chemical mediators |

| (B) | *Changes of alveolar ventilation* |
|---|---|
| | Alveolar hyperventilation (hypocapnia, alkalemia) or relative alveolar |
| | hypoventilation |

| (C) | *Changes of respiratory mechanics* | |
|---|---|---|
| | Reduced dynamic compliance | Decreased surfactant |
| | | Atelectasis |
| | | Bronchoconstriction |

| (D) | *Changes of diffusing capacity* |
|---|---|
| | Reduced capillary blood volume |
| | Reduced membrane permeability (?) |

| (E) | *Changes of ventilation/perfusion ratio* |
|---|---|

increased to 67% with involvement of the thigh, and up to 77% if the pelvic veins were involved. In severe PEs, most emboli arise from thrombi in the proximal veins. Many of these thrombi, however, originate in the calf and progress into the proximal vein before embolization [25].

The treatment modalities available are:

1. Hemodynamic support.
2. Respiratory support.
3. Anticoagulation with unfractioned heparin (UFH), low-molecular-weight heparins (LMWHs) and oral anticoagulants.
4. Thrombolysis.
5. Thromboembolectomy either percoutaneous catheter-guided or surgical.
6. Interruption of vena cava.

## Hemodynamic Support

A significant number of the deaths caused by massive PE occur within hours after the onset of symptoms. Initial supportive treatment could therefore have a major role in patients with PE and circulatory failure. The hemodynamic treatment must enhance RV contractility to improve cardiac output, overweighing the pulmonary occlusion arterial pressure, and to vasodilate the pulmonary region thereby reducing RV afterload without altering ventilation/perfusion ratio. It is also necessary to manage systemic hypotension to avoid hypoperfusion of coronary vessels with subsequent RV ischemia and cardiac failure.

The traditional first-line agent for treating hypotension is volume expansion. However, some evidence suggests that, in the setting of pulmonary hypertension and elevated RV volume, this approach increases RV myocardial wall stress, with an increase in RV myocardial oxygen consumption and a critical decrease in the RV supply/demand ratio, resulting in RV ischemia and deterioration in RV function. Nonetheless, Mathru *et al.* [26] found a favorable effect of volume expansion on myocardial performance. Clearly the response to volume expansion depends on different factors, including aggressiveness of volume administration, baseline cardiovascular status and extent of RV afterload [26-29]. This treatment must be undertaken cautionsly because RV function can deteriorate with volume even at relatively low right ventricular end-diastolic pressure and RV filling pressure may not predict the response to volume expansion when an increased RV afterload causes a low CO with or without systemic hypotension [30].

The available data seem to support the administration of norepinephrine to ensure adequate RV coronary perfusion pressure when CO and systemic blood pressure are decreased. In an animal study of PE in which profound hypotension was induced, norepinephrine administration was superior to isoproterenol [26, 31]. It may be that the positive inotropic effect of isoproterenol is outweighed by the peripheral vasodilation it causes. The resultant hypotension leads to decreased RV perfusion and RV ischemia. In contrast to isoproterenol, norepinephrine appears to reverse shock improving RV function and cardiac output and increasing systemic blood pressure. This effect occurs over a wide range of blood pressures and RV afterload, suggesting that beneficial effects are not limited to the subset of patients with frank shock [32]. Of note, when norepinephrine was titrated to a moderate increase in blood pressure, ventricular performance improved without increasing pulmonary vascular resistance and without detrimental effect on renal flow and function.

Amrinone and milrinone (which have inotropic as well pulmonary and systemic vasodilation properties with anticoagulant effects) administration caused, in an animal model of PE, a significant increase in mean systemic arterial pressure and CO and a decreased pulmonary arterial pressure [33]. Carefully attention must be paid to pulmonary vasodilatatory effects which may lead to worse oxygenation due to pulmonary shunting and to inhibition of hypoxic pulmonary vasoconstriction [34].

Only high doses of dopamine improve CO and RV ejection fraction, but at these doses a profound tachycardia resulted [26]. In patients with PE, dobutamine raised CO and improved oxygen transport and tissue oxygenation at constant $PaO_2$ [35, 36]. In some cases $PaO_2$ fell but arterial oxygen transport improved because the increase in CO was more than compensatory [35]. There is currently a controversy concerning the use of inotropes to raise CO to supraphysiologic value in order to improve oxygen transport in the critically ill. In the setting of acute PE, raising CO may worsen the ventilation/perfusion matching by the redistribution of flow from obstructed to non-obstructed vessels [35]. However, dobutamine may be more appropriate in patients with moderate systemic hypotension, provided there is close monitoring of systemic arterial resistance and mean arterial pressure to ensure that adequate RV coronary arterial pressure is maintained [37].

Intravenously administered pulmonary vasodilators decrease pulmonary arterial pressure and pulmonary arterial resistance but worsen oxygenation increasing intrapulmonary shunt and leading to concomitant systemic hypotension that requires phenylephrine or norepinephrine administration to maintain normotension [38, 39]. Transbronchial administration restricts vasodilator action to perfusing pulmonary vessels in well-ventilated areas, thereby decreasing pulmonary hypertension and reducing ventilation/perfusing mismatch [39, 40]. These agents have selective pulmonary vasodilating effects with improved arterial oxygenation. More recently, it has been shown in a few patients with PE that inhaled nitric oxide may improve hemodynamic status and gas exchange [41].

The combined use of various vasoactive agents to achieve optimal hemodynamic response deserves further evaluation. For example the combined use of the inotropic effects of dobutamine with a vasoconstrictor such as norepinephrine offers theoretical merit and warrants investigation in patients with massive and submassive PE [37]. In a recent study, Vizza *et al.* suggest the beneficial effects of the combination of dobutamine and inhaled nitric oxide in patients with mild-severe pulmonary hypertension [42]. The combination of both drugs causes an increase in cardiac index but no change in mean pulmonary arterial pressure. This suggests that the increase in the cardiac index induced by dobutamine is counterbalanced by the concomitant actual pulmonary vasodilation induced by nitric oxide. This interpretation is supported further by analysis of the pulmonary pressure-flow relationship: during administration of the combination of the two drugs the line has a slope intermediate between that of dobutamine and inhaled nitric oxide when each is given alone. The other relevant finding is that the favorable hemodynamic effects are not associated with a deterioration in gas exchange, but with an increase in $PaO_2$, probably because of the vasodilatory effect of inhaled nitric oxide, which is evident in well-ventilated areas of the lung. In accordance with their results, the Authors presented an algorithm (Fig. 2) as a guide in the management of patients with mild to moderate secondary pulmonary hypertension in cases of acute cardiorespiratory decompensation.

Inhaled aerosolized prostacyclin and inhaled prostaglandin E1 have been shown to induce a dose-dependent selective pulmonary vasodilation after heart surgical and heart transplantation [43] and to have beneficial effects on pulmonary vasculature and oxygenation in ARDS as well as other conditions associated with pulmonary hypertension [44]. The additive effects of the association of inhaled nitric oxide and inhaled prostacyclin in decreasing pulmonary hypertension and improving arterial oxygenation have been reported

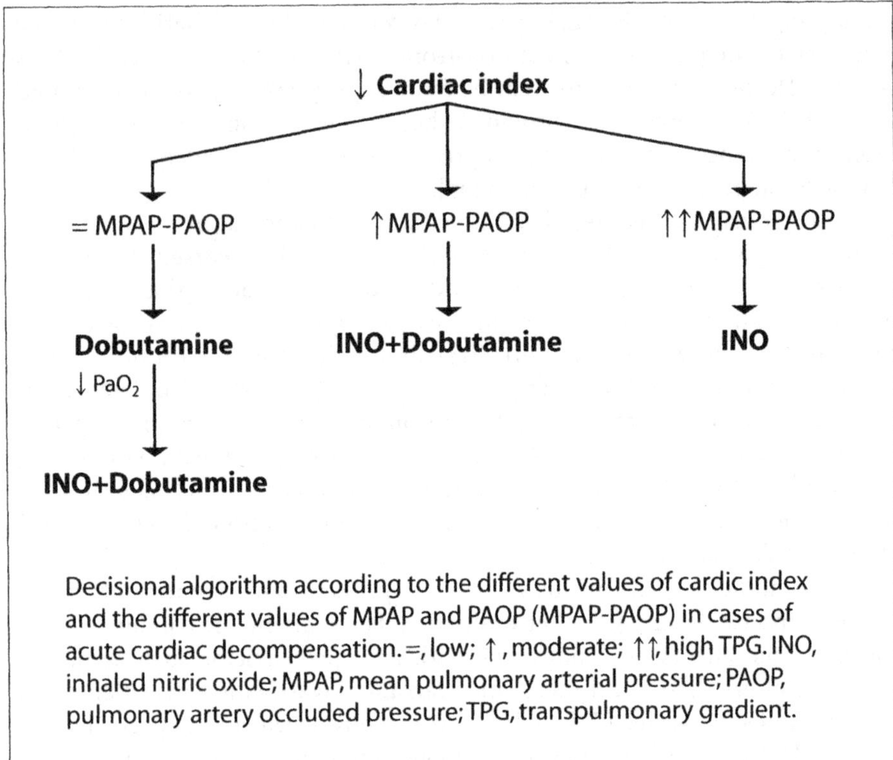



**Fig. 2.** Decisional algorithm

[45-47]. No studies have reported the use of prostaglandins during PE, although their administration during pulmonary hypertension could offer advantages in decreasing and improving right ventricular afterload.

## Respiratory Support

Supplemental oxygen to ameliorate hypoxic vasoconstriction is vital to the hemodynamic support of patients with PE. If mechanical ventilation is required, care should be given to limit its adverse effects. Positive intrathoracic pressures induced by mechanical ventilation reduce the venous return and increase pulmonary arterial pressure and thus worsen RV failure in patients with massive PE [1].

Different grades of clinical severity reflect the different extents of pulmonary thromboembolism. Individual patient management should be guided by hemodynamic and oxygenation parameters and by individual response to pharmacological treatment.

Otherwise in all the forms of PE, massive, submassive and non-massive, vasoactive support must be associated with thrombolytic therapy in order to reverse the cause of pathology and to prevent further embolization.

## Unfractioned Heparin, Low Molecular Weight Heparins, Oral Anticoagulants

In an hemodynamically stable patient who does not have contraindications, heparin therapy should be promptly instituted when PE is diagnosed or strongly suspected because rapid progression of embolization and heavy hemodynamic deterioration may occur while awaiting a definitive diagnosis. Heparin reduces the mortality of PE from 30% to less than 10% by preventing progression of clot formation, and reduces the risk of new embolic events.

The options for anticoagulation are: weight-adjusted continuous infusion of unfractioned heparin (UFH) and low-molecular-weight heparins (LMWHs) administred subcutaneously. LMWHs have been demonstrated to be at least as safe and effective as UFH in the treatment of PE, and are easier to manage because there is no need to perform laboratory tests. LMWHs have a longer half-life, greater bioavailability and a more predictable dose-response than UFH, and determination of aPTT is unnecessary unless overdosage occurs. Furthermore, there is better protection against recurrencies and less incidence of major bleeding during the treatment of DVT [48].

**Table 3.** Adjustments of UFH dose on the basis of aPTT [1]

| | |
|---|---|
| Initial dose | 80 IU/kg bolus |
| aPTT < 35 s (< 1.2 x mean normal) | 80 IU/kg bolus, then increase infusion rate by 4 IU/kg/h |
| aPTT 35 - 45 s (1.2 to 1.5 x mean normal) | 40 IU/kg bolus, then increase infusion rate by 2 IU/kg/h |
| aPTT 46 - 70 s (1.5 to 2.3 x mean normal) | No change |
| aPTT 71 - 90 s (2.3 to 3.0 x mean normal) | Decrease infusion rate by 2 IU/kg/h |
| aPTT > 90 s (3 x mean normal) | Stop infusion 1 h, then decrease infusion rate by 3 IU/kg/h |

After a baseline determination of aPTT, an initial dose 80-150 IU UFH /kg is administered, followed by a continuous infusion initially of 18 IU/kg/h (until a maximum dose of 1600 IU/h). Alternative regimens provide a bolus of 5000 IU followed by an infusion of 1280 IU/h or 40,000 IU/day. The rate of infusion is then adjusted to maintain an aPTT value at 1.5-2.5 times the basal value. The aPTT should be checked every 6 h until stable (Table 3).

Various LMWHs are currently available; the most widely used for the treatment of DVT and PE are enoxaparin (Clexane), reviparin (Clivarina), tinzaparin (Innohep), nadroparin (Fraxiparina, Seleparina). The doses are the following:

- Enoxaparin: 100 IU/kg, sc twice daily.
- Tinzaparin: 175 IU/kg, sc once daily.
- Nadroparin: 90 IU/kg, sc twice daily.
- Reviparin: 100 IU/kg, sc twice daily.

At day 1-3 of heparin treatment, oral anticoagulation can be started (e.g. warfarin 5-10 mg initially), and heparin can be suspended when INR value is between 2 and 3 for at least two determinations 24 h apart from one another. Heparin should be continued at least for 5-7 days, until all vitamin K-dependent factors have been depleted; otherwise, in the first few days, this relatively hypercoagulable state can induce recurrencies of PE [1, 48-50]. The optimal duration of oral anticoagulation is still uncertain, but some evidence suggests that 6 months are more efficacious than 6 weeks and 3 months without influencing the risk of bleeding, and might be sufficient for patients at the first episode of PE and with reversible risk factors (e.g. surgery, prolonged bed rest, trauma). For patients with both irreversible risk factors – either congenital or inherited (malignancy, lupus anticoagulant, protein C and protein S deficiency, activated protein C resistance) – and recurrent episodes of PE, longer duration of therapy, even lifelong, is advocated [48-51].

Heparin without oral anticoagulant, even in association with IVC interruption, is used in the management of PE during pregnancy [1, 52]. UFH is still the standard of care because the data regarding LMWHs are limited. After an initial 5-10 days of treatment, UFH may be given subcutaneously twice a day throughout pregnancy. After delivery, oral warfarin may replace heparin if needed [1].

## Thrombolytic Therapy

Thrombolytic therapy is indicated in patients with massive PE and hemodynamic instability and in those with limited cardiopulmonary reserves due to underlying disease; another possible field of application of thrombolysis is in patients with normal systemic arterial pressure and echocardiographic signs of right ventricular impairment, but in this situation the results are uncertain and the benefit must be weighed with the risk of bleeding complications [53, 54]. Table 4 lists the contraindications to fibrinolytic treatment.

Thrombolytic agents have been demonstrated to rapidly reverse right ventricular dysfunction, pulmonary hypertension and systemic hypotension; by dissolving the clots, they reduce recurrencies and prevent the development of chronic pulmonary hypertension [49-51, 55]. In patients with massive PE, a significant reduction in pulmonary hypertension and a significant increase in systemic arterial pressure could be seen soon after the initiation of therapy with thrombolytic agents but not with heparin alone. Locally administered drugs, via a pulmonary artery catheter, have not been demonstrated to be superior to systemic treatment regarding the incidence of bleeding, hemodynamic improvement and clot lysis [55], but further investigations are necessary. Heparin is not infused during thrombolytic treatment. After completion of the thrombolytic regimen, heparin infusion is started when aPTT returns to < 2.5 the control value, and then adjusted to reach the same range of forementioned values.

**Table 4.** Contraindications to fibrinolytic therapy [1]

*Absolute contraindications*

– Active internal bleeding
– Recent spontaneous intracranial bleeding

*Relative contraindications*

– Major surgery, delivery, organ biopsy or puncture of non-compressible vessel within 10 days
– Gastrointestinal bleeding within 10 days
– Serious trauma within 15 days
– Neurosurgery or opthalmologic surgery within 1 month
– Uncontrolled severe hypertension (systolic pressure > 180 mmHg; diastolic pressure > 110 mmHg)
– Recent cardiopulmonary resuscitation
– Platelet count < 100,000/mm$^3$, prothrombin time less than 50%
– Pregnancy
– Bacterial endocarditis
– Diabetic hemorragic retinopathy

**Table 5.** Thrombolytic regimens [55]

| Drug | Regimen |
| --- | --- |
| Streptokinase | 250,000 U over 30 min followed by 100,000 U/h for 24 h |
| Urokinase | 4,400 U/kg over 10 min followed by 4,400 U/kg/h for 12-24 h |
| rt-PA | 100 mg over 2 h |

Various therapy modalities and various drugs are available; in recent reviews of the literature, infusion of rt-PA was shown to produce a more rapid clot lysis and hemodynamic improvement than streptokinase and urokinase, and no augmented incidence of major bleeding (Table 5) [1, 55].

Accelerated regimens (e.g. rt-PA 0.6 mg/kg over 15 min) do not have advantages compared with standard regimens in producing faster hemodynamic improvement [1, 55, 56].

## Embolectomy

Percutaneous or surgical embolectomy is reserved for patients with massive PE and impending or overt shock despite supportive therapies, who have contraindications to thrombolysis or in whom thrombolysis has failed or PE is recurring despite appropriate treatment. Transvenous catheter embolectomy or fragmentation has lower perioperative mortality and morbidity, but this technique is still of limited availability. Surgical embolectomy (performed with media sternotomy, institution of normothermic cardiopulmonary bypass and incision of the main pulmonary artery) requires angiography for confirmation of diagnosis and for planning the procedure, although this delay in treatment may pose serious risks of further hemodynamic worsening and cardiac arrest, and thus contribute to the higher mortality rate. Normothermic bypass permits restoration of blood flow and oxygenation and offers circulatory assistance for patients with shock or cardiac arrest due to PE [49, 50, 57].

## Interruption of Vena Cava

The widely accepted indications for interruption of vena cava by placement of a filter are  patients with absolute contraindications for anticoagulation, those in whom anticoagulant therapy has failed and those that undergo surgical embolectomy (Table 6); other indications remain a matter of controversy. A possible field of application in the hospitalized population is prophylactic application of caval filters in patients scheduled for surgery who have contraindications to anticoagulation, or patients with head or spine trauma [1]. Some authors pro-

**Table 6.** Indications for filter placement [58, 59].

| Indications |
| --- |
| Contraindications to anticoagulation (absolute or relative) |
| Complications of anticoagulation<br>   – Failure: objectively documented extension of existing DVT or new DVT or PE while therapeutically anticoagulated<br>   – Hemorrhage: major or minor<br>   – Thrombocytopenia<br>   – Skin necrosis<br>   – Drug reaction<br>   – Evidence/probability of poor compliance |
| Prophylaxis: no thromboembolic disease |
| Prophylaxis with thromboembolism in addition to anticoagulation |
| Failure of previous device to prevent PE; central extension of thrombus through an existing filter or recurrent PE |
| In association with another procedure: thrombectomy, embolectomy or lytic therapy |

pose that the use of filters in addition to heparin therapy initially reduces the onset of PE in patients with DVT, but there are no additional positive effects on mortality [49-52].

These devices also have some risks and complications: perforation of the vena cava, duodenal perforation, penetration into vertebral bodies, distal migration of the filter, migration in the right atrium and pulmonary artery, aortic perforation, filter occlusion, bleeding from the insertion site and recurrent PE from small emboli that pass the filter [1, 52].

# References


1. (2000) Task force on Pulmonary Embolism. European Society of Cardiology. Guidelines on diagnosis and management of acute pulmonary embolism. Eur Heat J 21:1301-1336
2. Stein PD, Henry JW (1995) Prevalence of acute pulmonary embolism among patients in a general hospital at autopsy. Chest 108:78-81
3. Morpurgo M, Rustici A (1988) Lo spettro dell'embolia polmonare. Cardiologia 33:1105-1108
4. Morpurgo M, Schmid C (1980) Clinic-pathologic correlations in pulmonary embolism: a posteriori evaluation. Prog Res Dis 13:8-15
5. Pacouret G, Alison D, Pottier JM et al (1997) Free-floating thrombus and embolic risk in patients with angiographically confirmed proximal deep venous thrombosis: a prospective study. Arch Intern Med 157:305-308
6. Barrit DW, Jordan SC (1961) Clinical features of pulmonary embolism. Lancet 1:729-739
7. Goldhaber SZ, Hennekens CH, Evans D et al (1982) Factors associated with corrected antemortem major of pulmonary embolism. Am J Med 73:822-826
8. Kasper W, Konstantinides S, Tiede N et al (1997) Prognostic significance of right ventricular afterload stress detected by echocardiography in patient with clinically suspected pulmonary embolism. Heart 77:346-349
9. Ribeiro A, Lindmarker P, Jublin-Dannfelt A et al (1997) Echocardiography Doppler in pulmonary embolism: right ventricular dysfunction as a predictor of mortality. Am Heart J 134:479-487
10. Konstantinides S, Geribel A, Kasper W et al (1988) Patent foramen ovale is an important predictor of adverse outcome in patients with major pulmonary embolism. Circulation 97:1946-1951
11. Sasahara AA, MacIntyre KM, Cella G et al (1988) The clinical and the hemodynamic feature of pulmonary embolism. Curr Pulmonol 9:305-346
12. Kenneth E, Wood DO (2002) Review of a pathophysiologic apport to the golden hour of hemodynamically significant pulmonary embolism. Chest 121:877-905
13. McIntyre KM, Sasahara AA (1974) Determinants of right ventricular function and haemodynamics after pulmonary embolism. Chest 65:534-643
14. McIntyre KM, Sasahara AA (1974) Hemodynamic and ventricular responses to pulmonary embolism. Prog Cardiovasc Dis 17:175-190
15. Benis CE, Serur JR, Borkenaghen D et al (1974) Influence of right ventricular filling pressure on left ventricular pressure and dimission. Circ Res 34:498-504
16. Menzel T, Wagner S, Kramm T et al (2000) Pathophysiology of impaired right and left ventricular function in chronic embolic pulmonary hypertension. Chest 118:897-903
17. Belenkie I, Dani R, Smith ER, Tyberg JV (1988) Ventricular interaction during experimental acute pulmonary embolism. Circulation 78:761-768

18. Adam JE, Siegel BA, Goldstein et al (1992) Elevation of CK-MB following pulmonary embolism. Chest 101: 1203-1236
19. Ramirez-Rivera A, Gutierrez-Fajardo P, Jerjez-Sanchez C et al (1993) Acute right myocardial infarction without significant obstructive coronary lesions secondary to massive pulmonary embolism. Chest 104:80S
20. Konstantinides S, Geibel A, Olschewski M et al (2002) Importance of toponins I and T in risk stratification of patients with acute pulmonary embolism. Circulation 106:1263-1268
21. Manier G, Castaing Y, Guenard H (1985) Determinants of hypoxemia during the acute phase of pulmonary embolism in humans. Am Rev Respir Dis 132:332-338
22. Krivec B, Voga G, Zuran I et al (1997) Diagnosis and treatment of shock due to massive pulmonary embolism. Approach with transesophageal echocardiography and intrapulmonary thrombolysis. Chest 112:1310-1316
23. Palla A, Petruzzelli S, Donnamaria V et al (1995) The role of suspicion in the diagnosis of pulmonary embolism. Chest 107:21S-24S
24. Kohen H, Koenig B, Mostbeck A (1987) Incidence and clinical feature of pulmonary embolism in patients with deep vein thrombosis: a prospective study. Eur J Nucl Med 13:S11-S15
25. Kakkar VV, Flanc C, Howe CT, Clarke MB (1969) Natural history of postoperative deep-vein thrombosis. Lancet 2:230-232
26. Mathru M, Venus B, Smith R et al (1986) Treatment of low cardiac output complicating acute pulmonary hypertension in normovolemic goals. Crit Care Med 14:120-124
27. Ducas J, Prewitt RM (1987) Pathophysiology and therapy of right ventricular dysfunction due to pulmonary embolism. Cardiovasc Clin 17:191-202
28. Prewitt RM (1997) pharmacological hemodynamic support in massive pulmonary embolism. Chest 111:218-224
29. Mercat A, Diehl JL, Meyer G et al (1999) Hemodynamic effects of fluid loading in acute massive pulmonary embolism. Crit Care Med 27:540-544
30. Ghignone M, Girling L, Prewitt RM (1984) Volume expansion versus norephinephrine in treatment of a low cardiac output complicating an acute in righr ventricular afterloads in dogs. Anesthesiology 80:132-135
31. Molloy DW, Lee KY, Jones D et al (1985) Effects of noradrenaline and isoproterenol on cardio-pulmonary function in a canine model of acute pulmonary hypertension. Chest 88:432-435
32. Angle MH, Molloy DW, Penner B et al (1989) The cardiopulmonary and renal hemodynamc effects of norephinephrine in canine pulmonary embolism. Chest 95:1333-1337
33. Wolfe MW, Saad RM, Spence TH (1992) Hemodynamic effects of amrinone in a canine model of massive pulmonary embolism. Chest 102:274-278
34. Hill NS, Rounds S (1983) Amrinone dilates pulmonary vessels and blunts hypoxic vasoconstriction in isolated rat lungs. Proc Soc Exp Biol Med 173:205-212
35. Manier G, Castaing Y (1992) Influence of cardiac output on oxygen exchange in acute pulmonary embolism. Am Rev Respir Dis 145:130-136
36. Jardin F, Genevray B, Brun-Neg D et al (1985) Dobutamine: a hemodynamic evaluation in pulmonary embolism shock. Crit Care Med 13:1009-1012
37. Layish DT, Tapson VF (1997) Pharmacological hemodynamic support in massive pulmonary embolism. Chest 111:218-224
38. Triantafillou AN, Pohl MS, Okabayashi K et al (1995) Effect of inhaled nitric oxide and prostaglandin E1 on hemodynamic and arterial oxygenation in patients following single lung transplantation. Anesth Analg 80:SCA 40
39. Walmrath D, Schermuly R, Pilch J et al (1997) Effect of inhaled versus intravenous vasodilators in experimental pulmonary hypertension. Eur Respir J 10:1084-1092
40. Brienza A (1999) Strategies on management of pulmonary hypertension. Minerva Anestesiol 65:769-773

41. Capellier G, Jacques T, Balay P et al (1997) Inhaled nitric oxide in patients with pulmonary embolism. Intensive Care Med 1089-1092
42. Vizza CD, Della Rocca G, Di Roma A et al (2001) Acute hemodynamic effects of inhaled nitric oxide, dobutamine and a combination of two in patients with mild to moderate secondary pulmonary hypertension. Critical Care 5:355-361
43. Haraldsson A, Kieler-Jensen N, Ricksten SE et al (1996) Inhaled prostcyclin for treatment of pulmonary hypertension after cardiac surgery or heart transplantation: a pharmacodynamic study. J Cardiothorac Vasc Anesth 10:864-868
44. Olschewski H, Gofrani HA, Walmarath D et al (1999) Inhaled prostcyclin and iloprost in severe pulmonary hypertension secondary to lung fibrosis. Am J Respir Crit Care Med 160:600-607
45. Mirza I, Nagamine J, Pearl RG (1997) Additive effects of inhaled prostacyclin and inhaled nitric oxide in reducing experimental pulmonary hypertension. Anesthesiology 87:1122
46. Hill LL, Pearl RG (1999) Combined inhaled nitric oxide and inhaled prostacyclin during experimental chronic pulmonary hypertension. J Appl Physiol 86:1160-1164
47. Della Rocca G, Coccia C, Pompei L et al (2001) Hemodynamic and oxygenation changes of combined therapy with inhaled nitric oxide and inhaled areosolized prostacyclin. J Cardiothorac Vasc Anesth 15:224-227
48. Ginsberg JS (1996) Management of venous thromboembolism. N Engl J Med 335:1816-1828
49. Goldhaber SZ (1998) Pulmonary Embolism. New Engl J Med 339:93-104
50. Hyers TM, Russell DH, Weg JG (1995) Antithrombotic therapy for venous thromboembolic disease. Chest 108:335S-351S
51. Shulman S, Rhedin AS, Lindmarker P et al (1995) A comparison of six weeks with six months of oral anticoagulation therapy after a first episode of venous thrromboembolism. N Eng J Med 332:1661-1665
52. Ahearn GS, Hadjiadis D, Govert JA et al (2002) Massive pulmonary embolism during pregnancy succesfully treated with recombinant tissue plasminogen activator. A case report and review of treatment options. Arch Int Med 162:1221-1227
53. Hamel E, Pacouret G, Vinentelli D et al (2001) Thrombolysis or heparin therapy in massive pulmoanry embolism with right ventricular dilation. Chest 120:120-125
54. Konstantinides S, Geibel A, Olschewski M et al (1997) Association between throimbolytic treatment and the prognosis of hemodynamically stable patients with major pulmonary embolism. Circulation 96:882-888
55. Arcaoy Sm, Kreit JW (1999) Thrombolytic therapty of pulmonary embolism. Chest 115:1695-1707
56. Sors H, Pacouret G, Azarian R, Meyer G et al (1994) Hemodynamic effects of bolus vs 2-h infusion of alteplase in acute massive pulmonary embolism. A randomized controlled multicenter trial. Chest 106:712-717
57. Wood KE (2002) Major pulmonary embolism. Review of a patophysiologic approach to the Golden Hour of hemodynamically significant pulmoanry embolism. Chest 121:877-905
58. Girard P, Stern JB, Parent F (2002) Medical literature and the Vena Cava filters. Chest 122:963-967
59. (1999) Participants in the Vena Cava Filter Consensus Conference. Recommended reporting standards foe vena caval filter placement and patients follow-up. J Vasc Surg 30:573-579

# Chapter 17

# Pulmonary Infections in the Intensive Care Unit

A. Luzzani, E. Polati, S. Bassanini

Pulmonary infections in the intensive care unit (ICU) include two different entities: firstly, patients admitted with pneumonia, which may be either community (CAP)- or hospital acquired (HAP), and, second pneumonia developing in critically ill, mechanically ventilated patients (VAP or ventilator- associated pneumonia).

## Community- Acquired Pneumonia (CAP)

Community-acquired pneumonia (CAP) is defined as an acute inflammatory process of the pulmonary parenchyma caused by micro-organisms, occurring in non-hospitalized patients and associated clinical symptoms of infection and a chest radiography showing a new or progressive infiltrate, consolidation, cavitation or pleural effusion [1].

The incidence of CAP that needs hospitalization is 258/100,000 inhabitants in the United States [2-4], 300/100,000 habitants in Italy [5]. Mortality rates reported for CAP requiring hospitalization range from 2 to 30% [2-4, 6, 7]. A total of 10-36% of hospitalized patients for CAP are admitted to the intensive care unit (ICU) for severe CAP [2-4, 6, 7]. The incidence, aetiology, prognostic factors and outcome of these patients have been defined, and differ from those in the overall population of patients with CAP [8]. Cases of severe CAP have been separated from those of less severe pneumonia requiring hospitalization, because of the high mortality rate of the former illness (as much as 50%) [9].

Although there is no uniformly accepted definition of severe CAP, the original American Thoracic Society (ATS) guidelines [9] identified some criteria for severe illness, and the presence of at least one of these criteria used to define the CAP as severe (Table 1).

Subsequently, several studies showed that when only one of these criteria was used, as many as 65-68% of all admitted patients had severe CAP requiring ICU admission, indicating that the original definition was overly sensitive and not specific [8].

In a more recent study [10], the criteria for severe CAP were divided into five minor criteria that could be present at the admission and four major criteria that could be present at the admission or later in the hospital stay (Table 2). The presence of either two minor criteria or one major criteria defines the CAP as

**Table 1.** Criteria for definition of severe community-acquired pneumonia (CAP) (from [9])

Respiratory rate > 30

$PaO_2/FiO_2$ < 250

Intubation and VAM

Bilateral or multilobar X-ray infiltrate

Shock (SAP < 90 or DAP < 60)

Use of vasopressor for time > 4 h

Diuresis < 20ml/h or < 80ml in 4 h

**Table 2.** New criteria for definition of severe CAP (from [10])

*Minor criteria*

Respiratory rate > 30/min

$PaO_2/FiO_2$ < 250

Bilateral  X-ray infiltrate

Multilobar  X-ray infiltrate

Shock (SAP < 90 or DAP < 60)

*Major criteria*

Use of vasopressor for time > 4 h

Need for mechanical ventilation

Acute renal failure (urine output < 80ml in 4 h or serum creatinine > 2 mg/dl in absence of chronic renal failure)

Increase in size of infiltrate by > 50% within 48 h

severe and consequently the need for ICU admission. With this rule, the sensitivity was 78% and the specificity was 94% [10].

There are many factors that increase the incidence of CAP: age < 5 or > 65 years, alcohol addition, immune-suppressive illness (including therapy with corticosteroids) and coexisting illness, such as chronic obstructive pulmonary disease (COPD), diabetes mellitus, renal failure, congestive heart failure, coronary artery disease, malignancy, chronic neurological disease and chronic liver disease [1, 8].

A large number of pathogens have been associated with severe CAP (Table 3): *Streptococcus pneumoniae*, *Haemophylus influenzae*, and enteric gram-negative bacilli are the pathogens most frequently identified among patients with severe CAP [8, 9, 11]. In the ICU, the incidence of CAP caused by *Streptococcus*

**Table 3.** The most frequent etiologic agents of CAP in the ICU (from [11])

| Etiologic agents | % |
| --- | --- |
| *Streptococcus pneumoniae* | 32.6 |
| *Haemophylus influenzae* | 10.6 |
| Aerobic gram-negative bacilli | 6.8 |
| Polymicrobial infections | 6.8 |
| *Streptococcus species* | 5.3 |
| Respiratory viruses | 3.8 |
| *Staphylococcus aureus* | 3.0 |
| *Legionella* species | 2.3 |
| *Moraxella* species | 2.3 |
| *Coxiella burnetii* | 1.5 |
| *Mycoplasma pneumoniae* | < 1 |
| *Chlamydia psittaci* | < 1 |
| Anaerobic agents | < 1 |
| *Mycobacterium tuberculosis* | – |
| Fungi | – |
| Negative | 28 |

*pneumoniae* ranges from 10 to 36% [9]. Other important micro-organisms to be considered are *Legionella pneumophila*, *Staphylococcus aureus*, *Mycoplasma pneumoniae*, respiratory-tract viruses, and a group of miscellaneous pathogens (*Mycobacterium tuberculosis*, *Chlamydia pneumoniae*, *Moraxella* sp, *Coxiella burnetii*, and fungi).

There has been some debate about whether *Pseudomonas aeruginosa* can lead to severe CAP, and, although this micro-organism has been reported in some studies with an incidence of 1.5-5%, it is common opinion that this pathogen should be considered only when specific risk factors are present [8]. These risks include chronic or prolonged broad-spectrum antibiotic therapy (> 7 days within the past month), structural lung disease (bronchiectasis), malnutrition, and some medical comorbidities associated to neutrophil dysfunction (HIV infection, corticosteroid therapy) [8]. The frequency of *S. aureus* as a severe CAP pathogen is also variable; risks for infection with this micro-organism include recent influenza, diabetes and renal failure [8].

The diagnosis of CAP is based on the presence of new and persistent pulmonary infiltrates, associated to clinical and laboratory signs of systemic inflammation, including changes in body temperature, leukocytosis, tachypnea, and tachycardia. However, these signs may be noninfectious in origin and are neither specific nor sensitive for CAP. Critically ill patients often manifest a systemic inflammatory response syndrome (SIRS) without infection. A suitable marker that could distinguish the inflammatory response to infection from other types of inflammation would be of great clinical usefulness. While C-reactive protein (CRP) is commonly used as a marker of an acute inflammatory state, however the results of recent investigations suggest that these goals might be better achieved by monitoring procalcitonin (PCT) plasma concentrations, because they seemed to be closely related to the severity and evolution of infection [12].

Once the diagnosis of CAP is established or suspected, an effort should be made to identify a specific etiologic pathogen. Microbiological examinations should be carried out as soon as possible and before the administration of antibiotic therapy. An antibiotic therapy selected on the basis of microbiological data is likely to be more effective of than an empirically based therapy and often the initial empirical therapy requires to be changed when microbiological data are available [8, 13-15]. However, the usefulness of diagnostic testing in the management of CAP is a subject of controvers [15]. First of all, if diagnostic testing leads to delays in the initiation of appropriate therapy, there may be an adverse outcome for the patient [8]. Second, the value of a focused therapy, directed at a rapidly identified bacterial etiology is uncertain, since the possibility of co-infection with a bacteria and an atypical pathogen (which may take days or weeks to identify). Indeed, in large population studies, treatment that accounted for atypical pathogen co-infection, led to a better outcome than treatment that did not account for this possibility [16, 17].

One of the most controversial recommendations regards the performance of a sputum Gram stain and culture in all patients with CAP. Several studies suggest that the sputum Gram stain is an insensitive but specific early guide to diagnosis and treatment of CAP when interpreted by a skilled observer [15]. Indeed, the recent ATS guidelines too acknowledge the importance of the performance of a sputum Gram stain in patients with CAP [8]. A sample taken from the lower respiratory tract that is not heavily contaminated by oral secretions will have fewer than 10 squamous epithelial cells and more than 25 neutrophils per low-power field. In this sample, an evidence of a predominant bacterial morphotype of a likely pulmonary pathogen is helpful for choosing on an initial empirical therapy [8, 15]. Moreover, there are some micro-organisms, such as *Legionella pneumophila*, *M. tuberculosis*, influenzae, adeno-, coxsackie, and hanta viruses, *Pneumocystis carinii*, *Histoplasma capsulatum*, *Coccidiodes immitis* and *Blastomyces dermatitidis*, that, when identified, are recognised pathogens independent from the technique of respiratory sampling used [8, 9].

There is also a considerable controversy about the role and use of invasive techniques (bronchoscopy with a protected brush catheter, bronchoalveolar lavage, and fine-needle aspiration of the lung) to acquire lower-airway samples, uncontaminated by oropharyngeal flora. The use of bronchoscopy for diagnostic assessment of CAP patients who have failed initial management identified an infectious agent in less than 30% of patients [11, 15]. Moreover, retrospective data have shown that, with severe illness, outcome is not improved by identifying the etiologic agent [11, 18]. In the most recent guidelines for CAP management, these procedures are not indicated for most patients, being recommended only for particularly severe, selected cases [8, 13, 19].

Also the cost/effectiveness ratio of blood cultures in patients with CAP has been questioned, essentially for two reasons: the low percentage of patients with CAP who have bacteremia (the incidence of positive blood cultures in patients hospitalized with CAP is lower than 20%, with *S. pneumoniae* accounting for half of the positive cultures), and the clinical relevance of the culture for either modifying antibiotic therapy or predicting the outcome [15]. However, there is now a general agreement that two sets of blood cultures should be drawn before initiation antibiotic therapy, because they can provide useful informations on both the etiologic pathogen and its antibiotic sensitivity [8, 15]. The systematically execution of blood cultures in patients with severe CAP has been proved to be associated with a statistically significant reduction in 30-day mortality [20]. In addition, any significant pleural effusion should be sampled to rule out the possibility of empyema or complicated parapneumonic effusion [8]. Viral cultures, serologic testing and cold-agglutinin measurements are not useful in the initial assessment of patients with CAP and therefore should not be routinely performed [8], while the urine test for *Legionella* antigen is recommended in patients with severe CAP [15].

The Infectious Diseases Society of America published a set of guidelines for the management of CAP in adults: empirical antibiotic therapy is recommended before microbiological results are available and it is based on local epidemiology and patterns of resistance [13]. It is desirable to give as narrow a spectrum of therapy as possible, avoiding excessively broad antibiotic therapy, if it is not needed. This goal is easily achieved if a specific etiologic agent is identified, but this is impossible in at least half of all patients, making relatively broad-spectrum empirical therapy a necessity for most patients, at least initially [8]. Empirical therapy of severe CAP requires the use of an intravenous macrolide (clarithromycin, azithromycin) or an intravenous fluoroquinolone (levofloxacin), combined to a β-lactam (cefotaxime, ceftriaxone) that would be active against drug-resistant *S. pneumoniae* (DRSP) [8]. This therapy provides coverage for *S. pneumoniae* (also DRSP), *H. influenzae*, *Legionella* and other atypicals. In the presence of pseudomonal risk factors (chronic or prolonged broad-spectrum antibiotic therapy, bronchiectasis, malnutrition, corticosteroid therapy), therapy should include a selected intravenous antipseudomonal β-lactam (cefepime, imipenem, meropenem, piperacillin/tazobactam) plus an intravenous fluoroquinolone with an antipseudomonal activity (ciprofloxacin), or a selected intravenous antipseudomonal β-lactam plus an intravenous aminoglycoside plus either an intravenous macrolide or an intravenous fluoroquinolone without an antipseudomonal activity [1, 8, 13].

# Ventilator-Associated Pneumonia (VAP)

## Epidemology

Ventilator-associated pneumonia (VAP) is defined as a nosocomial pneumonia caused by infectious agents not present or incubating at the time when mechanical ventilation was started [21, 22]. There is no doubt that prolonged (more than 48 h) mechanical ventilation is the most important factor associated with VAP; however, VAP; may also occur within the first 48 h after intubation [22]. According to Langer *et al.* [23], we prefer to distinguish early-onset VAP, occurring within the first 4 days of mechanical ventilation, from late-onset VAP, occurring 5 or more days after the beginning of mechanical ventilation, because the etiologic agents are commonly different, the disease is less severe and the prognosis is better in early-onset than in late-onset VAP [22].

VAP is the most common ICU-acquired infection. In the majority of reports, its incidence ranges from 8 to 28% [22], but it can reach 67% in some specific settings [24]. The criteria used for diagnosis, terminology and definitions of VAP differ between studies, so that the epidemiology of VAP may resulted significantly affected. Incidence rates for VAP using a clinical definition average 7 cases per 1000 ventilator days [25]. Two large-scale studies conducted in 107 and 1417 European ICUs and evaluating 966 and 10,038 patients respectively, showed an overall ICU-acquired pneumonia incidence rate of 8.9% [26] and a point prevalence of 9.6% [27]. VAP is a common complication of the acute respiratory distress syndrome (ARDS) and, even if its diagnosis is often difficult in patients with ARDS, various clinical studies reported that it affects between 34 and more than 70% of patients with this condition [22]. VAP represents the main cause of morbidity and mortality among patients in the ICU and adds significant economic costs due to an increase in length of ICU stay [21, 27, 28]. The mortality rates for VAP have been reported to range from 24 to 50% and can reach 76% in some specific settings or when lung infection is caused by high-risk pathogens [22]. The risk of death for ICU-ventilated patients with VAP compared with that for patients without pneumonia is increased from two to ten-fold [21, 22].

## Risk Factors and Preventive Measures

Several risk factors for the development of pulmonary infections have been identified and they include both patient-related factors and intervention-related factors (Table 4).

Post-surgical patients, too, are at high risk for VAP, and the development of pneumonia is associated with preoperative markers of severity of underlying disease, such as low serum albumin level, and high ASA physical-status classification score; also, a history of smoking, longer preoperative stays, longer surgical procedures, and thoracic or upper abdominal surgery play a significant role in the occurrence of post-surgical pneumonia [22].

**Table 4.** Risk factors for pulmonary infections [22]

| Host factors | Intervention factors | Other factors |
| --- | --- | --- |
| Serum albumin < 2.2 g/dl | H2 blockers, antiacidics | Season: fall, winter |
| Age > 60 years | Paralytic agents | |
| ARDS | Continuous intravenous sedation | |
| COPD, pulmonary disease | > 4 units of blood products | |
| Coma, impaired consciousness | Intracranial pressure monitoring | |
| Burns, trauma | Prolonged mechanical ventilation (>2 days) | |
| Organ failure | Positive end-expiratory pressure | |
| Severity of illness | Frequent ventilator circuit changes | |
| Large-volume gastric aspiration | Nasogastric tube Reintubation | |
| Gastric colonization and pH | Supine head position | |
| Upper-airway colonization | Transport out of the ICU | |
| Sinusitis | Prior antibiotic or no antibiotic therapy | |

Patients-related illnesses predispose to pneumonia because of impairment of host defensive functions. These include severe acute or chronic conditions, such as hypotension, metabolic acidosis, respiratory and renal failure, chronic obstructive lung disease (COPD), diabetes, malnutrition, coma and central nervous system dysfunction, alcoholism. Severity of clinical conditions (APACHE > 16, SAPS > 9, GCS < 8), advanced age and prolonged hospitalization increase the risk of pneumonia [22, 25, 29].

Endotracheal tube and invasive ventilation represent important intervention-related risk factors for pulmonary infections in the ICU: an endotracheal tube can impair mucociliar clearance of the lower airways and prevent effective coughing [25]. In prospective studies, the incidence of ICU-acquired pneumonia is lower in non-invasively ventilated patients [22, 25]. The procedure of intubation itself increases significantly the risk of developing VAP, as demonstrated in patients requiring re-intubation, because there is an increased risk of tracheal aspiration of infected fluids during the intubation manoeuvres [30]. The role of early tracheotomy in VAP prevention remains controversial: whereas some studies found a reduction in the rate of VAP in patients with early tracheotomy, others could not demonstrate any benefit [22]. As regards the route of intubation, nasal intubation is associated with higher incidence of sinusitis than oral intubation [25]. However, we should consider that a diagnosis of sinusitis is more frequently a radiological finding than a real clinical and microbiological diagnosis, so that it is unclear whether nasal intubation represents a risk factor for VAP [22, 25]. Respiratory equipment itself may be a source of bacteria responsible for VAP: mechanical ventilators with cascade humidifiers have high rates of condensate formation in the ventilator circuit and this condensate can become contaminated with bacteria, and thereby leading to VAP [25]. Heated ventilator circuits markedly lower the rates of condensate formation, but there are no evidences that they reduce the rate of VAP [22]; rather, the use of heat-moisture exchangers is associated with lower incidence of VAP than the use of conventional heated-water humidification systems [22, 25]. However, some heat-moisture exchangers can increase dead-space and work of breathing [22, 25], and thus their use should be avoided during the weaning period in ARDS ventilated with a low tidal volume and in patients with COPD during the weaning period [22].

Nasogastric tube and early enteral nutrition increase the risk of aspiration of gastric content and pneumonia because they may promote reflux and aspiration of stomach contents, impairing the function of the lower esophageal sphincter, especially when patients are lying supine [22, 25, 29]. Post-pyloric placement of feeding tubes decreases neither the risk of aspiration nor of VAP [25]. Semi-recumbent body position (30-45°) reduces the incidence of pneumonia: prospective studies have demonstrated that supine position is associated with an higher risk of pneumonia when compared to semi-recumbent position in mechanically ventilated patients [31, 32]. Continuous sedation and paralysis reduce the normal airway reflexes and can prolong invasive ventilation, thereby representing important risk factors for the development of VAP [22, 25, 29, 31]. As regards the stress ulcer prophylaxis, drugs that raise the gastric pH, such as H2-receptor antagonists, could encourage bacterial colonization. The results of several studies [22, 25, 29] have indicated lower rates of pneumonia for patients given a gastroprotective drug (sucralfate) rather than drugs that neutralize or block gastric secretions (anti-acids or H2-receptor antagonists). However, this conclusion was not confirmed in the largest randomized controlled trials comparing ranitidine (50 mg every 8 h) to sucralfate (1 g every 6 h) for the prevention of upper gastrointestinal bleeding in 1200 mechanically ventilated patients: ranitidine was superior to sucralfate in preventing upper gastrointestinal bleeding (1.7% vs. 3.8%) and did not increase significantly the incidence of VAP (19.1% vs. 16.2%), as diagnosed by an adjudication committee using a modified version of the CDC criteria [33].

The prolonged use of antibiotics has been associated with an increased risk of nosocomial pneumonia and the selection of resistant pathogens [22, 25, 29, 31], even if a repeated rotation of empirical antibiotic therapy in the ICU may reduce some anti-microbial resistance rates and limit the emergence of new resistance profiles [34]. However, other investigators demonstrated a protective effect of antibiotic therapy in preventing early-onset VAP [35-37]. Moreover, a study conducted in 358 ICUs established that the absence of antibiotic therapy represents a significant risk factor for VAP onset [38]. The results of a multicentric Canadian study [39] on the incidence and risk factors for VAP indicated that antibiotic therapy conferred protection against VAP and that this protective effect disappeared after 2 to 3 weeks, suggesting that a higher risk for VAP cannot be excluded beyond this point. Therefore, it seems probable that antibiotics may eradicate susceptible micro-organisms early in a patient's stay or encourage the emergence of resistant micro-organisms later in the patient's stay [25]. Consequently, epidemiological studies have found that systemic antibiotics can either reduce or increase the risk for VAP [25, 39].

There are some effective preventive strategies that are widely recognised to reduce the incidence of ICU-acquired pneumonia. Safe, inexpensive, logical, but unproven interventions include general preventive measures, such as hand washing by the ICU personnel, including the use of gloves, and oral antiseptics; avoidance of indiscriminate antibiotic use and of excessive sedation and paralysis, and the use of non-invasive ventilation, and of semi-recumbent patient position are other important preventive measures [29]. The role of selective digestive decontamination (SDD) is a controversy question. SDD was developed to prevent nosocomial infections, especially pneumonia, by selectively eliminating aerobic, gram-negative, potentially pathogenic micro-organisms and fungi while preserving the endogenous anaerobic flora [40]. SDD consists of the topical administration of non-absorbable antibiotics in the mouth and the stomach, and it is optionally combined with systemic antibiotic prophylaxis during the patient's first few days in the ICU. The topical component usually includes tobramycin, polymyxin E, and amphotericin B and it is directed against the colonization of the aerodigestive tract. The systemic component consists of a third-generation cephalosporin, which is added to prevent early infections [40]. About 10 years ago, the members of the first European Consensus Conference on SDD [41] concluded that *the available information does not permit an unequivocal recommendation for the use of SDD in any particular population of patients*, basing this statement on the lack of evidence that mortality can be reduced by SDD. Since then, several controlled trials and meta-analyses have been published, demonstrating that the combination of topical and systemic antibiotics reduces the rate of both pneumonia and mortality, while SDD performed using topical antibiotics alone reduces only the incidence of pneumonia, but not of mortality [36, 42-44].

## Pathogenesis and Etiology

As regards the pathogenesis and the etiology of VAP, the postulated mechanism is the aspiration of contaminated secretions from the oropharynx into the lower respiratory tract, which is a common event in critically ill patients. Pneumonia can result when the inoculum is large, the microbes are virulent, or host defences are impaired [25]. Micro-organisms responsible for VAP may differ according to the population of patients in the ICU, the duration of mechanical ventilation and ICU stay, and the specific diagnostic methods used [22]. The data from a recent review [22] revealed that the dominant etiologic agents in VAP are gram-negative bacteria (accounting for 50-70% of all VAP episodes): the most common bacteria within this category are *Pseudomonas aeruginosa* (accounting for 24% of all VAP), Enterobacteriaceae such as *Escherichia coli*, *Klebsiella* spp., *Proteus* spp., *Enterobacter* spp., *Serratia* spp., *Citrobacter* spp. (accounting for about 14% of all VAP), *H. influenzae* (accounting for about 10% of all VAP), *Acinetobacter* spp. (accounting for about 8% of all VAP), and *S. maltophilia* (accounting for about 2% of all VAP). *S. aureus* is second to gram-negative bacteria, and it accounts for about 20% of all VAP episodes, with an increasing incidence, while *S. pneumoniae* is involved in about 4% of cases. *Legionella* spp., anaerobes, viruses, fungi, and even *P. carinii* should be mentioned as potential etiologic agents, but are not common in this context. However, these agents may be potentially underestimated because of difficulties involved with the diagnostic techniques used to identify them. In up to 40-50% of patients, the etiology is a polymicrobial infection [45]. The etiologic agents involved in early-onset VAP somewhat differ from those found in late-onset VAP. The pathogens that are most frequently associated with "early pneumonia" are methicillin-sensitive *S. aureus*, *H. influenzae*, *S. pneumoniae* and susceptible Enterobacteriaceae, whereas the pathogens most frequently associated with "late pneumonia" are *P. aeruginosa*, *Acinetobacter baumannii*, methicillin-resistant *S. aureus* (MRSA), and multiresistant gram-negative bacteria [22]. Patients with late pneumonia are at risk for infection with potentially resistant micro-organisms, and this different distribution pattern of etiologic agents between early- and late-onset VAP may also be due to the prior use of broad-spectrum antibiotics in many patients with late-onset VAP [22, 46, 47]. Underlying diseases may predispose patients to infection with specific micro-organisms. For example, patients with COPD are at increased risk for *H. influenzae*, *S. pneumoniae* and *Moraxella catarrhalis* infections. Cystic fibrosis and structural lung disease (bronchiectasis) increase the risk of *P. aeruginosa* and *S. aureus* infections, whereas trauma and neurologic patients are at increased risk for *S. aureus* infection [22].

## Diagnosis

VAP is the most common ICU-acquired infection, but also the most difficult to diagnose. The signs and symptoms of VAP are not specific and a gold-standard diagnostic test is not available [27, 48]. The International Conference on the diagnosis and treatment of VAP (Tarragona, May 2000) [21] defined pneumonia as the presence of new and persistent chest X-ray pulmonary infiltrates not otherwise explained, associated with at least two of the following clinical criteria: fever > 38 °C, leukocytosis, and purulent respiratory secretions. Microbiological criteria are not necessary for the diagnosis [21]. Pneumonia is considered to be ventilator-associated if it occurs in intubated patients and it is judged not to have incubated before intubation [21]. A post-mortem study [49] established 69% sensitivity and 75% specificity for a diagnosis of VAP based on these clinical criteria. Thus, available data indicate that the diagnosis of VAP based only on

**Table 5.** Clinical pulmonary infections score (CPIS) calculation (from [50])

---

Temperature (°C)

$\geq 36.5$ and $\leq 38.4$ = 0 points

$\geq 38.5$ and $\leq 38.9$ = 1 point

$\geq 39$ and $\leq 36$ = 2 points
Blood leukocytes

$\geq 4,000$ or $\leq 11,000$ = 0 points

$< 4,000$ or $> 11,000$ = 1 point + band forms $\geq 50\%$= add 1 point
Tracheal secretions

Absence of tracheal secretions = 0 points

Presence of nonpurulent tracheal secretions = 1 point

Presence of purulent tracheal secretions = 2 points
Oxygenation: $PaO_2/FiO_2$ (mmHg)

> 240 or ARDS (ARDS defined as $PaO_2/FiO_2 \leq 200$, pulmonary arterial wedge pressure $\leq 18$ mmHg and acute bilateral infiltrate) = 0 points

$\leq 240$ and no ARDS = 2 points
Pulmonary radiography

No infiltrate = 0 points

Diffuse (or patchy) infiltrate = 1 point

Localized infiltrate = 2 points
Progression of pulmonary infiltrate

No radiographic progression = 0 points

Radiographic progression (after CHF and ARDS excluded) = 2 points
Culture of tracheal aspirate

Pathogenic bacteria cultured in rare or light quantity or no growth = 0 point

Pathogenic bacteria cultured in moderate or heavy quantity = 1 point

Same pathogenic bacteria seen on Gram stain, add 1 point

---

*ARDS*, acute respiratory distress syndrome; *CHF*, congestive heart failure; *$PaO_2/FiO_2$*, ratio of arterial oxygen pressure to fraction of inspired oxygen

clinical criteria is associated with 30-35% of false negative and 20-25% of false positive results. An effort to improve the diagnostic yield of clinical parameters was made by Pugin *et al.* [50], who designed a score combining clinical, physiological, and microbiological parameters (Table 5).

A high clinical pulmonary infection score (CPIS), with a threshold value of 6, was found to correlate to a diagnosis of VAP [50]. Some investigators [51-53] demonstrated that CPIS [51, 52], or its simplified version [53], could be used to evaluate the response to therapy or to select patients for whom a short course of antibiotics may be appropriate. However, this scoring system is tedious to calculate and difficult to use in clinical practice, because several variables, such as purulence of tracheal secretions and progression of pulmonary infiltrates, can lead to different calculations depending on the observer [22].

Microbiological data may improve the precision of diagnosis and could also be useful for the choice of antibiotic therapy. A suspected diagnosis of VAP could be confirmed by isolation of a pathogenic micro-organism from blood and, eventually, pleural effusion cultures, or from respiratory secretions. Bacteriemia and positive pleural effusion cultures are generally considered to be able to identify the etiologic agent causing pneumonia, if no other source of infection is found. Therefore, two sets of blood cultures should be drawn and any significant pleural effusion should be sampled before initiating antibiotic therapy, even if spread to the blood or the pleural space occurs in less than 10% of VAP patients [22].

As regards the methods for obtaining samples from the respiratory tract, there is still much controversy. The debate centers on the cost and efficacy of the different techniques of respiratory-tract sampling. There essentially are two different diagnostic approaches:

- *Non-invasive techniques*: culture of endotracheal aspirate is the easiest, less expensive and most widely used microbiological technique. It is known to have a high sensitivity, and negative results virtually exclude pneumonia due to the common aerobic pathogens [22, 25]. The specificity is much lower, and qualitative culture has a high percentage of false-positive results because of bacterial colonization of the proximal airways [54]. Some investigations from several groups [55-59] showed that the specificity of unprotected tracheal aspirates may be improved by a quantitative analysis with a cut-off point of $\geq$ $10^6$ cfu/ml. Thus, tracheal aspirates have a role in diagnosing pneumonia, and, by adopting a quantitative analysis, may have an acceptable overall accuracy, similar to that of other, more invasive techniques [55-59]. Tracheal aspirate may be an adequate tool for the diagnosis when fiber-optic techniques are available [22].
- *Invasive techniques*: secretions of distal airways are collected through a bronchoscope to avoid contamination of the upper airways. Broncho-alveolar lavage (BAL) is a safe method for sampling secretions of a large and distal area of the lung; the cut-off point is $\geq$ $10^4$ cfu/ml [22]. Protective specimen brushing (PSB) collects uncontaminated specimens directly from the affected area; the cut-off point is $\geq$ $10^3$ cfu/ml [22]. These two invasive techniques have a specificity and sensitivity higher than 80% [22, 25].

The clinical usefulness of the different techniques of respiratory-tract sampling is still an open question. Many studies compared invasive and non-invasive techniques of respiratory sampling, and the conclusions were often contradictory [60, 61]. French researchers, Chastre and Fagon [61] advocated the use of invasive bronchoscopic sampling, such as PSB and BAL. On the other hand, ther researchers such as Niedermanand *et al.* [60] are in favour of non-invasive techniques, such as qualitative and quantitative examinations of tracheal aspirate. Some trials evaluated the impact of the different diagnostic techniques on antibiotic use and outcome of patients with suspected VAP. Three Spanish randomized trials [62-64] did not find any significant difference in patient morbidity and mortality when invasive (PSB or BAL) or non-invasive (quantitative endotracheal aspirate cultures) techniques were compared. However, these studies considered relatively few patients (51, 76, and 88, respectively), and antibiotics were continued in all of theme despite negative cultures. On the contrary, a large randomized trial comparing invasive to non-invasive techniques on 413 patients with suspected VAP found that the former reduced the antibiotic use and improved patient outcome, both in terms of mortality (16% vs. 25% on day 14) and morbidity (lower mean sepsis-related organ failure assessment scores on days 3 and 7) [65]. Similar results in terms of mortality (19% vs. 35%) were reported in a smaller trial [66]. Thus, we believe that the use of an invasive approach for the diagnosis of VAP may reduce antibiotic use and improve patient outcome. Furthermore treatment of VAP should be based on the results of reliable microbiological investigations whenever possible. However, we also believe that there are some reasons not to systematically use these invasive techniques in patients with suspected VAP: (1) their accuracy is questionable for patients who received new antibiotics after the onset of symptoms suggestive of VAP; (2) they may transiently worsen the patient's status; (3) a systematically invasive approach may increase the costs; (4) there is evidence that some physicians are reluctant to discontinue antibiotics for suspected VAP despite a negative culture [52, 60, 66, 67].

## Therapy

There is a general agreement that the appropriateness of the initial antibiotic regimen is a crucial determinant of outcome [21, 22, 25, 29], and several studies have shown that immediate initiation of appropriate antibiotic therapy is associated with a reduced mortality from pulmonary infections [68-72]. Therefore, empirical antibiotic therapy must be started before microbiological results are available and should be based on local microbial epidemiology and patterns of resistance [21, 25]. The choice of an empirical therapy is particularly difficult in critically ill, mechanically ventilated patients, for the following reasons: first, VAPs are likely to result from highly resistant micro-organisms, especially in patients previously treated with antibiotics [46, 47]; second, multiple micro-organisms are frequently cultured from pulmonary secretions of patients with suspected VAP [46, 54], thereby even an empirical broad-spectrum antibiotic therapy would not ensure an adequate coverage for all potential pathogens; finally, the use of an empirical broad-spectrum antibiotic therapy may contribute to the emergence of multiresistant pathogens and increase the risk of severe super-infections [22]. In 1996, ATS published a Consensus Statement [29] that provided guidelines on initial antimicrobial therapy based on assessments of disease severity, the presence of risk factors for specific micro-organisms, and time of onset of pneumonia. Because these guidelines have not been updated since their publication, they do not include newer antibiotics that may be effective and/or associated with less resistance rates, such as cefepime, meropenem and newer fluoroquinolones. Moreover, the risk stratification proposed by the ATS did not consider important variables, such as the previous use of antibiotics [47].

On the basis of these considerations and according to the kind of patients, as well as to the local microbiological etiology of VAPs and patterns of resistance, monotherapy with a second-generation cephalosporin (cefotetan, cefuroxime), or a third-generation cephalosporin without anti-pseudomonal activity (cefotaxime, ceftriaxone), or a β-lactam (amoxicillin) combined to a β-lactamase inhibitor (clavulanic acid), may represent an appropriate choice for most patients with an early-onset VAP who have not received prior antimicrobial treatment [22]. In patients with allergy to penicillin, a fluoroquinolone, or clindamycin plus aztreonam may be used [22, 29]. An early-onset VAP must be treated with a combination therapy like that used to treat a late-onset VAP, if it occurs after a prolonged hospitalization, or in COPD or malnutrited patients, or in patients with structural lung disease (bronchiectasis), or in patients who received antibiotic therapy in the last 3 months or a prolonged course of corticosteroids for a prolonged time [21, 22].

Patients with late-onset VAP should be treated with a combination antimicrobial therapy: aminoglycosides or ciprofloxacin combined with a broad-spectrum anti-pseudomonal β-lactam (piperacillina-/tazobactam) or with a third-generation cephalosporin with anti-pseudomonal activity (ceftazidime, cefepime), or with a carbapenem (imipenem, meropenem). A glycopeptide should be added in patients at risk of developing VAP due to MRSA. Indeed, *S. aureus*, usually methicillin-sensitive (MSSA), is a common pathogen in neurosurgical, head-trauma and comatose patients, or in patients who have a history of intravenous drug use, recent influenza, diabetes mellitus, and renal failure. If VAP develops after the patient has had a prolonged hospital stay or after the use of antibiotics, there is an increased risk of infection with MRSA [73].

The treatment of pulmonary infections in immunocompromised patients must take into account for different pathogens according to the type of immunodeficiency [74]. In severe neutropenia, the pulmonary infection may be due to fungi, such as *Candida* spp., or *Aspergillus* spp. In this situation, antifungal therapy should be considered. A defect of cell-mediated immunity increases the risk of infection due to *Legionella pneumophila*, *Pneumocystis carinii*, *Mycobacterium tubercolosis* and *M. avium*, and viruses [74]. Cytomegalovirus (CMV) is the major cause of pulmonary infection in patients undergoing solid-organ transplantation, while *Pneumocystis carinii* is the most common cause of pneumonia in HIV patients. Bronchoscopy with BAL plays a major role in diagnosis, particularly for *Pneumocystis carinii* and CMV [75]. Transbronchial biopsy must be used when clinical and radiological criteria are positive for pulmonary infection but microbiological results are negative. Empirical antibiotic therapy could be started before receiving microbiological results, and trimethoprim-sulfamethoxazole is the drug of choice if a *Pneumocystis carinii* is suspected. Macrolides or fluorquinolones are the drug of choice if pneumonia is suspected to be caused by *Legionella pneumophila*.

Recent data have revealed that consistent use of a few, broad-spectrum antibiotics in rotation reduces the prevalence of resistant strains [35, 76, 77]. In these protocols, a group of antibiotics is chosen for empirical treatment of all suspected infections according to the local patterns of resistance and is used exclusively for a several-month period and then avoided for the remainder of the year. In this way, the prevalence of resistant isolates in the face of new selection pressure increases linearly with time, while the loss of prevalence after the selection pressure is removed occurs by exponential decay [25].

Another important concept that should be kept in mind the concept of de-escalation therapy, which is based on the use of a broad-spectrum, high-dose, empirical antibiotic therapy, which is reassessed and reduced to a narrower-spectrum therapy when microbiological data are available, according to the results of the microbiological and susceptibility tests. Among physicians there is a general agreement with the concept of de-escalation therapy, because the use of broad-spectrum antibiotics for not more than 48 h, until the results of microbiological tests become available, does not seem to favour the development of multiresistance [21]. On the contrary, the duration of an established, definitive antibiotic therapy for a VAP is still a question under debate. The American Thoracic Society recommended that the duration of therapy should be based on the severity of pneumonia, the clinical response, and the causative pathogen [29]. As a general statement, patients infected with sensitive micro-organism may be treated for 7-10 days; patients infected with multiresistant pathogens may require 14-21 days of treatment; also patients with multilobar, necrotizing, or cavitary pneumonia require prolonged (2-3 weeks) treatment [29]. The majority of the experts participating in the International Conference on the diagnosis and treatment of VAP (Tarragona, May 2000) [21] recommended a duration of treatment for VAP of 7-10 days, but a consensus among the participants was not reached. During the discussion, it was agreed that the main factor for deciding the duration of therapy should be the time to clinical response and not the pathogen involved, and therefore that all patients should be treated for at least 72 h after clinical response [21]. From a conceptual point of view, there are three potential disadvantages for using prolonged antimicrobial therapy: (1) the emergence of multiresistant micro-organisms, (2) antibiotic toxicity, and (3) increased costs [22]. However, a regimen of insufficient duration may be associated with high rates of relapse and treatment failure. Thus, a short-term regimen has been rarely prescribed. Singh *et al.* [52] showed that patients with clinically suspected VAP who had a CPIS ≤ 6 (implying low likelihood of VAP) can be safely managed with a 3-day course of monotherapy. Similar results were obtained by Ibrahim *et al.* [78], who studied patients who were more likely to have VAP (mean CPIS of 6.9±1.2). This group found that a duration of antibiotic treatment limited to 7 days, unless persistent signs and symptoms of infection were present, was correlated with a better outcome. In conclusion, the complexities of diagnosing VAP, the escalating problems of antimicrobial resistance, and the importance of prescribing an appropriate initial antibiotic treatment to patients with VAP, might be responsible in part for with-holding, delaying, or overutilizing antimicrobial treatment in critically ill patients. Kollef [79] recently proposed an approach for the antibiotic management of VAP (Fig. 1), based on the overriding need to prescribe an appropriate

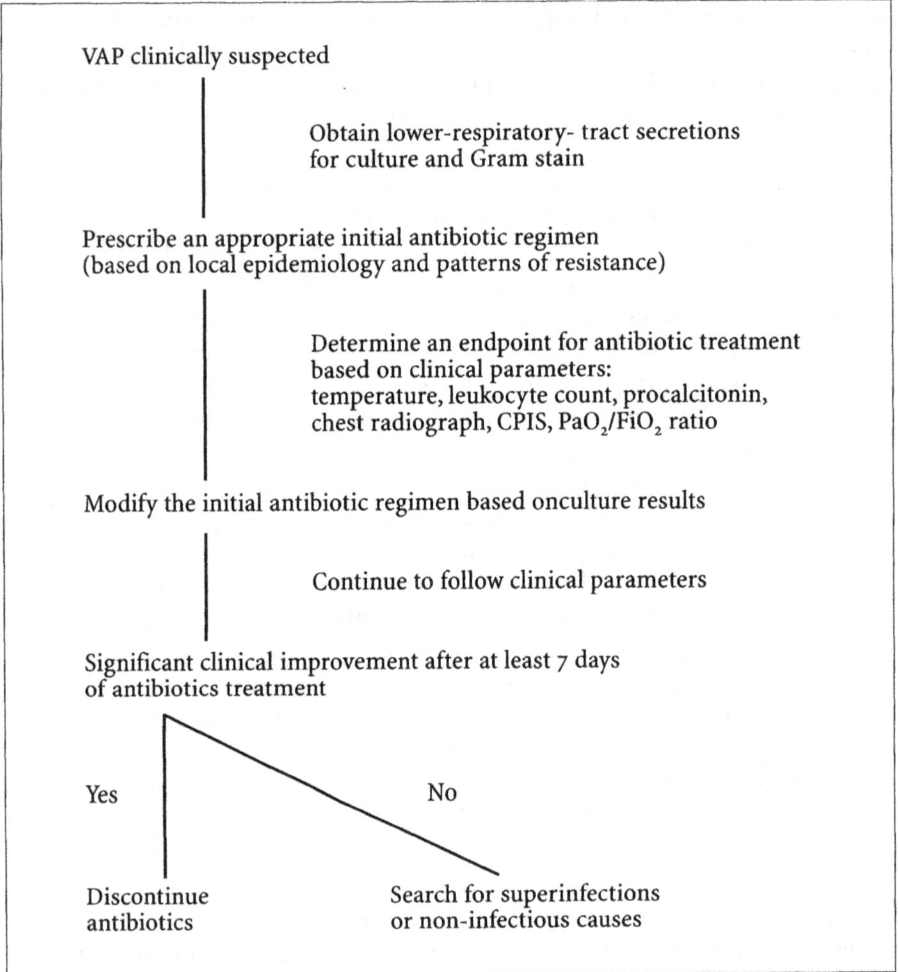



**Fig. 1.** Simple algorithm for the antibiotic management of ventilator-associated pneumonia (VAP), modified from [79]. *CPIS*, clinical pulmonary infection score

initial antibiotic treatment while attempting to minimize the occurrence of antibiotic resistance. This approach emphasizes the importance of obtaining lower-respiratory-tract secretions for both culture and Gram stain before the initiation of antibiotic therapy and of modifying the initial regimen according to the culture results, even if it is difficult to change a treatment that seems to be working with a narrower-spectrum one. Moreover, it stresses the concept that the elements of CPIS, especially the $PaO_2/FiO_2$ ratio (but we also add other elements, such as the trend of procalcitonin plasma levels in bacterial infections [12]), may be used to determine a logical endpoint for antibiotic treatment of VAP as opposed to arbitrary treatments that usually range from 10 to 21 days [77].

# References

1. (1999) Gruppo italiano di studio sulle infezioni gravi GISIG. Diagnostica e terapia del paziente con o senza deficit immunologico che entra con polmonite e grave insufficienza respiratoria. In: Infezioni in Terapia Intensiva, Langer M (ed) Effetti, Milano:49-67
2. Marrie TJ, Durant H, Yates L et al (1989) Community acquired pneumonia requiring hospitalisation: 5 year prospective study. Rev Infect Dis 11:586-599
3. (1997) Centers for desease control and prevention. Premature deaths, monthly mortality and monthly physicians contacts-United States. MMWR Morb Mortal Wkly Rep 46:556
4. Marston BJ, Plouffe JF, File TM et al (1997) Incidence of community-acquired pneumonia requiring hospitalization: results of a population based active surveillance study in Ohio. Arch Int Med 157:1509-1718
5. Blasi F (2002) Polmonite acquisita in comunità: epidemiologia e definizione. In: Polmoniti Clinica e Terapia, Blasi F (ed) Pharma Project Group, Saronno (VA):3-7
6. Fine MJ, Smith MA, Carson CA et al (1996) Prognosis and outcomes of patients with community-acquired pneumonia: a meta analysis. Jama 275:134-141
7. Torres A, El Ebiary M, Zavola E et al (1996) Severe community acquired pneumonia. Sem Respir Crit Care Med 17:265-271
8. (2001) American Thoracic Society Guidelines for the management of adults with community-acquired pneumonia. Diagnosis, assessment of severity, antimicrobial therapy, and prevention. Am J Respir Crit Care Med 163:1730-1754
9. (1993) American Thoracic Society Guidelines for the initial management of adults with community acquired pneumonia: diagnosis, assessment of severity and initial antimicrobial therapy (official ATS statement). Am Rev Respir Dis 148:1418-1426
10. Ewig S, Ruiz M, Mensa J et al (1998) Severe community acquired pneumonia: assessment of severity criteria. Am J Respir Crit Care Med 158:1102-1108
11. Moine P, Verken JB, Chevret S et al (1994) Severe CAP. Etiology, epidemiology and prognosis factors. French Study Group for CAP in ICU. Chest 105:1487-1495
12. Luzzani A, Polati E, Dorizzi R, Rungatscher A, Pavan R, Merlini A (2003) Comparison of procalcitonin and C-reactive protein as markers of sepsis. Crit Care Med 31 (in press)
13. Bartlett JG, Dowell SF, Mandell LA et al (2000) Practice guidelines for the management of community-acquired pneumonia in adults. Guidelines from the Infectious Diseases Society of America. Clin Infect Dis 31:347-382
14. Sorensen J, Forsberg P, Hakanson E et al (1989) A new diagnostic approach to the patient with severe pneumonia. Scand J Infect Dis 21:33-41
15. Rello J, Paiva JA, Dias CS et al (2003) Current dilemmas in the management of adults with severe community-acquired pneumonia. In: Yearbook of Intensive Care and Emergency Medicine, Vincent JL (ed) Springer-Verlag, Berlin, Heidelberg, New York, London, Milan, Paris, Tokyo 162-174
16. Gordon GS, Throop D, Berberian L et al (1996) Validation of the therapeutic recommendations of the American Thoracic Society (ATS) guidelines for community acquired pneumonia in hospitalized patients. Chest 110:55S
17. Gleason PP, Kapoor WN, Stone RA et al (1997) Medical outcomes and antimicrobial costs with the use of American Thoracic Society guidelines for outpatients with community-acquired pneumonia. JAMA 278:32-39
18. Leroy O, Santre C, Beuscart C et al (1995) A 5-year study of severe community-acquired pneumonia with emphasis on prognosis in patients admitted to an ICU. Intensive Care Med 21:24-31
19. (1998) European Study on Community-acquired pneumonia (ESOCAP) Committee. Guidelines for management of adult community-acquired lower respiratory tract infections. Eur Respir J 11:986-991

20. Arbo MDJ, Snydman DR (1994) Influence of blood cultures results on antibiotic choice in treatment of bacteremia. Arch Intern Med 154:2641-2645
21. Rello J, Paiva JA, Baraibar J et al (2001) International Consensus Conference for the Development of Consensus on the Diagnisis and Treatment of Ventilator-Associated Pneumonia, Chest 120:955-970
22. Chastre J, Fagon JY (2002) Ventilator-associated pneumonia, State of the Art. Am J Respir Crit Care Med 165:867-903
23. Langer M, Cigada M, Mandelli M et al (1987) Early onset pneumonia: a multicenter study in intensive care unit. Intensive Care Med 13:342-346
24. Kerver AJ, Rommes JH, Mevissen Verhage EA et al (1987) Colonization and infection in surgical intensive care patients: a prospective study. Intensive Care Med 13:347-351
25. Hubmayr RD (2002) Statement of the 4th International Consensus Conference in Critical Care on ICU-acquired pneumonia-Chicago, Illinois, May 2002. Intensive Care Med 28:1521-1526
26. Chevret S, Hemmer M, Carlet J, Langer M et al (1993) Incidence and risk factors of pneumonia acquired in ICU. Int.Care Med 19:256-264
27. Vincent JL, Bihari DJ, Suter PM et al (1995) The prevalence of nosocomial infection in intensive care units in Europe. Results of the European Prevalence of Infection in Intensive Care (EPIC) Study. EPIC International Advisory Committe. JAMA 274:639-644
28. Warren DK, Shukl SJ, Olsen MA et al (2003) Outcome and attributable cost of ventilator associated pneumonia among intensive care unit patients in a suburban medical centre. Crit Care Med 31:1312-1321
29. (1996) American Thoracic Society. Hospital acquired pneumonia in adults: diagnosis, assessment of severity, initial antimicrobical therapy, and preventive strategies. Am J Resp Crit care Med 153:1711-1725
30. Torres A, Gatell JM, Aznar E et al (1995) Re-intubation increases the risk of nosocomial pneumonia in patients needing mechanical ventilation. Am J Respir Crit Care Med 152:137-141
31. Kollef MH (1993) Ventilator-associated pneumonia. A multivariate analysis. JAMA 270:1965-1970
32. Drakulovic MB, Torres A, Bauer TT et al (1999) Supine body position as a risk factor for nosocomial pneumonia in mechanically ventilated patients: a randomised trial. Lancet 354:1851-1858
33. Cook D, Guyatt G Marshall J et al (1998) A comparison of sucralfate and ranitidine for the prevention of upper gastrointestinal bleeding in patients requiring mechanical ventilation. Canadian Critical Care Trials Group. N Eng J Med 338:791-797
34. Allegranzi B, Luzzati R, Luzzani A et al (2002) Impact of antibiotic changes in empiricalal therapy on antimicrobial resistance in intensive care unit-acquired infections. J Hosp Infect 52:136-140
35. Sirvent JM, Torres A, El-Ebiary M et al (1997) Protective effect of intravenously administered cefuroxime against nosocomial pneumonia in patients with structural coma. Am J Respir Crit Care Med 155:1729-1734
36. D'Amico R, Pifferi S, Leonetti C et al (1998) Effectiveness of antibiotic prophylaxis in critically ill adult patients: systematic review of randomised controlled trials. Br Med J 316:1275-1285
37. Rello J, Diaz E, Roque M et al (1999) Risk factors for developing pneumonia within 48 hours of intubation. Am J Respir Crit Care Med 159:1742-1746
38. George DL, Falk PS, Wunderink RG et al (1998) Epidemiology of ventilator-acquired pneumonia based on protected bronchoscopic sampling. Am J Respir Crit Care Med 158:1839-1847
39. Cook DJ, Walter SD, Cook RJ et al (1998) Incidence and risk factors for ventilator-associated pneumonia in critically ill patients. Ann Intern Med 129:433-440

40. Heinenger A, Krueger WA, Unertl KE (2003) A reappraisal of selective decontamination of the digestive tract. In: Yearbook of Intensive Care and Emergency Medicine, Vincent JL (ed) Springer-Verlag, Berlin, Heidelberg, New York, London, Milan, Paris, Tokyo: 199-208
41. Loirat P, Johanson WG, Van Saene HFK et al (1992) Selective decontamination in intensive care unit patients. Intensive Care Med 18:182-188
42. Nathens AV, Marshall JC (1999) Selective decontamination of the digestive tract in surgical patients. Arch Surg 134:170-176
43. Krueger WA, Lenhart FP, Neesen G et al (2002) Influence of combined intravenous and topical antibiotic prophylaxis on the incidence of infections, organ dysfunctions, and mortality in critically ill surgical patients. Am J Respir Crit Care Med 166:1029-1037
44. De Jonge E, Schultz M, Spanjaard L et al (2002) Effects of selective decontamination of the digestive tract on mortality and antibiotic resistance. Intensive Care Med 28 (Suppl 1):S12
45. Gruppo italiano di studio sulle infezioni gravi GISIG (1999) La polmonite nel paziente ventilato. In: Infezioni in Terapia Intensiva, Langer M (ed) Effetti, Milano: 68-97
46. Rello J, Ausina V, Ricart M et al (1993) Impact of previous antimicrobial therapy on the etiology and outcome of ventilator-associated pneumonia. Chest 104:1230-1235
47. Trouillet JL, Chastre J, Vaugnat A et al (1998) Ventilator-associated pneumonia caused by potentially drug-resistant bacteria. Am J Respir Crit Care Med 157:531-539
48. Aarts MA, Marshall JC (2003) Empirical antibiotics in critical illness: do they help or harm? In: Yearbook of Intensive Care and Emergency Medicine, Vincent JL (ed) Springer-Verlag, Berlin, Heidelberg., New York, London, Milan, Paris, Tokyo: 219-28
49. Torres A, El-Ebiary M, Padro L et al (1994) Validation of different techniques for the diagnosis of ventilator-associated pneumonia. Comparison with immediate postmortem pulmonary biopsy. Am J Respir Crit Care Med 149:324-331
50. Pugin J, Auckenthaler R, Mili N at al (1991) Diagnosis of ventilator-associated pneumonia by bacteriologic analysis of bronchoscopic and non- bronchoscopic "blind" bronchoalveolar lavage fluid. Am Rev Respir Dis 143:1121-1129
51. Singh N, Yu V (2000) Rational empirical antibiotic prescription in the ICU: clinical research is mandatory. Chest 117:1496-1499
52. Singh N, Rogers P, Atwood CW et al (2000) Short-course empirical antibiotic therapy for patients with pulmonary infiltrates in the intensive care unit: a proposed solution for indiscriminate antibiotic prescription. Am J Respir Crit Care Med 162:505-511
53. Luna MC, Blanzaco D, Niederman MS et al (2003) Resolution of ventilator-associated pneumonia: prospective evaluation of the clinical pulmonary infection score as an early clinical predictor of outcome. Crit Care Med 31:676-682
54. Torres A, Puig de la Bellacasa J, Xaubet A et al (1989) Diagnostic value of quantitative cultures of bronchoalveolar lavage and telescoping plugged catheters in mechanically ventilated patients with bacterial pneumonia. Am Rev Respir Dis 140:306-310
55. Torres A, Martos A, Puig de la Bellacasa J et al (1993) Specificity of endotracheal aspiration, protected specimen brush and bronchoalveolar lavage in mechanically ventilated patients. Am Rev Respir Dis 147:952-957
56. Marquette CH, Georges H, Wallet F et al (1993) Diagnostic efficiency of endotracheal aspirates with quantitative bacterial cultures in intubated patients with suspected pneumonia. Comparison with the protected specimen brushing. Am Rev Respir Dis 148:138-144
57. El-Ebiary M, Torres A, Gonzales J et al (1993) Quantitative cultures of endotracheal aspirates for the diagnosis of ventilator associated pneumonia. Am Rev Respir Dis 148:1552-1567

58. Marquette CH, Copin MC, Wallet F et al (1995) Diagnostic tests for pneumonia in ventilated patients: prospective evaluation of diagnostic accuracy using histology as a diagnostic gold standard. Am J Respir Crit Care Med 151:1878-1888
59. Cook D, Mandell L (2000) Endotracheal aspiration in the diagnosis of ventilator-associated pneumonia. Chest 117(S):195-197
60. Niederman MS, Torres A, Summer W et al (1994) Invasive diagnostic testing is not needed routinely to manage suspected ventilator-associated pneumonia. Am J Respir Crit Care Med 150:565-569
61. Chastre J, Fagon JY (1994) Invasive diagnostic testing should be routinely used to manage patients with suspected pneumonia. Am J Respir Crit Care Med 150:570-574
62. Sanchez-Nieto JM, Torres A, Garcia Cordoba F et al (1998) Impact of invasive and non invasive quantitative culture sampling on outcome of ventilator-associated pneumonia: a pilot study. Am J Respir Crit Care Med 157:371-376
63. Ruiz M, Torres A, Ewig S et al (2000) Noninvasive versus invasive microbial investigation in ventilator-associated pneumonia: evaluation of outcome. Am J Respir Crit Care Med 162:119-125
64. Sole Violan J, Fernandez JA, Benitez AB et al (2000) Impact of quantitative invasive diagnostic techniques in the management and outcome of mechanically ventilated patients with suspected pneumonia. Crit Care Med 28:2737-2741
65. Fagon JY, Chastre J, Wolff M et al (2000) Invasive and non-invasive strategies for management of suspected ventilator-associated pneumonia. A randomized trial. Ann Intern Med 132:621-630
66. Heyland DK, Cook DJ, Marshall J et al (1999) The clinical utility of invasive diagnostic techniques in the setting of ventilator-associated pneumonia. Canadian Critical Care Trials Group. Chest 115:1076-1084
67. Niederman MS (1998) Bronchoscopy for ventilator-associated pneumonia: show me the money (outcome benefit)! Crit Care Med 26:198-199
68. Alvarez-Lerma F (1996) Modification of empirical antibiotic treatment in patients with pneumonia acquired in the intensive care unit. ICU-Acquired Pneumonia Study Group. Intensive Care Med 22:387-394
69. Luna CM, Vujacich P, Niederman MS et al (1997) Impact of BAL data on the therapy and outcome of ventilator-associated pneumonia. Chest 111:676-685
70. Rello J, Gallego M, Mariscal D et al (1997) The value of routine microbial investigation in ventilator-associated pneumonia. Am J Respir Crit Care Med 156:196-200
71. Heyland DK, Cook DJ, Griffith L et al (1999) The attributable morbidity and mortality of ventilator-associated pneumonia in the critically ill patients. The Canadian Critical Care Trials Group. Am J Respir Crit Care Med 159:1249-1256
72. Kollef MH, Sherman G, Ward S, Fraser VJ (1999) Inadequate antimicrobial treatment of infections: a risk factor for hospital mortality among critically ill patients. Chest 115:462-474
73. Rello J, Torres A, Ricart M et al (1994) Ventilator-associated pneumonia by Staphylococcus aureus. Comparison of methicillin-resistant and methicillin-sensitive episodes. Am J Respir Crit Care Med 150:1545-1549
74. Palmer DL (1984) Microbiology of pneumonia in the patient at risk. Am J Med 76:53-60
75. Menon LR, Divate S, Achaya VN et al (2002) Utility of BAL in the diagnosis of pulmonary infections in immunosuppressed patient. J Assoc Physicians India 50:1110-1114
76. Kollef MH, Vlasnik J, Sharpless L et al (1997) Scheduled change of antibiotic classes: a strategy to decrease the incidence of ventilator-associated pneumonia. Am J Respir Crit Care Med 156:1040-1048
77. Raymond DP, Pelletier SJ, Crabtree TD et al (2001) Impact of a rotating empiric antibiotic schedule on infectious mortality in an intensive care unit. Crit Care Med 29:1101-1108

78. Ibrahim EH, Ward S, Sherman G et al (2001) Experience with a clinical guideline for the treatment of ventilator-associated pneumonia. Crit Care Med 29:1109-1115
79. Kollef MH (2003) Treatment of ventilator-associated pneumonia: get it right from the start. Crit Care Med 31:969-970

# Intravascular Catheter- Related Infections: An Update on Epidemiology and Prevention

M. Viviani, R. Dezzoni, L. Silvestri, H.K.F. van Saene

## Epidemiology

In modern-day medical care, the use of intravascular devices, especially in an intensive care (ICU) setting, is necessary because of the continuous increase in the numbers of catheters inserted, the possibility to administer various fluids and the use of invasive cardiovascular monitoring. However, extensive clinical use of central venous catheters (CVC) is associated with various iatrogenic diseases, particularly local and systemic infectious complications, such as local site infections, intravascular catheter-related bloodstream infections (CR-BSI), septic thrombophlebitis, endocarditis and metastatic infections (e.g., cerebral abscess, lung abscess, osteomyelitis).

The incidence of CR-BSI depends on numerous factors, particularly, illness severity with increasing co-morbidity (malignancy, neutropenia, shock), length of ICU stay, prolonged indwelling catheter time, insertion at the emergency scene without aseptic technique [1], type of catheter (multi-lumen, tunnelled, cuffed, anti-infective coating, etc.), frequency of catheter manipulation because of drug administration, total parenteral nutrition, fluids, and haemodynamic invasive monitoring [2].

Several studies showed a relationship between the use of CVCs and the potential increase of morbidity and mortality of ICU patients due to infective complications [2]. For this reason, a valid method of calculation is necessary to estimate the rate of catheter-associated BSIs. In general, the parameter commonly preferred is the number of new episodes of catheters-related BSIs per 1000 CVC days [3, 4] instead of rate of catheter-associated infections (number of episodes / 100 catheters). Also important is the standardization of definitions of clinical and microbiological catheter-related bloodstream infections to avoid possible reporting errors. In particular, the rate of true CR-BSI could be overestimated if all other sources of secondary bacteraemia (e.g., hospital-associated pneumonia, urinary tract infections, postoperative surgical sites, intra-abdominal infections) are not excluded and if the pathogens isolated from catheter (or catheter segment) and/or in the bloodstream samples are not the same [2]. Although in 1996 the HICPAC [5] consensus proposed an example of the appropriate definition of terms (Table 1), it is not still universally accepted. Therefore the estimation of CR-BSI varies depending on clinical data and methods employed for the diagnosis.

**Table 1.** Definition of microbiological complications related to central venous catheters.

| Infections | Definitions |
| --- | --- |
| Catheter colonization | Significant growth of a microorganism in a quantitative or semiquantitative culture of the catheter tip, subcutaneous catheter segment, or catheter hub |
| Phlebitis | Induration or erythema, warmth, and pain or tenderness around catheter exit site |
| Exit-site infection | |
| Microbiological | Exudate at catheter exit site yields a microorganism with or without concomitant bloodstream infection |
| Clinical | Erythema, induration, and/or tenderness within 2 cm of the catheter exit site; may be associated with other signs and symptoms of infection, such as fever or pus emerging from the exit site, with or without concomitant bloodstream infection |
| Tunnel infection | Tenderness, erythema, and/or induration > 2 cm from the catheter exit site, along the subcutaneous tract of a tunneled catheter (e.g., Hickman or Broviac catheter), with or without concomitant bloodstream infection |
| CR-BSI | |
| Infusate related | Concordant growth of the same organism from infusate and cultures of percutaneously obtained blood samples with no other identifiable source of infection |
| Catheter related | Bacteremia or fungemia in a patient who has an intravascular device and $\geq 1$ positive result of culture of blood samples obtained from the peripheral vein, clinical manifestations of infection (e.g., fever, chills, and/or hypotension), and no apparent source for bloodstream infection (with the exception of the catheter). One of the following should be present: a positive result of semiquantitative ($\geq 5$ cfu per catheter segment) or quantitative ($\geq 10^2$ cfu per catheter segment) catheter culture, whereby the same organism (species and antibiogram) is isolated from a catheter segment and a peripheral blood sample; simultaneous quantitative cultures of blood samples with a ratio of $\geq 5{:}1$ (CVC vs. peripheral); differential time to positivization (i.e., a positive result of culture from a CVC is obtained at least 2 h earlier than is a positive result of culture from peripheral blood) |

Catheter-associated bloodstream infections are related to increased morbidity and mortality rates (10-20%), prolonged hospitalization (7-14 days, 24 days in survivors) and a rise in costs (excess of $ 10000 per hospitalization) [1].

Every type of device is correlated with an increased risk of BSI, but CVC is the most frequent cause. Central venous catheters are involved in up to 75% of CR-BSIs; particularly, noncuffed CVCs, single or multi-lumen catheters, short-term devices and CVC inserted into subclavian or internal jugular vein cause CR-BSIs ranging from 3 to 5% [6].

The relative risk of CR-BSI was evaluated in a meta-analysis [7] which considered both BSIs per 100-catheter and BSIs per 1000-catheter days rates. These rates depended on patients-related parameters (type of illness, illness severity) and on catheter-related parameters such as the type of catheter and the situation in which the catheter was inserted. During the period 1992-2001, NNIS reported the CR-BSI rates in patients admitted to intensive care. The results of this study showed changes of incidence corresponding to different type of ICU [cardiothoracic 2.9/$_{oo}$, coronary 4.5/$_{oo}$, neurosurgical 4.7/$_{oo}$, medical/surgical major teaching 5.3/$_{oo}$, neonatal nursery high risk from 3.8/$_{oo}$ (> 2500 g/weight) to 11.3/$_{oo}$ (< 1000 g/weight) and paediatric ICU from 3.4/$_{oo}$ (medical respiratory patients) to 9.7/$_{oo}$ (burn patients)] [4].

Types of pathogens isolated in patients with diagnosis of CR-BSI varied over time: during 1986-1989, coagulase-negative *Staphylococcus* (CNS) was isolated in 27% of BSIs followed by *Staphylococcus aureus* (16%), gram-negative bacilli (19%), enterococci (8%), and *Candida* spp. (8%) [8], while during the period 1992-1999, CNS was isolated in 37% of cases, enterococci in 13.5% (resistant to vancomycin 0.5% in 1989, 25.9% in 1999), *Staphylococcus aureus* in 12.6% (methicillin resistant in > 50% of all *Staphylococcus aureus* isolated), gram-negative bacilli in 14%, *Candida* spp. in 8% (10% were resistant to fluconazole) [3]. Gram-positive bacilli and particularly CNS and methicillin-resistant *Staphylococcus aureus* (MRSA) seem to represent the major cause of CR-BSI in intensive-care settings. Also, in our experience regarding adult intensive-care, data collected over 6 years are in agreement with the current literature. In fact, 76 episodes of catheter-related infection were diagnosed in 841 patients mechanically ventilated more than 3 days (1998-2003), for a total CR-BSI rate of 9.7/$_{oo}$ (unpublished data). This rate reduced from 10.2/$_{oo}$ to 4.5/$_{oo}$ when standardized prevention policy was introduced 2 years ago. CNS (36 episodes, 47.4%) accounted for the main pathogen isolated in diagnosed CR-BSI, the other principal microorganisms were: MRSA (*n*=19, 25%), *Pseudomonas aeruginosa* (*n*=8, 10.5%), other gram-negative (*n*=6, 7.8%), *Candida albicans* (*n*=1, 1.3%).

The CDC, in recently published guidelines, reported the results of a meta-analysis of CR-BSI. The case-fatality rate was 14%, and 19% of these deaths were attributable to the catheter-related infections. The mortality rate attributed to CR-BSI was 8.2% for *Staphylococcus aureus* (the highest), but only 0.7% for CNS (the lowest) [2].

## Pathogenesis

It is possible to classify the pathogenesis of CR-BSI as follows [6]:
- Contamination of the fluids infused through the catheter, or *"infusate-related infection"* (the most frequent cause of epidemic CR-BSI).
- Colonization of the device, or *"catheter-related infection"* (responsible for most endemic CR-BSI).

In the case of catheter-related infection, microorganisms can adhere to the catheter extraluminally or intraluminally. They are then incorporated into a biofilm, colonizing the device and sustaining the infection with dissemination into the bloodstream.

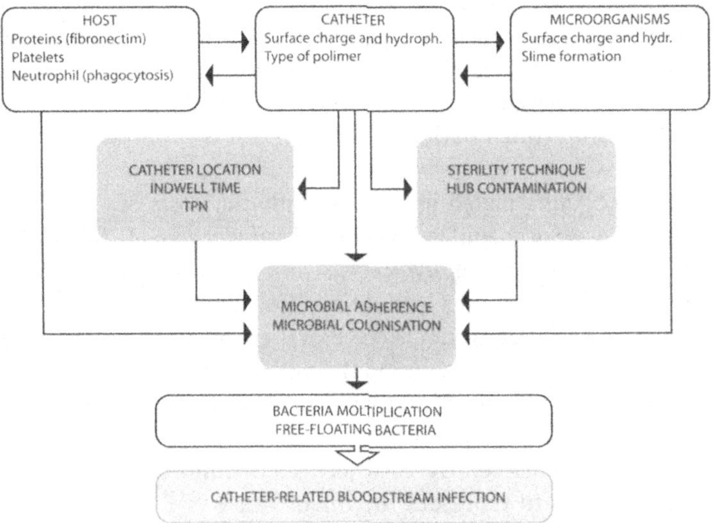


**Fig. 1.** Relationship between host, catheter surface and bacteria in the pathogenesis of CR-BSI

Three mechanisms (Figure 1) are implicated in this process [1, 2, 6]:
1. Skin microorganisms (usually gram-positive and resistant, especially in hospitalized patients) which are present around the insertion site of the catheter migrate into the percutaneous tract. Growth on the skin is favoured by local particular circumstances (lack of hygiene, warm, moist, foreign body) and allows invasion of the percutaneous tract at the time of insertion or after some days. The colonization and survival of the bacteria is facilitated if a thrombus (Table 2) has formed at the catheter tip or at the point in which the catheter penetrates the vessel wall. Substances produced by bacteria (adhesins, slime-associated antigen, etc.) determine the adherence and the cohesion on the catheter surfaces favoured by plasma proteins (fibrinonectin), platelets and leukocytes.

**Table 2.** Main characteristics of materials employed for catheter manufacture

| Material | Stiffness | Thrombogenesis |
| --- | --- | --- |
| Polyurethane | ++ | ++ |
| Polyurethane hydromers | + | + |
| Polyethylene | +++ | +++ |
| Polyvinylchloride | +++ | ++++ |
| Polypropylene | ++++ | ++++ |
| Nylon | +++ | +++ |
| Teflon | ++ | ++ |
| Silycon | o | + |

2. Microorganisms contaminate the catheter hub (and lumen) when the CVC is manipulated or is inserted through a percutaneous guidewire (extrinsic origin); otherwise the catheter can be contaminated by skin flora (intrinsic origin). This type of contamination is usually the cause of colonization of long-term catheters.
3. Haematogenous contamination of the intra-vascular device (IVD) from remote sources of infection (abscess, pneumonia, etc).

Another type of classification is based on indwelling time criteria [6]:
– *Short-term* IVDs (duration of insertion < 10 days): peripheral intravenous catheters, arterial catheters, noncuffed and nontunnelled CVCs. Most CR-BSIs are of cutaneous origin from the site of insertion (extraluminal origin).
– *Long-term* IVDs (duration of insertion ≥ 10 days): cuffed Hickman- and Broviac-type catheters, subcutaneous central venous catheter (Port), cuffed haemodialysis CVCs, peripherally inserted central catheters. Contamination of hub and lumen of catheter cause CR-BSIs (intraluminal origin).

Finally, it is important to understand two important pathogenic aspects of catheter-related infections [2]:
a. The *material* of which the catheter is made: some catheters present irregularities on their surface promoting adherence of a specific bacterial strain (e.g., CNS, *Pseudomonas aeruginosa, Acinetobacter calcoaceticus*) followed by colonization and infection (Fig. 1). Some *in vitro* studies have demonstrated that catheters made of Teflon, silicone elastomer or polyurethane are more resistant to colonization than those made of polyvinylchloride and polyethylene [9]. Furthermore, certain materials favour the formation of thrombi (polyvinylchloride, polyethylene) which predispose to colonization and infection (Table 2) [10].
b. *Intrinsic virulence factors*: some microorganisms, such as *Staphylococcus aureus*, which adhere to fibronectin (a host-derived protein deposited on the indwelling catheter surface) [11] and CNS (some strains produce an extracellular polysaccharide often defined as "slime") which attach to the polymer

surface of the catheters, have strong adherence properties. Adherence to the catheter surface and biofilm formation are the bioproducts of intrinsic phenotypic changes of the colonizing bacteria. CNS produce several enzymes that catalyze the production of exopolysaccharide, thus causing biofilm formation. The biofilm is made of free-floating bacteria which become adherent and resistant to antibiotics, especially glycopeptides, and to the host defence agents such as phagocytes and antibodies [12]. Also, certain *Candida* spp. produce slime similar to that produced by bacteria in the presence of glucose-containing fluids. This could be an explanation to account for increasing BSIs in patients receiving parenteral nutrition fluids [13].

## Strategies for Prevention of Catheter-Related Bloodstream Infections

1. Selection of catheter type (material, number of catheter lumen, tunnelled and totally implantable ports).
2. Insertion site of the catheter.
3. Skin antisepsis, topical anti-infective creams or ointments, antibiotic lock prophylaxis.
4. Catheter-site dressing regimen.
5. Replacement strategies.
6. Antimicrobial and antiseptic impregnated catheters.

1. Teflon and polyurethane catheters are involved in fewer infectious complications than those made of polyvinylchloride or polyethylene [9, 14, 15]. Although the relationship between catheter materials and the risk of CR-BSI was advocated in recent studies [16] and in the HICPAC guidelines, controversial conclusions about the contribution of catheter material to CR-BSI [5] were obtained. Thus, no additional evidence has to be provided about the risk of infection associated with different materials [17].

Considering the number of catheter lumens [18], the HICPAC correlated multi-lumen catheters with an increased risk of infection because of trauma during insertion manoeuvres and the presence of multiple ports which imply an increased frequency of CVC manipulation due to fluids administration, medication and invasive haemodynamic monitoring. Moreover, it was noted that, although multi-lumen catheters were inserted in more severely ill patients, the risk of infectious complications was independent of the patient's underlying morbidity [19]. The recommendations are [18]: (a) to insert a single-lumen catheter unless multiple ports are essential for the management of the patient; (b) to use one central venous catheter or dedicated line in case of total parenteral nutrition administration.

There are two types of catheters for  patients requiring long-term intravenous therapy: *tunnelled* CVC (e.g., Hickman catheters) and *totally implantable* intravascular devices. These are tunnelled in the subcutaneous tract and have a subcutaneous reservoir for needle puncture through the skin (e.g., Port-A-Cath). HICPAC examined various studies [5] comparing the rate of infections in patients with long-term tunnelled catheters (and/or totally implantable intravascular devices) versus non-tunnelled catheters. In general, most studies reported a reduction of infection in patients with tunnelled catheters but significant differences rarely were obtained [20]. A recent meta-analysis on short-term CVC showed a significant reduction of colonization (39%) and a decrease in CR-BSI (44%) when tunnelled devices were employed [21]. The use of tunnelled devices and totally implantable catheters are thus recommended only when long-term (> 30 days) vascular access is required.

2. The role of insertion site in minimizing the risk of CR-BSI is also extensively investigated. Multiple studies examined by HICPAC and CDC concluded that the subclavian site was less frequently correlated with catheter infections than the internal jugular and femoral sites (internal jugular vein is near oropharyngeal secretions and CVC may easily be moved from its site; femoral vein is near the high contaminated inguinal and genital zones) [22, 23], however, recent trials reported contradictory results about the relationship between the site of catheter insertion and CR-BSI [24]. A prospective study [17] concluded that there are not significant differences in the risk of infections between subclavian, internal jugular and femoral vein sites. Nonetheless, higher bacterial colonization and higher risk of deep vein thrombosis were found in patients with femoral catheters [25].

Insertion of the catheter into the superior vena cava by way of the cephalic or basilar veins of the antecubital space (peripherally inserted CVC, or PICCs) represents an alternative to the classical approach. HICPAC suggests that PICCs are correlated with a lower rate of infection than non-tunnelled CVC, probably because the antecubital zone is less colonized by microorganisms, less oily, and less moist than the neck and the chest [26]. Finally, HICPAC discussed about the duration of PICCs catheterization, but it was argued that further studies were necessary to establish the exact indwelling duration influencing the risk of infection [5].

According to the recent guidelines for preventing infections [22], the subclavian site is preferred to the jugular and femoral sites for non-tunnelled CVC, unless contraindicated. The insertion of PICCs represents a good alternative to subclavian and jugular vein catheterization.

3. Considering the importance of cutaneous microorganisms in the pathogenesis of short-term CR-BSI, the *disinfection* of the insertion site is one of the most important measures for preventing this type of infection. Products containing chlorhexidine are commercially available, in particular 2% tincture for skin antisepsis. Chlorhexidine (2%) was compared with preparations of povidone-iodine (the most widely used for clearing arterial catheter and CVC) and alcohol 70%. One study [27] demonstrated the superiority of 2% chlorhexidine tincture in preventing central venous and arterial CR infections. A recent trial [28] showed a significant reduction of CVC-related infections in the chlorhexidine-containing antiseptic group. An additional trial [29] confirmed the superiority of chlorhexidine in

reducing colonization of CVC when compared to povidone-iodine. Finally, a recent meta-analysis reporting the results of five trials on CVC and arterial catheters indicated that, currently, chlorhexidine-containing antiseptic represents the best choice in cutaneous antisepsis for vascular access sites [6].

Among anti-infective creams and ointments, three types have been investigated:

1. Polyantibiotic ointment, containing polymyxin, neomycin and bacitracin, periodically applied at the catheter insertion site did not show a clear benefit for the prevention of CR-BSIs, but this compound determined a five-fold increased risk of catheter colonization by *Candida* species [30].

2. Povidone-iodine ointment was tested in some studies particularly in patients with short-term haemodialysis catheter [31, 32]. Even if a reduction of CR-BSI due to *Staphylococcus aereus* was documented in one trial [33], no indication as to its use was recommended.

3. Topical mupirocin, an antistaphylococcal agent was effective in preventing colonization of short-term noncuffed CVCs [34] and in reducing significantly the rate of CR-BSI caused by *Staphylococcus aureus* [35]. However, the routine use of mupirocin as prophylaxis for CR-BSI in neonatal ICU resulted in 42% of resistance among CNS isolated [36], and a higher level of resistance among MRSA when used for control of outbreak of infection [37]. For these reasons, the HICPAC guideline discourages the routine use of mupirocin [6]. To prevent CR-BSI, antibiotic lock prophylaxis has been evaluated by flushing and filling the lumen of the catheter with solutions containing antimicrobials and leaving the solution to dwell in the lumen. Trials [38, 39] in which a solution containing vancomycin was employed showed a significant reduction of CR-BSI due to ram-positive microorganisms in neutropenic patients. This procedure should be used only in particular situations (immunodepressed cancer subjects, long-term catheters) as vancomycin is considered an independent risk factor for the acquisition of vancomycin-resistant *Enterococcus* [2].

4. A proper medication of the insertion site is considered a cornerstone in the management of CVC, consequently, the efficacy of many types of dressing preventing insertion-site colonization have been tested. In the last 15 years, transparent dressing has been extensively used. However, studies comparing standard semipermeable polyurethane dressing with a novel hyperpermeable type (permitting good escape of moisture) failed to show any advantage in reduction of catheter colonization and CR-BSI [40, 41]. More recently, chlorhexidine sponge applied to the insertion site under transparent dressing was investigated in patients with short-term CVC, showing a significant reduction (60%) in the rate of CR-BSI compared to standard polyurethane dressing [42]. Other types of dressing, including hydrocolloid dressing, polyurethane impregnated with povidone-iodine or ionized silver dressing, have failed to show any benefit [6]. Although the current literature and guidelines give conflicting results about the efficacy of transparent dressing in the prevention of catheter-related infection, it is well accepted that this

kind of device has some advantages. Transparent dressings allow continuous visual inspection of the insertion site, reduce the frequency of medication changes compared to standard gauze and tape dressings and permit more frequent bathing. With regard to substitution of dressings and medications, some authors suggest that changing them at least every 48 h can reduce the incidence of CR-BSI [1].

5. Some trials have evaluated the utility of routine catheter substitution at day 3 or 7 in patients carrying short-term devices [43, 44]. Unfortunately, mechanical complications and the risk of infection appeared to be slightly increased; therefore, this procedure is not currently supported if clinical signs of infection are absent. Otherwise, CDC guidelines recommend substitution with eventual de-novo replacement of pulmonary artery catheters on day 5, as the risk of CR-BSI increases after this period [4].

6. The rationale for the use of antiseptic- and antimicrobial-impregnated catheters relies on the large potential sources of infection, including the contact between the patient's skin with the catheter and the crucial role of bacteria adherence on the catheter surface. The development of devices coated with non-toxic antiseptic or antimicrobial drugs represents an important technological innovation for the prevention of CR-BSI.

Recent guidelines [1, 2, 18] suggested the use of antibiotic-impregnated catheters (chlorhexidine/silver-sulfadiazine-impregnated and minocycline/rifampin-coated devices) for adult patients who require short-term central venous catheterization and who are at high risk for CR-BSI. This consideration is argued by many studies and two meta-analyses [45, 46] showing a significant reduction rate (40%) of catheter-related infections when chlorhexidine/silver-sulfadiazine-impregnated device was used instead of polyurethane catheters. Furthermore, a multicenter trial [47] evaluating minocycline/rifampin-coated CVC versus chlorhexidine/silver-sulfadiazine-impregnated devices showed that antibiotic-coated catheters were less colonized at removal ($p < 0.001$) with a significant reduction of overall CR-BSI ($p < 0.001$) (Table 3). The superiority of this type of CVC was explained by the fact that both the external and internal surfaces of the catheter are coated compared with antiseptic-impregnated devices in which only the external surface is coated. Unfortunately, a recent review [48] evaluating the results of 11 trials testing this argument revealed several methodological flaws. McConnell *et al.* concluded that the reported success of antibiotic-impregnated catheters in preventing CR-BSI or improving patient outcomes is questionable and that more trials are needed for validation of this preventive measure. Apart from the methodological bias, the equivocal efficacy of these devices may be ascribed to the limited half-life of antimicrobial activity (3 days) of the chlorhexidine/silver-sulfadiazine-impregnated catheters, the *in-vivo* and *in-vitro* differences and the bactericidal activity toward different microorganisms. Finally, concern about the emergence of antimicrobial resistance and the possible serious acute anaphylactoid toxicity limit the large diffusion of these antiseptic- and antimicrobial-impregnated catheters [2, 6].

**Table 3.** Results of trials evaluating prevention measures for CR-BSI

| Variables | CR-BSIs/CVCs studied (n) | | | | |
| --- | --- | --- | --- | --- | --- |
| | Trials | Study technology | Control device | RR (95% CI) | P |
| Chlorhexidine (vs. povidone-iodine) cutaneous antisepsis | 5 | 14/931 | 33/1213 | 0.55 (0.22-1.15) | .07 |
| Povidone-iodine ointment | 3 | 10/212 | 23/228 | 0.47 (0.14-1.21) | .04 |
| Mupirocin ointment | 1 | 1/69 | 10/67 | 0.10 (0.00-1.24) | < .01 |
| Polyurethane (vs. gauze) dressing | 7 | 27/1070 | 20/725 | 0.97 (0.43-1.89) | .76 |
| Hydrocolloid dressing | 1 | 5/77 | 1/78 | 5.06 (0.38-> 50) | .12 |
| Hyperpermeable polyurethane dressing | 2 | 3/259 | 4/206 | 0.60 (0.02-8.73) | .70 |
| Chlorhexidine sponge | 1 | 8/665 | 24/736 | 0.37 (0.17-0.81) | .01 |
| Silver-impregnated cuff | 5 | 10/283 | 14/247 | 0.62 (0.28-1.38) | .30 |
| Benzalkonium chloride iCVC | 2 | 1/131 | 3/123 | 0.31 (0.00-22.90) | .36 |
| Chlorhexidine-silver sulfadiazine iCVC | 15 | 68/2100 | 107/2135 | 0.65 (0.45-0.90) | < .01 |
| Minocycline-rifampin iCVC | 1 | 0/130 | 7/136 | 0.00 (0.00-2.80) | .02 |
| Minocycline-rifampin (vs. chlorhexidine-silver sulfadiazine) CVC) | 2 | 1/394 | 14/418 | 0.08 (0.00-0.81) | < .01 |
| Silver-impregnated iCVC | 4 | 18/260 | 42/246 | 0.40 (0.24-0.68) | < .01 |
| Silver iontophoretic iCVC | 3 | 8/275 | 21/295 | 0.41 (0.18-0.91) | .02 |

Silver-coated or impregnated catheters represent an alternative to the antiseptic- and antimicrobial-impregnated devices. The first generation of silver catheters failed to reduce colonization and CR-BSI as the release of silver ions with bactericidal was inadequate [49]. A novel silver-impregnated CVC using oligodynamic iontophoresis technology seems to promote adequate local release of ions even if its efficacy declines rapidly in a short period of time. The few, small-sample-size studies failed to show a significant reduction of the risk of infection [6].

## Conclusions

CVC-related infections represent a major problem in intensive care as they are associated with important impact on clinical complications and mortality. An adequate preventive policy is necessary to significantly reduce the incidence of CR-BSI when the patients' illness severity induces extensive use of CVC, increasing the possibility of infection. Novel types of device are under investigation but mostly they have failed to significantly reduce colonization and the risk of catheter-related infective episodes because small-sample-size studies and methodological bias have curbed the validity of the results. Thus, more extensive trials and continuing educational support are required to improve the prevention of CR-BSI in the critical setting.

# References


1. Polderman KH, Girbes ARJ (2002) Central venous catheter use. Part 2: infectious complications. Intensive Care Med 28:18-28
2. (2002) Guidelines for the Prevention of Intravascular Catheter-Related Infections. MMWR. CDC 51(RR-10):1-30
3. CDC (1999) National Nosocomial Infections Surveillance (NNIS) System report, data summary from January 1990-May 1999, issue June 1999. Am J Infection Control 27:520-532
4. CDC (2001) National Nosocomial Infections Surveillance (NNIS) System report, data summary from January 1992-June 2001. Am J Infection Control 6:404-421
5. Pearson ML (1996) Hospital Infection Control Practices Advisory Committee. Guideline for Prevention of Intravascular device-related Infections. Infect Control Hosp Epidemiol 17:438-473
6. Crnich CJ, Maki DG (2002) The promise of novel technology for the prevention of intravascular device-related bloodstream infections. Pathogenesis and short-term devices. Clin Infect Dis 34:1232-1242
7. Kluger DM, Maki DG (1999) The relative risk of intravascular device related bloodstream infections in adults (abstract). In: Abstract of the 39th Interscience Conference on Antimicrobial Agents and Chemotherapy. San Francisco, CA: American Society for Microbiology, pp 514
8. Schaberg DR, Culver DH, Gaynes RP (1991) Major trends in the microbial etiology of nosocomial infection. Am J Med 91(Suppl) S72-S75
9. Sheth NK, Franson TR, Rose HD et al (1983) Colonization of bacteria on polyvinyl chloride and Teflon intravascular catheters in hospitalized patients. J Clin Microbiol 18:1061-1063
10. Nachnani GH, Lessin LS, Motomiya T et al (1972) Scanning electron microscopy of thrombogenesis on vascular catheter surface. N Engl J Med 286: 139-140
11. Herrmann M, Lai QJ, Albrecht RM et al (1993) Adhesion of Staphylococcus aureus to surface-bound platelets: a role of fibrinogen/fibrin and platelet integrins. J Infect Dis 167:312-322
12. Raad I (1998) Intravascular-catheter-related infections. Lancet 351:893-898
13. Branchini ML, Pfaller MA, Rhine-Chalberg J et al (1994) Genotypic variation and slime production among blood and catheter isolates of Candida Parapsilosis. J Clin Micrl 32:452-456
14. Maki DG, Ringer M (1987) Evaluation of dressing regimens for prevention of infection with peripheral intravenous catheters: gauze, a trasparent polyurethane dressing, and iodophor-trasparent dressing. JAMA 258:2396-2403
15. Maki DG, Ringer M (1991) Risk factors for infusion-related phlebitis with small peripheral venous catheters: a randomized controlled trial. Ann Intern Med 114:845-854

16. Tebbs SE, Sawyer A, Elliot TSJ (1994) Influence of surface morphology on in vitro bacterial adherence to central venous catheters. Br J Anaesth 72:587-591
17. Gil RT, Kruse JA, Thill-Baharozian MC, Carolson RW (1989) Triple- vs single-lumen central venous catheters. A prospective study in a critically ill population. Arch Int Med 149:1139-1143
18. (2001) Guidelines for preventing infections associated with the insertion and maintenance of central venous catheters. J Hosp Infection 47(Suppl.):S47-S67
19. Clark-Christoff N, Watters VA, Sparks W et al (1992) Use of triple-lumen subclavian catheters for administration of total parenteral nutrition. J Parent Enteral Nutrit 16:403-407
20. Andrivet P, Bacquer A, Ngoc CV et al (1994) Lack of clinical benefit from subcutaneous tunnel insertion of central venous catheters in immunocompromised patients. Clin Inf Dis 18:199-206
21. Randolph A, Cook D, Gonzales C et al (1998) Tunnelling short-term central venous catheters to prevent catheter-related infection: a meta-analysis of randomized controlled trials. Crit Care Med 26:1452-1457
22. Richet H, Hubert B, Nitenberg G et al (1990) Prospective multicenter study of vascular catheter related complications and risk factors for positive central catheter cultures in intensive care unit patients. J Clin Microbiol 28:2520-2525
23. Mermel LA, McCormick RD, Springman SR et al (1991) The pathogenesis and epidemiology of catheter-related infection with pulmonary artery Swan-Ganz catheters: a prospective study utilizing molecular subtyping. Am J Med 91(Suppl 3B)197S-205S
24. Fletcher SJ, Bodenham AR (1999) Catheter-related sepsis: an overview–Part 1. Br J Int Care 9:46-53
25. Trottier SJ, Veremakis C, O'Brien J et al (1995) Femoral deep vein thrombosis associated with central venous catherisation: results from a prospective, randomized trial. Crit Care Med 23:52-59
26. Ryder MA (1995) Peripheral access options. Surg Oncol Clin North Am 4:395-427
27. Maki DG, Ringer M, Alvarado CJ (1991) Prospective randomized trial of povidone-iodine, alcohol, and chlorhexidine for prevention of infection associated with central venous and arterial catheters. Lancet 338:339-343
28. Maki DG, Knasinski V, Narans LL et al (2001) A randomized trial of a novel 1% chlorhexidine-75% alcohol tincture versus 10% povidone-iodine for cutaneous disinfection with vascular catheters (abstract 142). In: Program and abstracts of the 31st Annual Society for Hospital Epidemiology of America Meeting (Toronto). Thorofare, NJ: Society for Hospital Epidemiology of America: 70
29. Mimoz O, Pieroni L, Lawrence C et al (1996) Prospective, randomized trial of two antiseptic solutions for prevention of central venous and arterial catheter colonization and infection in intensive care unit patients. Crit Care Med 24:1818-1823
30. Flowers RHD, Schwenzer KJ, Kopel RF et al (1989) Efficacy of an attachable subcutaneous cuff for the prevention of intravascular catheter-related infection: a randomized, controlled trial. JAMA 261:878-883
31. Maki D, Will L (1986) Study of polyantibiotic and povidone-iodine ointments on central venous and arterial catheter sites dressed with gauze or polyurethane dressing (abstract). In program and abstracts of the 26th interscience conference on antimicrobial agents and chemotherapy (New Orleans). Washington, DC: American Society for Microbiology: 311
32. Prager RL, Silva J (1984) Colonization of central venous catheters. South Med J 77:458-461
33. Levin A, Mason AJ, Jindal KK et al (1991) Prevention of haemodialysis subclvian vein catheter infections by topical povidone-iodine. Kidney Int 40:934-938
34. Hill RL, Fisher AP, Ware RJ et al (1990) Mupirocin for the reduction of colonization of internal jugular cannulae-a randomized controlled trial. J Hosp Infect 15:311-321

35. Sesso R, Barbosa D, Leme IL et al (1998) Staphylococcus aureus prophylaxis in hemodialysis patients using central venous catheter : effect of mupirocin ointment. J Am Soc Nephrol 9:1085-1092

36. Zakrzewska-Bode A, Muytjens HL, Liem HD et al (1995) Mupirocin resistance in coagulase-negative  staphylococci, after topical prophylaxis for the reduction of colonization of central venous catheters. J Hosp Infect 31:189-193

37. Miller MA, Dascal A, Portnoy J et al (1996) Development of mupirocin resistance among methicillin-resistant Staphylococcus aureus after widespread use of nasal mupirocin ointment. Infect Control Hosp Epidemiol 17:811-813

38. Carratalà J, Niubò J, Fernandez-Sevilla A et al (1999) Randomized, double-blind trial of an antibiotic-lock techinique for prevention of Gram-positive central venous catheter related infection in neutropenic patients with cancer. Antimicrob Agents Chemother 43:2200-2204

39. Henrickson KJ, Axtell RA, Hoover SM et al (2000) Prevention of central venous catheter-related infections and thrombotic events in immunocompromised children by the use of vancomycin/ciprofloxacin/heparin flush solution: a randomised, multicenter, double-blind trial. J Clin Oncol 1269-1278

40. Maki DG, Stolz SM, Wheeler SJ et al (1992) A prospective, randomized, three-way clinical comparison of a novel highly permeable polyurethane dressing with 442 Swan-Ganz catheter (abstract 825). In program and abstract 32nd interscience conference on antimicrobial agents and chemotherapy (Anaheim). Washington DC: American Society for Microbiology: 248

41. Wille JC, Blusse van Oud Albas A, Thewessen EA (1993) A comparison of two transparent film-type dressings in central venous therapy. J Hosp Infect 23:113-121

42. Maki DG, Mermel LA, Kluger DM et al (2000) The efficacy of a chlorhexidine-impregnated sponge (biopatch) for the prevention of intravascular catheter-related infection – a prospective, randomized, controlled, multicenter trial (abstract 1430). In program and abstract 40th interscience conference on antimicrobial agents and chemotherapy (Toronto). Washington DC: American Society for Microbiology: 422

43. Cobb DK, High K, Sawyer RG et al (1992) A controlled trial of scheduled replacement of central venous and pulmonary artery catheters. New Engl J Med 327:1062-1068

44. Snyder RH, Archer  FJ, Endi T et al (1988) Catheter infection: a comparison of two catheter maintainance techniques. Ann Surg 208:651-653

45. Mermel LA (2000) Prevention of intravascular catheter related infections. Ann Intern Med 132:391-402

46. Veenstra DL, Saint S, Saha S et al (1999) Efficacy of antiseptic-impregnated central venous catheters in preventing catheter-related bloodstream infection: a meta-analysis. JAMA 281:261-267

47. Darouiche RO, Raad II, Heard SO et al (1999) A comparison of two antimicrobial-impregnated central venous catheters. Catheter Study Group. N Engl J Med 340:1-8

48. McConnel SA, Gubbins PO, Anaissie EJ (2003) Do antimicrobial-impregnated central venous catheters prevent catheter-related bloodstream infection? Clin Infect Dis 37:65-72

49. Schierholz JM, Lucas LJ, Rump A et al (1998) Efficacy of Silver-coated medical devices. J Hosp Infec 40:257-262

# PALLIATIVE CARE

# Challenges in End-of-Life Care

F.M. Rubulotta, L. Serra, A. Gullo

## Introduction

It may seem rhetorical discussing an issue as universal and certain as human mortality. However, death is still the source of an enormous amount of ethical dilemmas and uncertainty in clinical decision-making regarding whether to withdraw and withhold care in terminal illnesses. Modern society is trying to approach and to standardize the dying process, while sometimes failing to recognize that it is an unpreventable and unavoidable phenomenon. Reliable and valid research on attitudes toward dying and death is surprisingly limited to academic debate and selected literature.

The most relevant studies refer to small samples, including patients enrolled in various countries [1-5]. As a matter of fact, worldwide surveys rarely focus on the dying process. The Study to Understand Prognoses and Preferences for Outcome and Risks of Treatments (SUPPORT) [6], conducted in the USA, is the most broad-ranged and expensive research ever performed in this field. It shows that it is extremely difficult to assess how current proposals in end-of-life practices may affect social attitudes. Researchers and clinicians interested in end-of-life care assume that the development of knowledge in the dying process involves everyone around the world. Current opinion shows that there is no single way to live ones life, and many people think that there is no single way to die. The experiences of humans while dying are variously shaped according to the nature of the illness and to the patient's physical and psychological compliance towards the clinical approach, appropriate pharmacological treatments and palliative care. Dying is a dynamic and ineluctable process in terminal patients; palliative care represents a strategic multi-modal approach to assess discomfort, to manage pain and, finally, to improve quality of life/death.

## Values, Attitudes, Cultures and the Dying Process

Currently, up to 20% of Americans die in acute-care units [7], but 90% of them would prefer to die at home. Most Americans rarely think about death [8], but, despite characterizations of the USA as a "death-denying society", evidence for this assumption is remarkably sparse [9]. Patients may actively be involved in their own life-sustaining care discussions, according to the 14th Amendment and recognized by The Supreme Court of the United States [10]. Similarly, the European Convention on Human Rights states that the right to live shall be protected by law, and each individual should be free to decide regarding health-care treatments [11]. Unfortunately, some evidence suggests that education to improve patients end-of-life decision-making attitudes may arouse death anxiety rather than reduce it [12-14]. When questioned about whom they would prefer to make the final choices about their care if they are seriously ill, 67% of Americans answered they would prefer to make the decisions themselves, whereas 28% would ask their doctor to decide on their behalf [2]. Everyone may use the right to refuse health-sustaining treatments only after having understood bioethical problems, alternative courses of the disease, and the significance of tools such as advanced directives. For this reason, clinicians must engage patients and families in information exchanges before asking them to make a decision.

A century ago, communicable diseases, such as influenza, tuberculosis, and diphtheria, were the leading causes of death [15]. Today in the USA, and in industrialized nations in general, the three main causes of death are heart diseases, cancer, and stroke [16]. In 1995, estimates suggested that these diseases (which primarily affect older people) accounted for 62% of all deaths [15-17].

In 1939, national statistics revealed that 37% percent of deaths occurred in general hospitals. In 1989, the percentage of patients dying in nosocomial structures rose to 85% [18]. In 1983, two main events changed the trend in hospital mortality: Medicare began to offer financial support to hospice services [19], and nursing-home death rates increased [20]. By 1992, the main sites-of-death in the USA were hospitals (57%), followed by nursing homes and residences (17% and 20%), while only 6% of the total population died elsewhere [18]. Nonetheless, percentages on site-of-death tell only a part of the story about the end-of-life [21]. Little is known about where and how dying patients spend their last hours, but one in five americans die using intensive care services [16].

In 1996, considering all deaths at regional hospitals in Australia, Hillman [22] found that, in over 60% of patients transferred to the intensive care unit, potentially life-threatening abnormalities were documented during the 8 h before their admission. The most common antecedents recorded were hypotension ($n=199$), tachycardia ($n=73$), tachypnoea ($n=64$), and sudden change in level of consciousness ($n=42$). Hillman suggested that this may be a patient population who could benefit from improved resuscitation and care at an earlier stage.

The results also indicated that a large proportion of preventable hospital deaths were attributable not to willful negligence on the part of doctors or nurses, but to institutionalized neglect of "people who the system thought were salvageable". Professor Hillman wrote in the Australian Journal of Internal Medicine that "apart from a cardiac arrest team, there is little in the way of a systematic response that crosses geographical and functional boundaries to seriously ill patients in acute hospitals". Nowadays, the Australian New Zealand Commonwealth-funded study is the first in the world to examine what happens to patients immediately before they die in hospital. The study by Professor Hillman might result in procedures to select and treat vulnerable patients sooner. By 2030, the doubling of persons over the age of 65, will require a system wide expansion in ICU CARE for dying patients [16].

In Asia, Singapore is one of the most representative areas involved in end-of-life care. It is a small country with a total land area of 659.9 sq km, and a population in 1999 of about 4.0 million. Only 11% of the total population is above 60 years of age. Eighty percent of the primary health-care services are provided by private practitioners while the government polyclinics provide the remaining 20% [23]. For the more costly hospital care, including end-of-life care, it is the reverse situation with 80% of the hospital care being provided by the public sector and the remaining 20% by the private sector. In 1999, Singapore spent about $5.3 billion, meaning that per capita health care spending was approximately $1,347 [23]. Palliative care, and on some occasions hospice services, may provide more support and comfort for the dying patient and the family than traditional care. For those dying at home, hospice personnel are more intensively trained than other hospital personnel to provide physical, psychological, spiritual, and practical support.

Important cultural differences in end-of-life care exist within the USA [8, 16, 24-26]. In fact, behaviourism in the dying process is affected by a number of variables, such as race, ethnicity, and religious, legal and economic aspects [10, 17-20, 22, 27]. As a consequence, it is easy to extend this concept, assuming that deep differences in end-of-life care must characterize each country and each continent, according to the above-mentioned reasons.

## Transoceanic Point of View

In the current literature, the incidence of patients dying with full aggressive measures may range from 4 to 79%, while the percentage of withholding or withdrawing of life-support varies from 0 to 90% in different ICUs around the world [8, 28, 29].

Challenges in physicians' skills and attitudes are emphasized by comparing data collected from studies carried out 20 years ago with current standards of terminal patients' care. In the same way, several differences may be pointed out matching USA palliative care with regular medical practice in countries lacking the possibility of withdrawal treatments. In 1983, 73% of American physicians believed that intravenously administered fluids should be provided to a comatose, terminally ill patient with no hope of recovery [30]. In 1992-1993, 90% of deaths in the ICU involved withholding or withdrawing at least one life-supporting intervention [29].

In 1994, only 53% of American physicians admitted ICU patients with no hope of survival for more than a few weeks [31, 32]. In contrast, 73% of European ICU physicians in 1999 still hospitalized patients with no chance of recovery, and 33% of them believed that patients with no hope of recovery should be kept in an ICU [31]. The SUPPORT trial showed that a substantial majority of patients had not discussed with physicians preferences for life-sustaining treatments after 14 days [6]. A large survey among several American Thoracic Critical Care Units reported that 34% of physicians continued life-sustaining treatments contrary to patients' or surrogates' wishes, while 25% of those who withheld or withdrew care did not ask for consent and 14% did not even inform patients or their surrogates [33].

The involvement of family members in the end-of-life decision making processes varies widely in Europe. As a matter of fact, while in Europe family members are informed of 50% of end-of-life care [31], in the United States family members participate in 70-80% of end-of-life decisions [33-34]. Directives in end-of-life care are more commonly made by physicians in Italy, Greece, and Portugal and by ICU staff in the UK and Switzerland. 69% of IC Societies in Europe have an ethics committee or working group on ethics subjects. Only 56% of IC Societies have adopted an official statement on end of life care [35] there is an obvious need for an international consensus conference and also for a joint european statement. On 24-25 april 2003 in Brussels, Belgium, a jury of ten intensivist attended the presentations of 30 experts in the field of end  of life care. The statement of this international consensus conference has recently been published [36]. Devictor *et al.* [37] showed that in France approximately 94% of parents and 54% of bedside nurses are excluded from meetings in which withdrawal-of-life sustaining treatments in paediatric intensive care are discussed. Worldwide, aggressive clinical and pharmacological treatments can be limited following different patterns [25, 38-41]. In Japan, life support can be withdrawn if the patient or surrogates request it [39, 40]. In Israel, withholding care is permitted, while hastening death by withdrawing life-support is prohibited [42]. In New Zealand, withdrawal of therapy involves medical consensus followed by family discussion. However, the clinician considers death decisions more as a medical responsibility than as a patient's choice [22]. In Asia, aspects belonging to both Chinese and Western medicine coexist [43] DNR orders are rarely used, and doctors hardily discuss advanced directives. Euthanasia is prohibited, and the withdrawal of life support is mainly decided by doctors. In Australia, attitudes in end-of-life care are in between those of Europe and America [22]. It is surprising to know that Harvard Brain Death Criteria are formally not accepted in Australia. In Saudi Arabia, a religious representative usually joins physicians and families in end-of-life discussions [44]. In South Africa, very few studies have investigated the limit of care, but one article reported that reductions in the level of provided care are often imposed, especially in ICU patients or just before death [45]. Extremely limited health care resources are a major problem in this area. In India, withholding life support is allowed while the withdrawal of care without evidence of brain death is illegal [46]. In Canada, several studies reported the same scenarios characteristic of Europe and the USA [42, 47-48]. In the Netherlands, doctors are likely to involve patients, families, and ICU staff in end-of-life decision-making processes [49]. Euthanasia is legal in the Netherlands and Belgium [49, 50], as is physician-assisted suicide in Oregon [51].

In many countries, medical decisions are still made in a paternalistic way, while in other nations in an absolutely autonomous manner. The problem of objectively defining the role of the physician in different cultural realities and scenarios is still unsolved. Since an increasing number of countries are moving from paternalism to patient autonomy, from unquestioned decision making to informed withholding or withdrawal of life-support, caregivers need to assess the use of new technologies within the broad confines of bioethical principles [36, 52].

## Challenges in End-of-Life Care

Challenges in end-of-life care have existed for decades. Major advancements in the USA regarding end-of-life care followed the statement of the Patients Self-Determination Act, in December 1990 [10].

During the 1990s Medicare and Medicaid funded caregivers to inform patients of their right to complete advanced directives and to refuse medical treatment. This process encouraged patient-physician interaction and the practical involvement of family members in critical- and terminal-care decision-making issues. Major challenges and main differences in end-of-life care are better evidenced by case reports. For this reason, the end-of-life approaches used to solve similar case scenarios in two different countries are briefly examined:

*Case report number 1.* A 34-year-old Caucasian male, diagnosed with kidney cancer, was transferred from the regular ward to the medical intensive care unit (MICU) at Rhode Island University Hospital in Providence, USA. His past medical history was positive for surgery and repeated trials of chemotherapy. Follow-up tests showed that the cancer had spread to lungs and bone. The patient received home medication to control depression, migraine syndrome, chronic mild neurological impairment, partial complex seizure disorder, and hypothyroidism.

He was receiving a round of chemotherapy in the regular ward when he developed hypotension, tachycardia, tachypnoea, and pulmonary oedema. He was transferred to the MICU, where he was sedated and intubated. Laboratory findings reported severe hypoalbuminaemia, anaemia, leucopoenia and thrombocytopoenia. His neck was thick, the extremities were oedematous, but pulses were palpable. A chest radiograph revealed left lower lobe moderate infiltrates, and CT scans showed bilateral pleural effusions. The patient's oxygen saturation was low (91%) and refractory to continuous suctioning of thick yellow secretions from the upper respiratory tract and repeated slow intravenous bolus of albumin. The proxy, identified as the patient's wife, agreed to withhold aggressive antibiotic therapy and to stop chemotherapy. Family members daily questioned ICU physicians about which treatment would best meet the patient's interests. The treating physician stated that no aggressive therapy could reverse the course of the disease. The patient was not scheduled for any further diagnostic procedure, and drugs, fluids, and nutrition were gradually withdrawn. The physician and the proxy decided to change the code status from full to comfort measure only. The morning after the family meeting, the patient was terminally extubated. He died in a private room, surrounded by his family members.

*Case report number 2.* A 38-year-old Caucasian male diagnosed with pancreatic cancer was admitted to the regular ward at Trieste Cattinara University Hospital, Trieste, Italy. His past medical history was positive for surgery and repeated trials of chemotherapy. Follow-up tests showed that the cancer had spread to brain, lungs and bone. The patient received home medication to control depression and morphine to manage chronic pain. The patient was cachetic, icteric and lethargic. The anaesthesiologist in charge of the Pain Clinic was alerted to reassess chronic pain management.

The patient was obnubilated, but was never asked whether he wanted to be admitted to the ward nor was he permitted to discuss with the physicians the level of desired care. The patient complained of severe pain, and during the day the physicians could barely control the symptoms with intravenous morphine bolus. The following morning, oxygen saturation was low (95%), and respiratory exchanges were poor. The mother questioned physicians why he could not die at home. The treating physician stated that aggressive therapy could reverse the course of the disease, and "everything" must be done in the hospital. The patient was scheduled for further expensive and burdensome diagnostic procedures. The physician and the proxy decided to continue full care while the anaesthesiologist responsible for pain control continued to provide palliative measures. Two days later, the patient suffered a cardiac arrest refractory to cardiopulmonary resuscitation manoeuvres. He died in the presence of practitioners, nurses and his mother.

## Key Points in Palliative Care

*Teaching Points.* The patients considered in both scenarios were similar in age, kind of disease and site of death. The ward of admission was different because the first patient was transferred to an ICU, while the second was in a regular ward. Kollef [53] found that, for patients who were cared for by a university-based ICU, the attending physicians were more likely to choose active withdrawal of life-sustaining treatment than were private attending physicians. Intensivists are more skilled in limiting life-support because of their experience in recognizing terminal illness.

In both scenarios, comfort measure were provided by critical care doctors, but the course of the acute episode ended in a profoundly different way. ICUs have been recognized in the USA as the best ward for acquiring end-of-life skills and attitudes. Starting in 1996, a long process allowed end-of-life care to become part of the Internal Medicine USA National Board [54]. In Italy and in some other countries the legislation is unclear and superficial in defining the legal approach to terminal patients [35]. Ideally, physicians themselves should be well versed in ethical questions or should be equipped to guide lawyers. Critical care professionals should decide where they want to draw the line between legal and illegal aid in dying and morally justified and unjustified cases of hastening death in their country [30]. Withdrawing life-support care, in the case of the second patient, would have required coordination of an interdisciplinary team. Internists were moving toward aggressive treatment of a clearly terminal patient, while the anaesthesiologist was providing comfort measures only. Sometimes, patients or family members do not understand the gravity of the disease, and the confusing information provided by caregivers may raise anxiety [55, 56].

Given the growing tendency in creating an educational multidisciplinary team, it seems intuitive that the complexity of end-of-life discussions would increase. New scenarios would assume the need of training or coordinating different experts for the same palliative care goals.

In conclusion, the basic tenets of palliative care, including symptom control, psychological and spiritual well being, and care of the family, should aim to help patients to die with dignity [57, 58]. Cardiopulmonary resuscitation in the regular ward is distressful and painful for both patients and proxies [56].

Dignity must be restored at the end of life by providing privacy and solemnity during the dying process [8, 57, 58]. Nowadays, the major challenge in American hospital care is identifying better ways to cure illnesses while avoiding needless physical and emotional harm to terminal patients. In the mean time, several industrialized countries are witnessing a high level of uncertainty in end-of-life decision-making issues, due to the slow progression of the learning curve. However, it is simplistic to suggest that some nations should follow the leading ones, regarding correctly withholding or withdrawing life-support from their patients. Dying is a biological, psychological and social process that occurs in a cultural context. Ethical problems should be resolved with solutions tailored to each geographical area. As a result, end-of-life care goals should fit different hospital realities, starting from the patient-physician relationship. Fundamental guidelines are necessary, and those are well established by the current USA literature [23, 59-66]. However, end-of-life guidelines must be adapted to legal and economic variables present in different nations [36].

Throughout the past four decades, social beliefs, physicians' attitudes, and laws have profoundly changed. As a result, the public has become interested in an increasing number of medical-ethical issues, while physicians have become more concerned with social needs. As the use of technology has increased, the field of ethics has changed from being a philosophical pursuit to a practical discipline. Traditionally, physicians were guided primarily by the principle of beneficence (*"primum non nocere"*) rather than by the principle of patients' autonomy. The ascendance of this new bioethical concept is revealed in the significant attention paid to issues such as patient preferences and informed consent [67].

An enormous amount of health-care resources are delivered to dying patients [65, 68], and the considerable number of intensive interventions used before death is a troubling finding that critics have argued might not be appropriate nor consistent with patients' wishes. Nevertheless, nearly half of all patients who die in the hospital are transferred to an ICU 3 days before death [16], and the incidence of distress and discomfort seems to increase proportionally with aggressive care administration [69]. A national survey in Canada showed that ICU health-care workers make different choices about withdrawal of life support when they are presented with the same patient scenarios [47]. The patient could theoretically receive full aggressive intensive care from one health care provider and only comfort measures from another. According to these data, it is possible to assume that the same, or even a worse scenario could characterize end-of-life care delivery in different countries [8, 36].

Walter *et al.* [47] hypothesized that a lack of confidence in end-of-life decision-making procedures might be a contributing factor to the variability of recommended level of care in Canadian ICUs. The SUPPORT study suggests that uncertainty is a primary reason for the admission of patients in American ICUs. The ineffectiveness in determining the timing for the shift from primarily curative care to primarily palliative care is the main reason why several patients receive numerous invasive and expensive procedures just before death [69]. Similarly, a national survey of 80% of American academic centres found that students, residents, and academic leaders evaluate themselves as inadequately prepared to provide compassionate end-of-life care [70]. On the other hand, physicians working in poor countries have more problems in making the triage of patients to admit to ICUs rather than in limiting life-sustaining treatments [71]. Withholding care in this scenario requires different competences when compared to industrialized areas, because it endorses a different ethical meaning.

Practitioners may state that end-of-life dilemmas are caused by "the capitalistic" use of health-care resources in rich countries. The physician's primary responsibility is traditionally centered on the patient's best interests, without regard to costs or social considerations. Nevertheless, this duty is increasingly criticized in relation to the re-evaluation of critical-care costs, standards and outcome results [16, 36, 64].

The lack of established "standards of care" even at the end of a critical patient's life suggests that high health-care costs and limited resources may have had a leading role in the national evolution of ethical dilemmas. Thus, strategies for reducing the use of costly life-sustaining care should focus as much attention on the preferences of terminal patients and the concerns of their families, as on the experience of physicians [36].

## Conclusions

Palliative medicine includes clinical palliative care, education, and research that focus on the quality of life of patients with advanced disease and on their relatives [72]. The image describing the process of dying provided by Roger Bone is impressive. This author wrote that dying can be a peaceful event or a great agony when it is inappropriately sustained by life support. Dunstan [73] encouraged further state-of-the-art evolutions in end-of-life care stating that the success of intensive care is not to be measured only by the statistics of survival, as though each death were a medical failure. It is to be measured by the quality of lives preserved or restored, the quality of the dying of those in whose interest it is to die, and by the quality of relationships involved in each death. The basic tenets of palliative care may be summarized as the goal of helping patients to die with dignity [74]. Nursing interventions, palliative care networks and other models aimed at promoting a coordinated approach to care delivery have been shown to decrease costs and improve the quality of care [75]. According to the critical appraisal of international advancements on end-of-life care, it is desirable that new generations focus not only in giving days to a patient's life, but also to giving a better quality of life to a patient's days.

## References


1.  Reilly BM, Magnussen CR, Ross J, et al (1994) Can we talk? Inpatient discussions about advance directives in a community hospital. Attending physicians' attitudes, their inpatients' wishes, and reported experience. Arch Intern Med 24 154:2299-2308
2.  McLeod GA, Saika G (1986) Patient attitudes to discussing life-sustaining treatment. Arch Intern Med 146:1613-1615
3.  Everhart MA, Pearlman RA (1990) Stability of patient preferences regarding life-sustaining treatments. Chest 97:159-164
4.  Curtis JR, Patrick DL, Caldwell ES, Collier AC (2000) Why don't patients and physicians talk about end-of-life care? Barriers to communication for patients with acquired immunodeficiency syndrome and their primary care clinicians. Arch Intern Med 160:1690-1696
5.  Hallenbeck J, Goldstein M, Mebane E (1996) Cultural considerations of death and dying in the United States. Clin Geriatr Med 12:393-405
6.  (1995) A controlled trial to improve care for seriously ill hospitalized patients. The study to understand prognoses and preferences for outcomes and risks of treatments (SUPPORT). JAMA 274:1591-1598
7.  Field MJ, Cassel C (1997) Approaching death improving care at the end of life. National Academy Press. Washington DC
8.  Levy MM (2004) Dying America. Crit Care Med 32:879-880
9.  Van Brunt E (1991) Concerned patient. West J Med 155:88-89
10. Omnibus Reconciliation Act 1990. Title IV, Section 4206, Congressional Record 1263-64
11. Appelbaum PS, Lidz CW, Meisel A (1987) Informed consent. New York, OUP
12. McClam T (1980) Death anxiety before and after death education: negative results. Psychol. Rep 46:513-514
13. Durlak CM, Rose E, Bursuck WD (1994) Preparing high school students with learn-

ing disabilities for the transition to postsecondary education: teaching the skills of self-determination. J Learn Disabil 27:51-59

14. Testa JA (1981) Group systematic desensitization and implosive therapy for death anxiety. Psychol Rep 48:376-378

15. Gardner P, Rosenberg HM, Wilson RW (1996) Leading causes of death by age, sex, race, and Hispanic origin: United States, 1992. Vital Health Stat 20 29:1-94

16. Angus DC, Barnato AE et al ( 2004) Use of intensive care at the end of life in the United States: an epidemiologic study. Crit Care Med 32:638-643

17. Caralis PV, Davis B, Wright K, Marcial E (1993) The influence of ethnicity and race on attitudes toward advance directives, life-prolonging treatments and euthanasia. J Clin Ethics 4:155-165

18. De Vita MA, Grenvik A (2000) Forgoing life-sustaining therapy in Intensive Care. IV Edition. WC Shoemaker, PR Holbrook, A Granvik. Philadelphia, W B Saunders, Textbook of Critical Care Medicine Section XV: 2110-2116

19. Sager MA, Easterling DV, Kindig DA, Anderson OW (1989) Changes in the location of death after passage of Medicare's prospective payment system. A national study. N Engl J Med 16 320:433-439

20. Brock DB, Foley DJ, Salive ME (1996) Hospital and nursing home use in the last three months of life. J Aging Health 8:307-319

21. Wallis CB, Davies HTO, Shearer AJ (1997) Why do patients die on general wards after discharge from intensive care units? Anaesthesia 52:9-14

22. Hillman KM, Bristow PJ, Chey T et al (2002) Duration of life-threatening ante-cedents prior to intensive care admission. Intensive Care Med 28:1629-1634

23. Vigano A, Watanabe S, Bruera E (1994) Anorexia and cachexia in advanced cancer patients. Ann Acad Med Singapore 23:197-203

24. Voltz R, Akabayashi A, Reese C, Ohi G, Sass HM (1998) End-of-life decisions and advance directives in palliative care: a cross-cultural survey of patients and health-care professionals. J Pain Symptom Manage 16:153-162

25. Koenig BA, Gates-Williams J (1995) Understanding cultural difference in caring for dying patients. West J Med 163:244-249

26. Prendergast TJ, Claessen MT, Luce JM (1998) A national survey of end-life care for critically ill patients. Am J Resp Crit Care Med 158:1163-1167

27. Klessig J (1992) Cross-cultural medicine a decade later: The effect of values and cul-ture on life-support decisions. West J Med 157:316-322

28. Knaus WA, Wagner DP, Zimmerman JE, Draper EA (1993) Variations in mortality and length of stay in intensive care units. Ann Intern Med 15 118:753-761

29. Prendergast TJ, Luce JM (1997) Increasing incidence of withholding and withdrawal of life support from the critically ill. AJRCCM 155:15-20

30. Sprung CL, Eidelman LA, Pizov R (1996) Changes in forgoing life-sustaining treat-ments in the United States: Concern for the future. Mayo Clin Proc 71:512-516

31. Vincent JL (1999) Forgoing life support in Western European intensive care units: The result of an ethical questionnaire. Crit Care Med 27:1626-1633

32. (1994) Society of Critical Care Medicine Ethics: Attitudes of critical care medicine pro-fessionals concerning distribution of intensive care recourses. Crit Care Med 22:358-362

33. Smedira NG, Evans BH, Grais LS et al (1990) Withholding and withdrawal of life support from the critically ill. N Engl J Med 322:309-315

34. Zimmerman JE, Knaus WA, Sharpe SM et al (1986) The use and implications of do not resuscitate orders in intensive care units. JAMA 17 255:351-356

35. Boles JM (2004) End-of-life care in the ICU professional society statements from european countries. Intensive Care Med (in press)

36. Carlet J, Thijs LG, Antonelli M et al (2004) Challenges in end-of-life care in the ICUStatement of the 5th International Consensus Conference in Critical Care: Brussels, Belgium, April 2003. Intensive Care Med 30:770-784

37. Devictor DJ, Nguyen DT (2001) Foregoing life sustaining treatments: how the deci-

sion is made in French pediatric intensive care units. Crit Care Med 29:1356-1359
38. Kalish R (1980) Death & Dying: Views From Many Cultures. Farmingdale, NY, Bay wood 39-46
39. Asai A, Ohnishi M, Nishigaki E et al (2002) Attitudes of the Japanese public and doctors towards use of archived information and samples without informed consent: preliminary findings based on focus group interviews. BMC Med Ethics 3:1-3
40. Asai A, Fukuhara S, Inoshita O et al (1997) Medical decisions concerning the end of life: a discussion with Japanese physicians. J Med Ethics 23:323-327
41. Sehgal AR, Weisheit C, Miura Y et al (1996) Advance directives and withdrawal of dialysis in the United States, Germany, and Japan. JAMA 276:1652-1656
42. Sprung J, Oppenheim A (1998) End-of-life decisions in critical care medicine. Where are we headed? Critical Care Medicine 26:201-202
43. Gilligan T, Koenig B, Raffin TA (1998) Ethical decision-making in critical care in Hong Kong. Crit Care Med 26:447-451
44. Saeed KS (1999) How physician executives and clinicians perceive ethical issues in Saudi Arabian hospitals. J Med Ethics 25:51-56
45. Tangwa GB (1996) Bioethics: an African perspective. Bioethics 10:183-200
46. Bilimoria P (1992) The Jaina ethic of voluntary death: a report from India. Bioethics 6:331-355
47. Walter SD, Cook DJ, Guyatt GH, Spanier A, Jaeschke R, Todd TRJ, Streiner DL (1998) The Canadian Critical Care Trials Group. Confidence in life-support decisions in the intensive care unit: A survey of healthcare workers. Critical Care Medicine Vol 26:44-49
48. Cook DJ, Guyatt GH, Jaeschke R et al (1995) Determinants in Canadian health care workers of the decision to withdraw life support from the critically ill. Canadian Critical Care Trials Group. JAMA 273:703-708
49. Van der Maas PJ, van der Wal G, Haverkate I (1996) Euthanasia, physician-assisted suicide, and other medical practices involving the end of life in the Netherlands, 1990-1995. N Engl J Med 335:1699-1705
50. Deliens L, Mortier F, Bilsen J et al (2000) End-of-life decisions in medical practice in Flanders, Belgium: a nationwide survey. Lancet 25 356:1806-1811
51. Sullivan AD, Hedberg K, Hopkins D (2001) Legalized physician-assisted suicide in Oregon, 1998-2000. N Engl J Med 344:605-607
52. Curtis JR, Wenrich MD, Carline JD et al (2001) Understanding physicians' skills at providing end-of-life care perspectives of patients, families, and health care workers J Gen Intern Med 16:41-49
53. Kollef MH (1996) Private attending physician status and the withdrawal of life-sustaining interventions in a medical intensive care unit population. Crit Care Med 24:968-975
54. (1996) American Board of Internal Medicine: Caring for the Dying: Identification and Promotion of Physician Competency. Philadelphia, PA. American Board of Internal Medicine
55. Pochard F, Azoulay E, Chevret S et al (2001) Symptoms of anxiety and depression in family members of intensive care unit patients: ethical hypothesis regarding decision-making capacity. Crit Care Med 29:1893-1897
56. Azoulay E, Pochard F, Chevret S et al (2003) Family participation in care to the critically ill: opinions of families and staff. Intensive Care Med 29:1498-1504
57. Chochinov HM (2002) Dignity-Conserving Care. A new model for palliative care. JAMA 287:2253-2260
58. Levy MM (2001) End-of-life care in the intensive care unit: can we do better? Crit Care Med(2 Suppl):N56-61
59. (1989) The Appleton Consensus: Suggested international guidelines for decisions to forgo medial treatment. J Med Ethics 15:129-136
60. (1994) Society of Critical Care Medicine Ethics: Attitudes of critical care medicine

professionals concerning distribution of intensive care recourses. Crit. Care Med 22:358-362

61.  (1991) Council on Ethical and Judicial Affairs, American Medical Association: Guides for the appropriate use of do-not-resuscitate orders. JAMA 265:1868-1871

62.  (1991) American Thoracic Society: Withholding and withdrawing life-sustaining therapy. Am Rev Respir Dis 144:726-731

63.  (1996) Council on Scientific Affairs, American Medical Association: Good care of the dying patient. JAMA 275:474-478

64.  Rubenfeld GD, Angus DC, Pinsky MR et al (1999) Outcomes research in critical care: results of the American Thoracic Society Critical Care Assembly Workshop on Outcomes Research. The Members of the Outcomes Research Workshop. Am J Respir Crit Care Med 160:358-367

65.  Lee K, Angus DC, Abramson NS (1996) Cardiopulmonary resuscitation: What cost to cheat death? CCM 24:2047-1053

66.  (1982) President's Commission for the Study of Ethical Problems in Medicine and Biomedical and Behavioral Research. Making Health Care Decisions. Washington, DC: US Government Printing Office

67.  Lemaire FJ, ESICM Task Force (2003) A European directive for clinical research. Intensive Care Med 29:1818-1820

68.  Cher DJ, Lenert LA (2001) Method of Medicare reimbursement and the rate of potentially ineffective care of critically ill patients. JAMA 278:1001-1007

69.  Chloe Bawter, Mark G. Brennan, Yvette Coldicott (2002) The Practical Guide to Medical Ethics & Law. Pastest edition. G. Ramsay, F.M. Rubulotta, MM Levy. Case Description 182-187

70.  Block SD, Sullivan AM (1998) Attitudes about end of life care: a national cross sectional study. J Palliat Med 1:347-355

71.  McLean RF, Tarshis J, Mazer CD, Szalai JP (2000) Death in two Canadian intensive care units: Institutional difference and changes over time. Crit Care Med 28:100-103

72.  Abrahm JL (2003) Update in palliative medicine and end-of-life care. Annu Rev Med 54:53-72

73.  Dunstan GR (1985) Hard questions in intensive care. A moralist answers questions put to him at a meeting of the Intensive Care Society. Anaesthesia 40:479-492

74.  Chochinov HM (2002) Dignity – conserving care – A new model for palliative care. JAMA Vol 287, No 17:2253-2260

75.  Reb M (2003) Palliative and End-of-life Care: Policy analysis. Oncol Nurs Forum 30:35-50

# Subject Index


*Acinetobacter baumannii* 192
*Acinetobacter calcoaceticus* 209
Acute lung injury 61-64, 66-68
Acute pancreatitis 61
Acute respiratory distress syndrome 61,
    62, 67-70
Acute respiratory failure 88, 95, 98
Afterload 20
Airflow obstruction 74, 76, 80, 81, 82, 92
Airway 146-149, 151, 154-156
Aminocaproic acid 20
Amoxicillin 196
Amphotericin B 191
Amrinone 172, 180
Amynophilline 92
Anaesthesia 29, 85, 87, 90, 91, 93, 113-121,
    123, 124, 126, 130, 145, 147, 149, 150,
    154-156
    cardiothoracic 20
    department 11, 12
    general 113, 116-121, 145
Anaesthesiologist 11, 13, 51, 84, 134, 135,
    145, 149, 226, 227
Anaphylaxis 124, 126, 128
Anatomy 4
Aorta 21
Aprotinin 20
Arginine vasopressin 56
Asphyxia 50, 83
Aspiration 49, 61, 68
Asthma 85, 92-94, 97, 146, 153, 154
Atelectasis 113-115, 117, 119, 120, 149
Atracurium 126-128
Atropine 21
Azathiprine 23
Azithromycin 187
Aztreonam 196

Bacitracin 212
Barbiturates 115, 119, 146, 152
Barotrauma 89, 93
Benzodiazepines 115, 119
Bernoulli's theorem 36, 45
Beta-blockers 159, 162
Blood transfusion 61
Blunt trauma 96
Boyle's law 29
Bradycardia 138
Brain death 20
Breathing 145-147, 151, 155
Bronchiolitis 85, 91, 97
Bronchitis 149
    chronic 74, 75, 80-82
Bronchoalveolar lavage 186, 201
Bronchoscopy 186, 196, 202
Bronchospasm 74, 149, 153-155
Budget 11

Cancer 222, 225, 226, 230
*Candida albicans* 207
*Candida* spp. 207, 210
Cardiac
    arrest 55, 56, 57, 58, 59
    resynchronisation therapy 159
    transplantation 22
Cardiomyopathy 18
Cardiopulmonary
    bypass 20
    resuscitation 86, 226, 227, 232
Caspases 20
Cefepime 187, 195, 196
Cefotaxime 187, 196
Cefotetan 196
Ceftriaxone 91, 187, 196
Cefuroxime 196, 200

Chagas' disease 18
Charles' law 29
Children 83-90, 92-98
*Chlamydia pneumoniae* 185
Chlorhexidine 211-217
Chronic Obstructive Pulmonary disease 73, 80-82, 153-155
Ciprofloxacin 187, 196
Circulation 147
Cisatracurium 125-131
*Citrobacter* spp 192
Citrus 7
Clarithromycin 187
Clavulanic acid 196
Clindamycin 196
Coagulase-negative staphylococcus 207
Collagen 62-70
Colonization 206, 208, 209, 211, 212, 214, 215-217
Communication 4
Confusion 150
Congestive heart failure 165, 166
Coronary
    angiography 19
    blood flow 55
Corticosteroids 75, 92
Cough 74, 75, 77
*Coxiella burnetii* 185
Crycothiroctomy 50
Croup 85, 88, 90, 91
Curricula 3
Cyanosis 150

Dalton's law of partial pressure 31
Death 221-224, 226-232
Diabetes
    insipidus 19
    mellitus 18
Diaphragm 76, 79, 80, 82, 113, 114, 117, 119, 120
Difficult intubation 125, 129
Diuretics 162
Dobutamine 21, 23, 172, 173, 180, 181
Donor 17
Drugs 145, 147, 148, 154, 156
Dynamic hyperinflation 75, 76
Dysphagia 91
Dysrhythmias 138

Echocardiography 167, 169, 179, 180
Education 6
Elastin 63-67, 69, 84
Embolectomy 171, 178
Emphysema 73-76, 78-82
End-of-life care 221, 223-232
Endotracheal intubation 23, 85, 90, 91, 93, 123, 129
Enoxaparin 175, 176
Entactins 66
Enterobacter 192
Enterobacteriaceae 192
Enterococcus 212
Epidural analgesia 149
Epiglottitis 85, 88, 90, 91
Epinephrine 22, 23, 55-59
*Escherichia coli* 66, 192
Etomidate 115, 120
Euthanasia 224, 230, 231

Fentanyl 20, 116, 119-121
Fever 91, 94, 95
Fibroblast 62-64, 67, 69, 70
Fibronectin 63, 66, 69
Fluid dynamics 33
Fluoroquinolone 187, 195, 196
Fluoroscopy 113
Fungi 185, 191, 192, 196

Gay-Lussac's law 30
Graham's law 31, 45

*Haemophylus influenzae* 184, 185
Haemorrhage 139, 140
Heart
    diseases 222
    failure 18, 163
    transplant 17, 19, 20, 23
Hemoptysis 96
Henry's law 31
Heparin 171, 175-177, 179, 181
Hepato-renal dysfunction 127, 129
Histamine 124, 127, 128
Hyaluronic acid 63
Hypercapnia 76, 79, 89, 92, 93, 95, 138
Hypercarbia 88, 89
Hyperinflation 74, 76, 81, 92, 93
Hypertension 137, 149, 150, 155

Hyperthermia 139
Hypnomidate 20
Hypocapnia 92
Hypotension 138, 140
Hypothermia 138, 139
Hypoventilation 146, 149, 152, 153
Hypovolemic shock 61
Hypoxemia 43, 83, 84, 86, 88, 90, 92, 93, 97, 137, 143, 146, 149-151, 154-156, 169
Hypoxia 79

Imipenem 187, 196
Infants 83-86
Inferior vena cava 21
Informed consent 99-107, 110
    conflict 67
    interest 99, 107, 109
    legislation 102
    patient information 103-106, 109, 110
    sociological aspects 99, 110
Intensive care unit 222, 225, 230-232
Ipatropium 92
Ischemic heart disease 163
Isoflurane 20, 118, 121
Isoproterenol 22, 172, 180

Ketamine 93, 94, 116, 119-121
*Klebsiella* spp 192

Laminar flow 42
Laminin 63, 66
Laryngeal oedema 151
Laryngitis 91
Laryngomalacia 90
Laryngoscopy 85, 90, 91
Laryngospasm 90, 137, 151
Larynx 85, 90, 97
Laudanosine 128
Learning 13
Left atrium 21
*Legionella pneumophila* 185, 186, 196
Leonardo's law 36
Levofloxacin 187
Lidocaine 93
Liquid ventilation 95
Lung
    hyperinflation 76
    parenchyma 61, 63, 64, 68, 69

trauma 61

Macrophages 63, 64
Magnesium sulfate 94
Malignant hyperthermia 125, 127, 128, 131
Mechanical ventilation 61, 68, 89, 92, 93, 95, 113-115, 119
Meropenem 187, 195, 196
Methoxamine 56, 58
Methylprednisolone 23
Midazolam 93
Milrinone 18, 22, 172
Mivacurium 123, 125-127, 130
Mole 30
*Moraxella* spp 185
Morphine 93
Mupirocin 212, 214, 216, 217
Muscle relaxation 123, 124
*Mycobacterium tuberculosis* 185
*Mycoplasma pneumoniae* 185
Myocardial dysfunction 55, 57, 58
Myocardial ischemia 138, 143
Myocytes 55

Nadroparin 175, 176
Naloxone 152
Neomycin 212
Nephropathy 19
Neuromuscular junction 124
Neuropathy 19
Nitric oxide 22, 89
Nitrogen monoxide 32
Nitroglycerin 22
Norepinephrine 172, 173

Operating theatre 133, 135-137, 139, 141
Opioids 116, 118, 152
Oxygen 18, 85, 86, 88-93, 95, 162
Oxygenation 50

Paediatrics 88
Pain 221, 226, 230
Pain clinic 226
Palliative care 221, 223, 227-232
Pancuronium 125-128
Paraquat 64, 65
Pascal's law 34
Patient care 4

Patient care 4
Pediatrics 130
Perioperative care 11, 17
Perioperative medicine 145
Permissive hypercapnia 89, 93
Pharmacology 4
Pharynx 151
Phenylephrine 55, 58, 59
Physiology 4
Piperacillin 187, 196
Pituitary dysfunction 19
Plasmapheresis 22
*Pneumocystis carinii* 186, 196
Pneumonia 23, 61, 149, 183-185, 187-192,
        194-203
    aspiration 95, 97
    community-acquired 199
Pneumothorax 96
Poiseuille's law 42, 44
Polymyxin E 191
Positive end-expiratory pressure 117
Post-resuscitation 55-58
Povidone-iodine 211, 212, 214, 216
Practice-based learning 4
Pregnancy 126, 129
Preload 20
Professionalism 4
Propofol 115, 118, 119, 120, 121
Propranolol 57, 59
Prostacyclin 173, 181
Prostaglandin 18
    E1 22, 173, 180
Proteoglycans 63, 66
*Pseudomonas aeruginosa* 207, 209
Pulmonary
    artery 21
    catheter 20
    contusion 96
    embolism 167, 168, 179-181
    hypertension 168, 170
    perfusion 114

Recovery room 133, 136, 143, 144
Remifentanil 116, 120
Residents 13
Respiratory
    acidosis 92
    failure 83, 85, 86, 88-90, 92, 95, 149

mechanics 61, 62, 69
    system 145, 150
Restlessness 150
Resuscitation 55-59
Retinopathy 19
Reviparin 175, 176
Reynold's number 43, 45
Ribavirin 92
Rocuronium 125-127, 129-131
Rofecoxib 12

Scurvy 7
Sellick manoeuvre 93
Sepsis 61, 62, 68
Sevoflurane 20, 91, 93
Smoke inhalation 61
Sodium nitroprusside 18, 22
*Staphylococcus aureus* 207, 209, 212, 215,
    217
Stoke's law 44
Streptokinase 177
Stroke 222
    volumes 55
Succinylcholine 123-131
Sufentanil 20
Superior vena cava 21
Surgeon 12
Surgery 89, 90, 97, 123, 124, 130
Surgical embolectomy 178
Suxametonium 93
Sweating 150

Tachycardia 149, 150
Tachypnea 95
Teaching 13
Terminal illnesses 221
Thiopentone 129
Thoracic trauma 96, 98
Thoracotomy 51, 149
Thrombolysis 171, 176, 178, 180, 181
Tinzaparin 175, 176
Tongue 150, 151
Trachea 85, 89, 90, 91, 97
Tracheostomy 90, 91
Training 13
Trauma patients 49
Trendelemburg position 117

Urokinase 177

Vancomycin 207, 212, 217
Vasopressin 20
Vecuronium 125-128, 130, 131
Vena cava 169, 171, 178, 179, 181
Ventilator-associated lung injury 61
Venturi
    mask 41
    tube 39

Wheezing 75, 77, 81

Made in the USA
Monee, IL
07 July 2026

56653406R00142